Case Studies in Psychopathology

Louis Diamant

University of North Carolina
at Charlotte

Charles E. Merrill Publishing Company
A Bell & Howell Company
Columbus, Ohio

RC
465
D52

International Standard Book Number: 0-675-09247-7

Library of Congress Catalog Card Number: 75-140674

1 2 3 4 5 6 7 8 9 10—75 74 73 72 71

Printed in the United States of America

Preface

Abnormal psychology is rapidly becoming one of the most vital as well as popular fields of study. The abundance of literature in the area attests to its dynamic character. Excellent theoretical and research reports, as well as several textbooks, have appeared in recent years. A number of books of readings and case studies in psychopathology have also been published.

It is felt, however, that there is an unmet need in abnormal psychology for a collection of case studies specifically designed to complement the available texts and supplement the student's understanding of the field.

Case histories as presented in this book have a number of unique functions. In a very practical way they demonstrate in depth many of the emotional disorders covered in the textbooks on abnormal psychology. They enable one to develop broader insights into the causes and treatment of mental illness. By careful selection of the studies, the reader will be exposed to the theories and techniques of outstanding practitioners. By the discussions of the diverse theoretical orientations, comparisons among practitioners can be made, and the application of the various personality theories in the field of psychopathology and the clinical validation of these theories can be seen.

In order to provide a meaningful organization and ordering of the diagnostic categories, it was decided to rely most heavily upon the classification system in the *Diagnostic and Statistical Manual of Mental Disorders* prepared by the Committee on Nomenclature and Statistics of the American Psychiatric Association (2nd edition, 1968). There is a controversy, it is true, among psychologists as to the validity of concepts such as mental illness and the realistic value of diagnostic classifications; and there is criticism by the behavioral theorists of the medical or disease model of psychopathology. Nevertheless, the American Psychiatric Association's classification system is most widely used clinically and will relate best to the most frequently used textbooks in abnormal psychology and psychiatry.

I am indebted to the authors and publishers of these case studies for allowing me to reprint their work. I wish to thank Julia Talbutt, Michael Stockton, Art Skibbe, and Carolyn Wall for reading and offering valuable comments on the selections. Also, Mrs. Lorraine Penninger, Reference Librarian at UNCC, was most helpful in obtaining source materials.

L. D.

Charlotte, North Carolina
November, 1970

Contents

I. Introduction

Theory in psychology, as in all sciences, is indispensable, and a number of theoretical positions have been advanced to explain abnormal behavior. Among the more influential are the analytic theories which attempt to explain behavior in intrapsychic terms. Perhaps the most familiar is the psychoanalytic theory of Sigmund Freud which is concerned with the role of the id (primitive drives), the ego (reality relationships) and the superego (morality and conscience), and with infantile sexuality and its function in shaping personality. In addition, there is the analytic theory of Carl Jung whose explanation of abnormal behavior is found in such ideas as the concept of the collective unconscious and its relationship to personality growth. There is also the individual psychology of Alfred Adler and the role he gives to the strivings for superiority, compensation, and the life style in the etiology of emotional disorders which seem to be the stepping-stone towards an interpersonal and socially-oriented explanation of psychopathology, as typified by the work of Harry Stack Sullivan, Erich Fromm, and Karen Horney.

A second grouping encompasses the behavioral theorists. These clinicians seek the development and treatment of emotional disorders within the framework of learning theory. They disagree with the disease theory of mental disorder which requires finding a cause for the disorder and aiming treatment at that cause rather than the symptom (counting the symptom as secondary). Rather, the behavioral theorists feel that the principles of conditioning account for the symptom and can account for the removal of the symptom. Thus, they are against hypothesizing an unconscious conflict. They seem to be most influenced by the learning

1

theories of C. L. Hull and B. F. Skinner. Currently active in research on behavior modification are Wolpe, Salter, Ullmann, and Krasner.

A third group of theorists show the influence of humanistic philosophy and their theories are sometimes referred to as phenomenological, existential, ontoanalytic. Historically, their roots are to be found in the writings of the phenomenologist Edmund Husserl, the existentialists Søren Kierkegaard and Martin Heidegger, and some are indebted to the Gestaltists for wholistic thinking. In clinical practice they are currently represented by May, Combs, Binswanger, and Rogers.

A fourth group feels that organic defect based on constitutional inferiority, body build, or some kind of physical trauma, is responsible for the physical symptoms that comprise abnormal behavior. Among this group are Kretschmer, Sheldon, Hoffer, Osgood, and others who work in the organic descriptive framework of Emil Kraepelin.

Finally, in addition to the purists, a great body of psychologists have adopted an eclectic position from many theories in their diagnostic and psychotherapeutic work. They organize within their own theoretical framework ideas from a number of positions. A great part of contemporary psychiatry and clinical psychology, while basically influenced by Freud, is still quite adoptive and eclectic.

CLASSIFICATION

It is reasonable to state that the inchoate stages of classification in mental disorders are more than two thousand years old and were probably begun by the Greek physician, Hippocrates (460-377 B.C.), who had taken the ruminations and speculations of the philosophers of medicine and developed the clinical method. He formulated sensible descriptions of mental illness and emphasized the importance of the brain in man's behavior. Hippocrates is usually credited with having inaugurated the first rational classifications of mental illness. His efforts included attempts to describe epilepsy, melancholia, paranoia, and what is now considered postpartum psychosis.

It was the years after the Renaissance, however, during the great era of modern scientific inquiry, that produced the men who expounded and organized the classifications in abnormal psychology. Although there was an intensification in the classifications of scientific phenomena, the classifiers in psychiatry were not concerned with the dynamics of these nosologies but nevertheless added diagnostic categories that currently remain in the jargon of psychiatry and abnormal psychology.

George Cheyne (1671-1743) provided an explanation for neurotic behavior by using the Hippocratic theory of humors and their effect on emotions. William Cullen (1712-1790) was perhaps the most comprehensive of the classifiers of the time and many of his descriptions of neuroses are remarkably accurate by current standards. Cullen was the first physician to use the term "neuroses" somewhat in line with current descriptions of neuroses as psychopathology. Later, Robert Whytt (1714-1766) divided neuroses into hysteria and hypochondriasis and while these classifications resemble present clinical description, they were not based on any valid psychological principles and did not attempt to explain emotional disturbance in dynamic fashion.

By the close of the eighteenth century, Phillippe Pinel (1745-1826), who became famous for his reform of mental institutions, advanced the cause of diagnosis and classification by separating the psychotic illnesses from dementia and describing many symptoms of psychosis that are still used in the diagnosis of this disorder. Pinel strongly advocated a psychological approach to the problems of mental illness and while he developed no strong theoretical framework within which to describe mental illness, he deplored the purely anatomical approach and campaigned against the unsupported use of bloodletting and drugs.

Jean Étienne Dominique Esquirol (1772-1840), a student of Pinel, followed in his master's footsteps by developing an elaborate classification of clinical syndromes. He was a tireless recorder and possibly the first psychiatrist to use statistics in his observations. His book, *Des Maladies Mentales* (1838), is said to be one of the first published volumes relating emotions in a causative way to mental illness. Esquirol introduced the term "hallucination" into psychiatric diagnosis and separated it from the term "delusion." While Esquirol's classifications are not currently in use, his contribution towards a unified diagnostic and classification approach cannot be underestimated.

The next important landmark in description and classication in abnormal psychology resulted from the work of Karl Kahlbaum (1828-1899). Kahlbaum introduced a number of terms which are still used in current classifications—"cyclothymia," related to the alternation of moods, and "catatonia." However, for the most part, Kahlbaum's students and their contemporaries related emotional disorders to degeneration of the brain.

Benedict Augustin Morel (1809-1873) was of the opinion that the psychiatrists of his day placed too much emphasis on the organic aspect of mental illness. Nevertheless, he suggested that a psychosis which appeared at adolescence was an hereditary disease with concomitant deterioration which he labeled "dementia praecox." The term "dementia praecox" was relabeled "schizophrenia" in 1911 by Eugen Bleuler who observed that dementia praecox did not leave a permanent dementia and that a number of patients recovered.

It remained the task of Emil Kraepelin (1856-1926), however, to make the most comprehensive classification of mental illness to that time. It is interesting to note that Kraepelin studied under Wilhelm Wundt, the famous physiological psychologist who is considered the founder of modern experimental psychology. Kraepelin classified dementia praecox into catatonic, hebephrenic, and paranoid subvarieties and in doing so he utilized the clinical observations gathered from thousands of patients' case histories. Kraepelin based his diagnoses on the classifications of observable, descriptive behavior. He also lent some clarification to the muddle of diagnoses by separating the psychoses into the manic-depressive psychoses and dementia praecox, and by developing separate prognostic evaluations for these entities. While Kraepelin's diagnostic classifications and descriptions were a landmark of clarity after an era of confusion related to the diagnosis of mental disorders, they lacked what a number of psychopathologists call the dynamic approach, since they were sterile in their descriptive character. The change in the study of psychopathology from a near description of manifest behavior with a supposition that an organic malfunction lay behind the behavior, to the dynamic psychological point of view with the consideration of emotional disorders as related to past and present experiences showing themselves in psychological conflict and symptomatology, waited upon the genius of Sigmund Freud (1856-1939).

Freud's unification of a theory of unconscious motivation as revealed in the patient's description of his personal history, memories, and feelings provided a framework for the treatment of emotional disorder that was later called "dynamic psychology." However, while Freud and his followers made attempts to uncover the "person" beneath the diagnosis, Freud himself did little to change the diagnostic classification system.

In Europe, other analysts dissatisfied with Freudian psychoanalytic theory branched off into theoretical frameworks of their own. Carl Jung (1875-1961) and Alfred Adler (1870-1937), for example, contributed themes to the dynamic interpretation of emotional disturbance. In the United States, Adolph Meyer (1866-1950), whose psychobiological theory challenged Kraepelin's classification rigidity, introduced terminology which he felt was more flexible. However, while Meyer's personalistic and dynamic attitude influenced those who followed, his classifications were not published and thus did not exert the influence on the system of classifications as did Kraepelin's.

By World War II, the classifications were largely Kraepelinian but bore the twentieth century dynamic influence of the psychoanalysts. However, their utilization depended more or less on an individual psychiatrist's predilection or some institutional bias.

Problems of classification had become acute in the United States Armed Forces during and immediately after World War II. As a result of this chaotic condition of classification, a Committee on Nomenclature and Statistics of the American Psychiatric Association was charged with the task of classification and organization. The results of their work were published in 1952 as the *Diagnostic and Statistical Manual of Mental Disorders,* revised in 1968. It is both dynamic and descriptive and appears to have synthesized a long history of contributions from the descriptive, organic, and analytic theorists. While there is current controversy over the validity of these classifications, the American Psychiatric Association system is still the most widely utilized.

2. Mental Retardation*

Mental retardation refers to subnormal general intellectual functioning which originates during the developmental period and is associated with impairment of either learning and social adjustment or maturation, or both. Classifications according to degree of retardation, as related to IQ, include borderline (IQ 68-85), mild (IQ 52-67), moderate (IQ 36-51), severe (IQ 20-35), or profound (IQ under 20).

In addition, cases are classified by etiology or cause. Categories include mental retardation following infection and intoxication, i.e., in which the retardation is the result of residual cerebral damage from intra-cranial infections, serums, drugs, or toxic agents, such as congenital rubella or syphilis, or encephalopathy associated with maternal toxemia of pregnancy; mental retardation following trauma or physical agent such as encephalopathy due to prenatal injury or mechanical injury at birth; mental retardation associated with metabolism, growth, or nutrition, such as phenylketonuria; and mental retardation associated with gross brain disease; chromosomal abnormality; prematurity; or psycho-social (environmental) deprivation.

---

*The descriptions of the various mental disorders are from the *Diagnostic and Statistical Manual of Mental Disorders.* (2nd ed.) Washington, D.C.: American Psychiatric Association, 1968.

1. Behavior in Phenylketonuria*

Jon Bjornson

Phenylketonuria (PKU) is a disturbance of protein metabolism that has been found to be associated with mental retardation. Bjornson cites generously from research literature to substantiate the genetic-biochemical determinance of this disorder. Succinctly, studies indicate that PKU is an inherited condition transmitted by a single autosomal recessive gene. The child with PKU is unable to convert the amino acid phenylalanine to tyrosine resulting in an accumulation of phenylpyruvic acid which is excreted in the urine. The detection of phenylpyruvic acid in the urine and the recently developed Guthrie Test, which measures phenylalanine levels in the bloodstream, provide an opportunity for treatment by special diet. The current case study presents an excellent sample of what would seem to be a purely physiological basis of a mental disorder. However, according to Bjornson, the relationship of biochemical functions seems better established to mental retardation than to behavioral characteristics. He suggests a similarity of research in the biochemistry of schizophrenia and PKU and believes that in neither has a relationship been established between behavioral characteristics and a biochemical etiology.

The eleven-year-old girl discussed in this case study had been diagnosed as mentally retarded from the age of seven, but no explanation for the retardation had been found. At age eleven, psychological evaluation indicated serious emotional disturbance in addition to mental retardation. At this time, a positive ferric chloride test for PKU was made.

---

*Reprinted by permission of the author and the American Medical Association from the *Archives of General Psychiatry*, 1964, **10**, 65-69.

The child had had an unstable homelife and her parents were seen as having considerable emotional problems. The patient had two sisters, one of whom had PKU and was severely retarded. The sisters with PKU exhibited the physical characteristics of blue eyes and blond hair typical of phenylketonurics. The third sister appeared developmentally normal although she too had some emotional problems.

The author's work dealing with the behavioral aspects of PKU is an innovative research study on this form of mental retardation. Although other studies have described behavioral symptoms of a psychotic nature, no detailed reports of schizophrenic-like symptoms in phenylketonuria were in the literature prior to Bjornson's report. He could find no specific behavioral pattern in PKU, and feels that the non-specific patterns are psychological rather than physiological and are probably, in part at least, related to the child's and family's adaptation to the retardation.

Perhaps no inherited disorder has been evaluated more thoroughly, nor demonstrated more decidedly gene-enzyme specificity dependent on specific environmental conditions and stimulus, than phenylketonuria. Yet many questions remain unanswered, one of the important of these being specific behavioral aspects of the disease, if any, and their biopsychogenesis.

Discovered in 1934 by Dr. Asbjörn Fölling of Oslo, with the help of a perspicacious Norwegian mother who noted a peculiar odor from the urine of two of her offspring, phenylketonuria has now become a preventable form of mental retardation(8). Approximately 700 cases have been mentioned in the literature which abounds with articles concerning various aspects of the disease. The abnormality, the result of homozygous recessive autosomal inheritance(6, 21) occurs once per 25,000 to 40,000 births in the United States(21), or in a ratio of 2 to 6 per 100,000 population (21, 37), accounting for 0.6% to 1% of institutionalized mental defectives(19, 25). Heterozygity for the disease is said to be one per 100 population as demonstrated by loading tolerance tests(17, 19), but whether this state is diathetic towards intellectual or emotional disturbance is unknown(25). The biochemical disturbance is that of the hydroxylation of phenylalanine to tyrosine due to the absence or inactivity of the necessary hepatic enzyme system(21, 22) resulting in a rise of phenylalanine in the serum as well as body tissues including the brain(21, 22, 35). Many secondary or metabolically compensatory aromatic metabolites in serum, urine, and body tissue result, including: phenylpyruvic acid, phenylacetic acid, phenylacetyl glutamine, p- and o-hydroxyphenyl-acetic acid and others(25, 35). While there is some contradiction, the concensus of opinion of investigators is that these metabolites are not directly toxic to the brain(25, 35) nor is there a direct correlation of blood levels with the degree of mental deficiency(7, 21, 25) though some authors disagree on clinical grounds(5, 38, 39). It has been postulated that there are more widespread metabolic dysfunctions via direct genetic effects or more likely through indirect inhibition by the secondary metabolites(25, 35) especially in view of the fact that no ketoacids have been demonstrated in spinal fluid(21). Possible affected enzyme systems include: tyrosinase and dihydroxyphenylalanine (DOPA) decarboxylase necessary for the formation of adrenalin and noradrenalin; 5-hydroxytryptophane decarboxylase necessary for the formation of 5-hydroxy-tryptamine and glutamic acid decarboxylase (35). These latter enzyme systems all appear to play a part in normal cerebral functioning. It is also of special importance that these enzyme systems with their biochemical products have all been implicated and studied as playing a role in the production of schizophrenia, though the literature in this latter regard remains a mass of conflictual data. A deficiency of adrenalin and noradrenalin in phenylketonuria was suggested by increased hypertensive responses to intravenous adrenalin, but this finding was based on only two cases(25). Low plasma adrenalin and noradrenalin as well as decreased urinary output of 3-methoxy-4-hydroxy-mandelic acid, one of the main excretion products of adrenalin and noradrenalin has been reported in phenylketonuria(33, 40). Abnormal "psychotomimetic" degradation products of adrenalin have been suggested as possibly being endogenously produced by schizophrenics(20, 26) with refutation(14, 23). In phenylketonuria, the impedance of the decarboxylation of 5-hydroxytryptophane has been supported by in vivo and in vitro inhibition with phenylalanine metabolic by-products and patients have been shown to have low blood 5-hydroxytryptamine, the decarboxylation product, as well as low urinary 5-hydroxyindolacetic acid(35). Presumably, 5-hydroxytryptophane, the probable precursor of serotonin (5-hydroxytryptamine), would accumulate resulting perhaps in some type of behavioral response as has been suggested(13, 15) and refuted(14, 23) in the search for a biochemical etiology of schizophrenia. Lowered cerebral blood oxygen uptake has also been reported in both diseases(16, 23). The similarity of research in these two diseases is striking.

Clinically the disease is characterized by an equal sex distribution (21, 37), blondness and blue eyes in 90% of the cases(21), photosensitivity in 33%(21), seizures in 25 to 33%(21, 25, 34), slight reduction in head size (21, 34) (no figures available), and IQ below 50 in 98%, below 30 in 84%(21). The EEG shows nonspecific abnormalities in 65% to 80% of the cases(21, 34) and neurological exam reveals unusual dyskinetic movements in approximately 66%(34). Serum phenylalanine rises as high as 60 mg%, spills at 6 to 8 mg%(21, 25). Diagnosis may be made with a simple screening test following sufficient ingestion of phenylalanine(1, 9) usually about the third neonatal day(9). The earlier the disease is treated with a restrictive diet the greater the salvage of intellectual function(10, 24, 32, 36). Prognosis and efficacy for treatment decreases with time, promotes little or no improvement after the age of three according to most authors(24), though some authors feel behavior may benefit from treatment(38); however, the attention given the child and thereby improved self-image with the treatment regimen was not considered. Decreased longevity with the disease is unproven and must take into account epidemics of hepatitis, dysentery, and respiratory diseases common in mental institutions. Pathological reports are scanty and inconclusive. One excellent review of 24 autopsies(35) suggested a tendency towards microcephally and diffuse fibrous gliosis of the centrum semiovale, mainly based on three of the authors' four cases, but as this finding is common in other types of mental retardation as mongolism or idiopathic amentia, the authors could only conclude that postnatal developmental arrest or loss of neurons resulted in a nonspecific gliosis.

Behavioral characteristics appear to be an untouched area of this illness. Perhaps this is because there is such a wide variation in behavior. But it is even more disconcerting that some conclusions or observations of these patients totally exclude the psychosocial effect upon the total adaptive pattern of these patients. For instance, it is perfectly reasonable to assume regression of intellectual functions can occur completely or in part with the isolation, rejection and loss of identity implied with placement in a large overcrowded undersupervised mental institution for the retarded. This would explain findings in the disease as "catatonic posture" or "mute-like facies," occasionally reported.

The following case histories illustrate some of the pervasive psychological effects of environment upon these children, the variation of emotional makeup of two siblings with the syndrome, a third sibling's responses to psychological tests for comparison, and the not unusual maladaptive family response to a child with mental retardation.

The patient, an 11-year-old girl, was referred to the Child Guidance Clinic of an Army General Hospital because of assaultive behavior, irritability, lability of mood, and "nervous jerks and prances." Recently she had been spitting in other people's food and jabbing or threatening other children with eating utensils. Numerous evaluations since the age of seven by psychologists, psychiatrists, and educational specialists had failed to provide an explanation for the girl's borderline IQ, full scale WAIS ranging from 65 to 70. Her past history revealed that she had been born by cesarean section, premature, and underweight. Growth and development up through the second year of life were within normal limits. When the child was two, her mother gave birth to the family's third daughter. This event was followed by a postpartum depression, necessitating that the patient go to the home of her paternal grandparents for approximately two months. At the same time arrangements had been made to place the patient's sister, four years older, in an institution for the mentally retarded. Patient "fell back six months," could not talk, walk, or use the bathroom. Subsequent development was slow and there were recurrent separations from the mother every two to three years when the mother was hospitalized with psychotic episodes characterized by depression and withdrawal requiring shock treatment. A peripatetic family contributed further to environmental instability. Retardation was suspected when the child was six, though the parents felt emotional difficulties were contributing to her inability to learn. When the child was eight, her mother was hospitalized for three months, after discovering that the child's father had been carrying on an extramarital affair. Following this one of many trips to foster homes, the child became markedly more hyperactive, unpredictable, and rivalrous with her sibling. Since roughly the age of five she had difficulty making friends, was ubiquitously rejected by other children and was increasingly isolated. Adjustment to special schools was poor with frequent aggressive acting out.

Clinical evaluation in the playroom and psychological tests concurred that the child was a tall attractive blue-eyed blond, who was hyperkinetic with frequent choreoathetoid movements, talked incessantly with loose pathological arbitrary associations and obsessive preoccupations with primarily violent themes (eg, "The Alamo" repeatedly associated out of context or coherency). Concrete in response to direct questions, she would easily become detached from the social situation and talk in a rambling bizarre disconnected manner, felt by all observers to indicate primary process thinking. Her responses to projective tests, including DAP, CAT, and Object Relations, contained disorganized or tangential themes, concern with violence, and fear of loss of mother or self. Reality testing was tenuous at best. Later she had a positive ferric chloride screen test for phenylketonuria and a serum phenylalanine of 32 mg% (normal less than 1.5 mg%).[1]

The parents, seen together and separately, were both found to be unspontaneous, communicated poorly with each other, and repeatedly rationalized. The mother was passive, insecure, guilt-ridden, lenient with the children, and schizoid, using the embarrassment over her two mentally retarded offspring as her reason for withdrawing from social contacts. The father, though obsequious and overcontrolled with authoritarian

---

[1]Test done by Dr. Harold Harper, University of California Medical Center.

figures, was rigid, punitive, and demanding of the two daughters at home, easily frustrated and dissatisfied with anything he considered amiss. Reared an only child of separated parents, the father repeatedly held his wife and children to account for his inability to accomplish worldly ambitions. Both the patient's parents had a positive history of mental illness but not retardation. Her older sister died at the age of 16, within the year that the patient's family started therapy. The autopsy report stated the sister died of pneumonia and myocarditis and also included findings of genitourinary tract congenital abnormalities and the brain showing "a nonspecific malformation of arrested development and a deficiency of melanin pigment in the substantia nigra." Review of the sister's hospital records from Sonoma State Hospital, Calif., revealed that she had three positive ferric chloride tests of her urine for phenylketonuria. The sister was strikingly similar to the patient in appearance with hazel eyes and blond hair but was profoundly retarded. Despite estimated IQ level below 10, she was ambulatory but could not dress herself, feed herself or talk, and was only partially toilet trained. Extracted descriptions by observers, varying little during nine years in the hospital, included: "mean to other people," "repeated biting of other patients," "plays with feces," "uncontrolled hostility . . . . . frequent restraining necessary." There was no history of sexual acting out. This child, the parent's first born, was delivered by cesarean section, unplanned, unwanted, and delivered when the father was overseas ten months after the marriage. The inlaws made repeated real or supposed criticisms about the mother's difficulty feeding the child, while pediatricians were contradictory in diagnosing her condition. The mother doctor-shopped, and the family moved repeatedly at her insistence. Gradually the child became more of a problem with grunting, hypo- or hyperactive behavior, was destructive of self and property, was untrainable and abusive to her sibling. The parents blamed themselves or each other. Despite positive professional assertions of mental retardation, the parents' denial persisted and their social contacts diminished to nil.

The "normal" 10-year-old sibling, the youngest of the three, had a negative urine test for phenylketonuria, as did the parents. Administered a battery of psychological tests, she was an attractive prim proper extremely inhibited overcontrolled child who frequently utilized denial, responding to the examiner and to the tests in a relevant but constricted manner. Her full scale WAIS was 107 without significant subtest scatter. Though avoiding mention of her emotional reaction to the family situation, from her projective story telling tests, it was clear that she felt a generalized hostility towards both parents, expected to be frustrated by her mother, feared the loss of her father, and desired to leave her home.

COMMENT

Reported behavioral disturbances in phenylketonuria are sparse in detail, at best, and to the best of my knowledge, the case reported above is the only reported case with a concomitant schizophrenic-like thinking disturbance; however, from a few case reports similar symptoms might be suspected, for example, the following description, "Labile, at times almost catatonic, at others emotional outbursts with intense expressions of fear"(21). The same author comments that only 10% of patients with the disease show "psychotic" behavior without any established relationship to excretion of phenylketones(21); however, since these "psychotic episodes" were characterized by restlessness, destructiveness, and noisy behavior, use of the word "psychotic" is highly questionable. In 1954, Jervis made brief comments on behavior in an otherwise exhaustive analysis of 330 cases (21) which are arbitrarily placed in groups as follows: Of those with IQ's of less than 30 ("idiot" or "low grade"), 112 were found to be "passive," "quiet," "apathetic," or "even tempered"; 77 were described as "excitable," "restless," "destructive" or "uncooperative"; and 12 as generally cooperative with occasional outbursts of temper. Of those with IQ's of 30 or above ("imbecile" or "high grade"), 62 were in the apathetic well-behaved group, 9 in the hyperactive, excitable group and 5 as generally well behaved with emotional instability or occasional outbursts of temper. No mention of behavior was made in 50 of the cases. Furthermore, 53 families with two or more siblings affected had a similar breakdown as the above with wide variations in those of the same family without apparent relationship of behavior to IQ, sex or these two variables in combination. These figures, though based on superficial descriptions, tend to show no specific behavioral pattern. A somewhat contradictory paper (38) based on two cases and descriptions of eight other cases suggests that phenylketonuria should be suspected, despite dull normal IQ, with a combination of dull expressionless facies, negativistic behavior, unrealistic fears, emotional outbursts, and speech disturbances. While such a conclusion may have justification, these symptoms are far from universal in all cases. Of the 35 untreated cases with borderline IQ levels that I found reported in the literature, and there are probably many more, there was no consistent behavior pattern described (2, 3, 11, 12, 18, 24, 27, 28, 29, 31, 34, 39, 41). If a specific categorizable psychological defect exists, it has escaped discovery. It is also to be considered that Bleuler's primary symptoms and other aspects of disordered perceptive-integrative-cognitive functions as depersonalization or referential thinking may be impossible to affirm or negate in the severely retarded, if one is to make an analogy of biochemical defects in this disease playing any role in the production of schizophrenic symptoms. It would appear also that induced "model psychoses" (30) might better be evaluated in terms of "primary symptoms," rather than secondary. Apparently phenylketonurics, who have a number of cerebrophysiological impairments, neither hallucinate nor have a proclivity towards persecutory delusions. Whether they have a specific type of disordered thinking is an important question. On the other hand the nonspecific behavioral defects of phenylketonuria may be partially, if not wholly, the result of psychological factors, especially the patient's and the family's adaptation to the retardation.

CONCLUSION

A case of a borderline-retarded phenylketonuric child with schizophrenic-like thinking was discussed. Some analogies to the observed biochemical defects in phenylketonuria with postulated biochemical defects in schizophrenia were noted. Probability of nonspecific behavioral patterns in phenylketonuria as the result of total adaptation with psychosocial factors playing the major role is suggested. Behavior in phenylketonuria appears not to be related to IQ or sex. The avoidance of exploration or investigation of the thinking-feeling aspects of phenylketonurics is noted. Prevention of retardation with early diagnosis and treatment is again urged. Some emphasis should be placed on behavioral characteristics in this early stage of research to evaluate treatment.

REFERENCES

1. Allen, R. J.: The Detection and Diagnosis of Phenylketonuria, *Amer. J. Pub. Health* 50:1662-1666, 1960.
2. Allen, R. J.; Gibson, R. M.; and Sutton, H. E.: Phenylketonuria with Normal Intelligence, *Amer. J. Dis. Child* 100:563-564, 1960.
3. Armstrong, M. D., and Tyler, F. H.: Studies on Phenylketonuria: Restricted Phenylalanine Intake in Phenylketonuria, *J. Clin. Investigation* 34:565-580, 1955.
4. Berman, P. W.; Graham, F. K.; Eichman, P. L.; and Waisman, H. A.: Psychologic and Neurologic Status of Diet-Treated Phenylketonuric Children and Their Siblings, *Pediatrics* 28:924-935, 1951.
5. Berry, H. K.; Sutherland, B. S.; Guest, M. D.; and Umbarger, B.: Chemical and Clinical Observations during Treatment of Children with Phenylketonuria, *Pediatrics* 21:926-939, 1958.
6. Blattner, R. J.: Phenylketonuria: Phenylpyruvic Aciduria, *J. Pediat.* 59:294-298, 1961.
7. Borek, E.; Brecher, A.; Jervis, G. A.; and Waelsch, A.: Oligophrenia Phenylpyruvica, Constancy of the Metabolic Error, *Proc. Exper. Biol. Med.* 75:86-89, 1950.
8. Centerwell, W. R., and Centerwell, S. A.: Phenylketonuria (Föllings Disease) the Story of Its Discovery, *J. Hist. Med.* 16:292-296, 1961.

9. Centerwell, W. R.; Chinnock, R. F.; and Pusavat, B. A.: Phenylketonuria Screening Programs and Testing Methods, *Amer. J. Public Health* 50:1667-1677, 1960.

10. Coates, S.: Results of Treatment in Phenylketonuria, *Brit. Med. J.* 5228:767-771, 1961.

11. Coates, S.; Norman, A. P.; and Woolf, C. I.: Phenylketonuria with Normal Intelligence and Gower's Muscular Dystrophy, *Arch. Dis. Child* 32: 313-317, 1957.

12. Cowie, V. A.: An Atypical Case of Phenylketonuria, *Lancet* 260:272, 1957.

13. Fazekas, J. F.: Pathologic Physiology of Cerebral Dysfunction, *Amer. J. Med.* 25:89-96, 1958.

14. Fazekas, J. F.; Toupin, H.; and Alman, R. W.: Physiologic and Pharmacologic Basis for the Chemotherapy of Psychiatric States, *Amer. J. Med.* 21: 825-831, 1956.

15. Himwich, H. E.: Psychopharmacologic Drugs, *Science* 127:59-71, 1958.

16. Himwich, H. E., and Fazekas, J. F.: Cerebral Arteriovenous Oxygen Differences: II. Mental Deficiency, *Arch. Neurol. Psychiat.* 51:73-77, 1944.

17. Hsia, D. Y-Y.: Medical Genetics, part 4, *New Engl. J. Med.* 262:1318-1323, 1960.

18. Hsia, D. Y-Y.; Knox, W. E.; and Paine, R. S.: A Case of Phenylketonuria with Borderline Intelligence, *J. Dis. Child* 94:33-39, 1957.

19. Hsia, D. Y-Y.; Driscoll, K. W.; Troll, W.; and Knox, W. E.: Detection of the Heterozygous Carrier for Phenylketonuria by Phenylalanine Tolerance Tests, *Nature* (London) 178:1279, 1956.

20. Hoffer, A.; Osmond, H.; and Smythies, J.: Schizophrenia: II. A New Approach, *J. Ment. Sci.* 100:29-45, 1954.

21. Jervis, G. A.: *Phenylpyruvic Oligophrenia (Phenylketonuria) in Genetics and the Inheritance of Integrated Neurological and Psychiatric Patterns,* Baltimore: Williams & Wilkins Co., 1954, pp. 259-282.

22. Jervis, G. A.: Studies on Phenylpyruvic Oligophrenia Phenylpyruvic Acid Content of Blood, *Soc. Exp. Biol.* 81:715-720, 1952.

23. Kety, S. S.: Biochemical Theories of Schizophrenia: Parts I and II, *Science* 129:1528-1532, 1590-1596, 1959.

24. Knox, W. E.: An Evaluation of the Treatment of Phenylketonuria with Diets Low in Phenylalanine, *Pediatrics* 26:1-11, 1960.

25. Knox, W. E., and Hsia, D. Y-Y.: Pathogenetic Problems in Phenylketonuria, *Amer. J. Med.* 22:687-702, 1957.

26. Leach, B. E., and Heath, R. G.: The in Vitro Oxidation of Epinephrin in Plasma, *Arch. Neurol. and Psychiat.* 76:444-450, 1956.

27. Leonard, S. A., and McGuire, F. L.: Phenylketonuria: An Unusual Case, *J. Pediat.* 54:210-214, 1959.

28. Lewis, I. C.: An Unusual Case of Phenylketonuria, *Med. J. Aust.* 47:811-813, 1960.

29. Low, L. L.; Armstrong, M. D.; and Carlisle, J. W.: Phenylketonuria: Two Unusual Cases, *Lancet* 2:917-918, 1956.

30. Luby, E. D.; Gottlieb, J. S.; Cohen, B. D.; Rosenbaum, G.; and Domino, E. F.: Model Psychoses and Schizophrenia, *Amer. J. Psychiat.* 119:61-67, 1962.

31. McLean, W. T.: Phenylketonuria with Borderline Intelligence, *N. Carolina Med. J.* 22:528-530, 1961.

32. Moncrieff, A., and Wilkinson, R. H.: Further Experiences in the Treatment of Phenylketonuria, *Brit. Med. J.* 5228:763-767, 1961.

33. Nadler, H. G., and Hsia, D. Y-Y.: Epinephrine Metabolism in Phenylketonuria, *Proc. Soc. Exp. Biol. Med.* 107:721-723, 1961.

34. Paine, R. S.: The Variability in Manifestations of Untreated Patients with Phenylketonuria (Phenylpyruvic Aciduria), *Pediatrics* 20:290-301, 1957.

35. Pare, C. M. B., and Crowe, L.: Phenylketonuria: Report of Pathological Findings in Four Cases, *J. Ment. Sci.* 106:862-883, 1960.

36. Partington, M. W.: The Early Symptoms of Phenylketonuria, *Pediatrics* 27:465-473, 1961.

37. Partington, M. W.: Observations of Phenylketonuria in Ontario, *Canad. Med. Ass. J.* 84:985-991, 1961.

38. Sutherland, B. S.; Berry, H. K.; and Shirkey, H. C.: A Syndrome of Phenylketonuria with Normal Intelligence and Behavior Disturbances, *J. Pediat.* 57:521-525, 1960.

39. Tapia, F.: Phenylpyruvic Oligophrenia: Report of a Case with Normal Intelligence, *Dis. Nerv. Syst.* 22:465-466, 1961.

40. Weil-Malkerbe: The Level of Adrenalin in Human Plasma and Its Relation to Mental Activity, *J. Ment. Sci.* 107:733-755, 1955.

41. Woolf, L. I.; Ounsted, C.; Lee, D.; Humphrey, M.; Cheshire, N. M.; and Steed, G. R.: Atypical Phenylketonuria in Sisters with Normal Offspring, *Lancet* 2:464-465, 1961.

42. Woolf, L. I.; Griffiths, R.; Moncrieff, A.; Coates, A.; and Dillistone, F.: The Dietary Treatment of Phenylketonuria, *Arch. Dis. Child* 33:31-45, 1958.

2. The Wild Boy of Aveyron: Development of the Intellectual Functions*

Jean-Marc-Gaspard Itard

Victor, the wild boy of Aveyron, was one of a number of feral children that have been reported throughout history. Some of these children were reputedly reared by wild animals, and among the most recent and celebrated was the "Indian Wolf Girl." In recent years, a number of scientists have cast doubt upon the possibility of such children having been nursed and reared by wild animals.

Victor was seen by Dr. Phillippe Pinel, famed for striking the chains from the mentally ill at Bicêtre Asylum in Paris, who diagnosed him almost immediately as mentally defective and not as a "wild boy." When Victor was first viewed by Itard in 1799, he looked not at all like Rousseau's noble savage but instead was a ragged, filthy child of age ten or eleven who walked on all fours, could not judge heat or cold, and showed little evidence of civilized or social behavior. Itard, who had already gained some distinction as a physician working with the deaf and the mute, did not agree with Pinel's diagnosis of mental deficiency, but felt that Victor was suffering from inadequate development of his sensory apparatus. He thought that corrective environmental stimulation could reestablish sensory efficiency and he undertook the task of making Victor a normal individual. When Victor died at about the age of 40 (in 1828), he was far from normal but he did evidence judgment, communication, appropriate emotions, social awareness, and some vocabulary.

*From: *The Wild Boy of Aveyron* by Jean-Marc-Gaspard Itard, and translated by George & Muriel Humphrey with an Introduction by George Humphrey. Copyright, 1932, by The Century Co. Copyright © 1962 by Meredith Publishing Company. Reprinted by courtesy of Appleton-Century-Crofts, pp. 67-86.

While it has been reported that Itard was disappointed in his progress with Victor, history has borne out the importance of his work as a landmark in the education of the mentally retarded. His techniques and efforts with his young student demonstrated a potential for learning on the part of the mentally retarded, with the aid of appropriate teaching. The chapter reprinted here, excerpts from Itard's full report to the French government, gives the reader interesting glimpses into his efforts, through stimulating learning experiences, to encourage Victor's intellectual and abstract thinking. The passages describing the experiments designed to help Victor develop concept formation are informative as well as charming. While Itard had limited educational success because of Victor's retarded functioning, he was not amiss in assessing environmental deprivation in childhood as an important contributing factor in retardation. It could be said, however, that perhaps he was wrong to give it total responsibility and too optimistic about the remediability of this type of intellectual deficiency.

XVIII. Although presented separately, the facts which have just been related are connected in many ways with those which will form the subject matter of the following sections. For such, my Lord, is the intimate relation which unites physical with intellectual man that, although their respective provinces appear and are in fact very distinct; yet the borderline between the two different sorts of function is very confused. Their development is simultaneous and their influence reciprocal. Thus while I was limiting my efforts to the exercise of the senses of our savage, the mind took its share of the attention given exclusively to the education of these organs and followed the same order of development. In fact it seemed that in instructing the senses to perceive and to distinguish new objects, I forced the attention to fix itself on them, the judgment to compare them, and the memory to retain them. Thus nothing was immaterial in these exercises. Everything penetrated to the mind. Everything put the faculties of the intelligence into play and prepared them for the great work of the communication of ideas. I was already sure that this would be possible by leading the pupil to the point where he would designate the thing he wanted by means of letters arranged in such a way as to spell the name of the thing he desired. In my pamphlet upon this child I have given an account of the first step made in recognizing written signs, and I am not afraid to signalize it as an important epoch in his education, as the sweetest and most brilliant success that has ever been obtained upon a creature fallen as was this one, into the lowest extremity of brutishness. But subsequent observations, by throwing light upon the nature of this result, soon came to weaken the hopes that I had conceived from it. [I noticed that Victor did not use words which I had taught him for the purpose of asking for the objects, or of making known a wish or a need, but employed them at certain moments only, and always at the sight of the desired things. Thus for example, much as he wanted his milk it was only at the moment when he was accustomed to take it and at the actual instant when he saw that it was going to be given him that the word for this favorite food was expressed or rather formed in the proper way.] In order to clear up the suspicion that this restricted employment of the words awoke in me I tried delaying the hour of his breakfast but waited in vain for the written expression of my pupil's needs although they had become very urgent. It was not until the cup appeared that the word *lait* (milk) was formed. I resorted to another test. In the middle of his lunch and without letting it appear in any way to be a punishment, I took away his cup of milk and shut it up in a cupboard. If the word *lait* had been for Victor the distinct sign of the thing and the expression of his want of it, there is no doubt that after this sudden privation, the need continuing to make itself felt, the word would have been immediately produced. It was not, and I concluded that the formation of this sign, instead of being for the pupil the expression of his desire, was merely a sort of preliminary exercise with which he mechanically preceded the satisfaction of his appetite. It was necessary then to retrace our steps and begin again. I resigned myself courageously to do this, believing that if I had not been understood by my pupil it was my fault rather than his. Indeed, in reflecting upon the causes which might give rise to this defective reception of the written signs, I recognized that in these first examples of the expression of ideas I had not employed the extreme simplicity which I had introduced at the beginning of my other methods of instruction and which had insured their success. Thus although the word *lait* is for us only a simple sign, for Victor it might be a confused expression for the drink, the vessel which contained it, and the desire of which it was the object.

XIX. Several other signs with which I had familiarized him showed the same lack of precision in application. An even more considerable defect was inherent in the method of expression we had adopted. As I have already said, this consisted in placing metal letters on a line and in the proper order, in such a way as to form the name of each object. But the connection which existed between the thing and the word was not immediate enough for his complete apprehension. In order to do away with this difficulty, it was necessary to establish between each object and its sign a more direct connection and a sort of identity which fixed them simultaneously in his memory. The objects first submitted to a trial of this new method of expression had therefore to be reduced to the greatest simplicity, so that their signs could not in any way bear upon their accessories. Consequently I arranged on the shelves of a library several simple objects such as a pen, a key, a knife, a box, etc., each one on a card upon which its name was written. These names were not new to the pupil. He already knew them and had learned to distinguish them from each other, according to the method of reading which I have already indicated.

XX. The problem then was merely to familiarize his eyes with the respective display of each of these names under the object which it represented. This arrangement was soon grasped as I had proof when, displacing all the things and instantly replacing all the labels in another order, I saw the pupil carefully replace each object upon its name. I varied my tests, and the variation gave me the opportunity to make several observations relative to the degree of the impression which these written signs made upon the sensory apparatus of our savage. Thus, leaving all the things in one corner of the room and taking all the labels to another, I wished by showing them successively to Victor to make him fetch each thing for which I showed him the written word. On these occasions, in order for him to bring the thing it was necessary that he should not lose from sight for a single instant the characters which indicated it. If he was too far away to be able to read the label, or if after showing it to him thoroughly I covered it with my hand, from the moment the sight of the word escaped him he assumed an air of uneasiness and anxiety and seized at random the first object which chanced to his hand.

XXI. The result of this experiment was not very reassuring and would in fact have discouraged me completely if I had not noticed that after frequent repetitions the duration of the impression upon the brain of my pupil became by imperceptible degrees much longer. Soon he merely needed to glance quickly at the word I showed him, in order to go without haste or mistake to fetch the thing I asked for. After some time I was able to extend the experiment by sending him from my apartment into his own room to look in the same· way for anything the name of which I showed him. At first the duration of the perception did not last nearly so long as that of the journey, but by an act of intelligence worthy of record, Victor sought and found in the agility of his legs a sure means of making the impressions persist longer than the time required for the journey. As soon as he had thoroughly read the word he set out like an arrow, coming back an instant later with the thing in his hand. More than once, nevertheless, the name escaped him on the way. Then I heard him stop in his tracks and come again towards my apartment, where he arrived with a timid and confused air. Sometimes it was enough for him to glance at the complete collection of names in order to recognize and retain the one which had escaped him. At other times the image of the word was so effaced from his memory that I was obliged to show it to him afresh. This necessity he indicated by taking my hand and making me pass my index finger over the whole series of names until I had shown him the forgotten one.

XXII. This exercise was followed by another which by offering his memory more work contributed more powerfully to develop it. Until then I had limited myself to asking for only one thing at a time. Then I asked for two, then three, and then four by showing a similar number of the labels to the pupil. He, feeling the difficulty of retaining them all, did not stop running over them with eager attention until I had entirely screened them from his eyes. Then there was no more delay or uncertainty. He set off hurriedly on the way to his room whence he brought the things requested. On his return his first care before giving them to me was to look hastily over the list, comparing it with the things of which he was the bearer. These he gave me only after he had reassured himself in this way that he had neither forgotten anything nor made a mistake. This last experiment gave at first very variable results but finally the difficulties which it offered were in their turn surmounted. The pupil, now sure of his memory, disdained the advantage which the agility of his legs gave him and applied himself quietly to this exercise. He often stopped in the corridor, put his face to the window which is at one end of it, greeted with sharp cries the sight of the country which unfolds magnificently in the distance, and then set off again for his room, got his little cargo, renewed his homage to the ever-regretted beauties of nature, and returned to me quite sure of the correctness of his errand.

XXIII. In this way memory, reëstablished in all its functions, succeeded in retaining the symbols of thought while at the same time the intelligence fully grasped their importance. Such, at least, was the conclusion that I thought I could draw when I constantly saw Victor, wishing to ask for various things, either in our exercises or spontaneously, making use of the different words of which I had taught him the meaning by the device of showing or giving him the thing when we made him read the word, or by indicating the word when he was given the thing. Who could believe that this double proof was not more than sufficient to assure me that at last I had reached the point to gain which I had been obliged to retrace my steps and make so great a detour? But something happened at this juncture which made me believe for a moment that I was further from it than ever.

XXIV. One day when I had taken Victor with me and sent him as usual to fetch from his room several objects which I had indicated upon his list of words, it came into my head to double-lock the door and unseen by him to take out the key. That done I returned to my study, where he was, and, unrolling his list, I asked him for some of the things on it, taking care to indicate none which were not also to be found in my room. He set out immediately, but finding the door locked and having searched on all sides for the key, he came beside me, took my hand and led me to the outer door as if to make me see that it would not open. I feigned surprise and sought for the key everywhere and even pretended to open the door by force. At last, giving up the vain attempt, I took Victor back into my study and showing him the same words again, invited him by signs to look about and see if there were not similar objects to be found there. The words designated were stick, bellows, brush, glass, knife. All these things were to be found scattered about my study in places where they could easily be seen. Victor looked at them but touched none of them. I had no better success in making him recognize them when they were brought together on a table and it was quite useless to ask for them one after the other by showing him successively their names. I tried another method. With scissors I cut out the names of the objects, thus converting them into single labels which were put into Victor's hands. By thus bringing him back to our original procedure, I hoped that he would put upon each thing the name which represented it. In vain. I had the inexpressible grief of seeing my pupil unable to recognize any of these objects or rather the connection which joined them to their signs. With a stupefied air which cannot be described he let his heedless glance wander over all these characters which had again become unintelligible. I felt myself sinking under a weight of impatience and discouragement.

I went and sat at the end of the room and considered bitterly this unfortunate creative reduced by the strangeness of his lot to such sad alternatives. Either he must be relegated as an unmistakable idiot to one of our asylums, or he must, by unheard-of labor, procure a little education which would be just as little conducive to his happiness. "Unhappy creature," I cried as if he could hear me, and with real anguish of heart, "since my labors are wasted and your efforts fruitless, take again the road to your forests and the taste for your primitive life. Or if your new needs make you dependent on a society in which you have no place, go, expiate your misfortune, die of misery and boredom at Bicêtre."

Had I not known the range of my pupil's intelligence so well, I could have believed that I had been fully understood, for scarcely had I finished speaking when I saw his chest heave noisily, his eyes shut, and a stream of tears escape through his closed eyelids, with him the signs of bitter grief.

XXV. I had often noticed that when such emotions had reached the point of tears, they formed a kind of salutary crisis that suddenly developed the intelligence which immediately afterwards was often able to overcome a difficulty that had appeared insurmountable some moments before. I had also observed that if at the height of this emotion I sud-

denly left off reproaching him and substituted caresses and a few words
of affection and encouragement, I obtained an increase of emotion which
doubled the expected effect. The occasion was favorable and I hastened
to profit by it. I drew near to Victor. I made him listen to a few kind
words which I spoke in such terms as he could understand and which I
accompanied by evidences of affection still more intelligible. His tears redoubled and were accompanied by gasps and sobs, while I myself redoubled the caresses, raising his emotion to the highest intensity and
causing him, if I may thus express myself, to vibrate to the last sensitive
fiber of his mentality. When all this excitement had entirely calmed down
I placed the same objects again under his eyes, and induced him to indicate them one after the other as soon as I successively showed him the
names. I began by asking him for the book. He first looked at it for rather
a long time, made a movement towards it with his hand while trying to
detect in my eyes some signs of approval or disapproval which would
settle his uncertainty. I held myself on guard and my expression was
blank. Reduced then to his own judgment he concluded that it was not the
thing asked for, and his eyes wandered, looking on all sides of the room,
pausing, however, only at the books which were scattered upon the table
and mantelpiece.

This examination was like a flash of light to me. I immediately
opened a cupboard which was full of books and took out a dozen among
which I was careful to include one exactly like the one Victor had left in
his room. To see it, quickly carry his hand to it and give it to me with a
radiant air was for Victor only the affair of a moment.

XXVI. Here I stopped the experiment. The result was enough to
revive the hopes which I had too easily abandoned and to make clear to
me the difficulties which this experiment had brought to light. It was evident that my pupil, far from having conceived a wrong idea of the meaning of the symbols, had only made too rigorous an application of them.
He had taken my lessons too literally and as I had limited myself to giving
him the nomenclature of certain things in his room he was convinced that
these were the only things to which it was applicable. Thus every book
which was not the one he had in his room was not a book for Victor, and
before he could decide to give it the same name it was necessary that an
exact resemblance should establish a visible identity between the one and
the other. This is a very different procedure in nomenclature from that
of children, who, when beginning to speak, give to particular terms the
value of general ones but keep the restricted meaning of the particular
term.[1]

---

[1]E.g., a child calling all men daddy (particular term) will really think of them
all as father (tr.).

What could account for this strange difference? If I am not mistaken it grew out of an unusual acuteness of visual observation which was the inevitable result of the special education given to his sense of sight. By the method of analytical comparison I had trained this sense organ so thoroughly in the recognition of the visible qualities of objects and the differences of dimension, color and conformation, that he could always detect between two identical things such points of dissimilarity as would make him believe there was an essential difference between them. With the source of the error thus located, the remedy became easy. It was to establish the identity of the objects by demonstrating to the pupil the identity of their uses or their properties. It was to make him see common qualities which earned the same name for things apparently different. In a word, it was a question of teaching him to consider things no longer with reference to their differences but according to their similarities.

XXVII. This new study was a kind of introduction to the act of comparison. At first the pupil gave himself up to it so completely that he was inclined to go astray again by attaching the same idea and giving the same name to things which had no other connection than the conformity of their shapes or uses. Thus under the name of book he indicated indiscriminately a handful of paper, a note book, a newspaper, a register, a pamphlet. All straight and long pieces of wood were called sticks. At one time he gave the name of brush to the broom, and at another that of broom to the brush, and soon, if I had not repressed this abuse of comparison, I should have seen Victor restricted to the use of a small number of signs which he would have applied indiscriminately to a large number of entirely different things which had only certain general qualities or properties in common.

XXVIII. In the midst of these mistakes, or rather fluctuations, of an intelligence tending ceaselessly to inaction but continually provoked by artificial means, there apparently developed one of those characteristic faculties of man, and especially thinking man, the faculty of invention. When considering things from the point of view of their similarity or of their common qualities, Victor concluded that since there was a resemblance of shape between certain objects, there ought in certain circumstances to be an identity of uses and functions. Without doubt this conclusion was somewhat risky. But it gave rise to judgments which, even though obviously found to be defective, became so many new means to instruction. I remember that one day when I asked him in writing for a knife, he looked for one for some time and contented himself with offering me a razor, which he fetched from a neighboring room. I pretended it would do and when his lesson was finished gave him something to eat as usual. I wanted him to cut his bread instead of dividing it with his fingers as was his custom. And to this end I held out to him the razor which he had given me under the name of knife. His behavior was consistent, he tried to use it as such, but the lack of stability of the blade prevented this. I did not consider the lesson complete. I took the razor and, in the actual presence of Victor, made it serve its proper use. From than on the instrument was no longer and could not be any longer in his eyes a knife. I longed to make certain. I again took his book and showed him the word *couteau* (knife) and the pupil immediately showed me the object he held in his hand and which I had given him a moment ago when he could not use the razor. To make the result convincing it was necessary to reverse the test. If the book were put in Victor's hand while I touched the razor, it was necessary that he should fail to pick out any word, as he did not yet know the name of this instrument. He passed this test also.

XXIX. At other times his substitutions were evidence of much more bizarre comparisons. One day when he was dining in town he wished to receive a spoonful of lentils offered him at a moment when there were no more plates and dishes on the table, I remember that he had the idea of going and taking from the mantelpiece and holding it out as if it were a plate, a little circular picture under glass, set in a frame, the smooth and projecting edge of which made it not at all unlike a plate.

XXX. But very often his expedients were happier, more successful and better deserving the name of invention. Quite worthy of such a name was the way by which he provided himself one day with a pencil case. Only once in my study had I made him use one to hold a small piece of chalk too short to take up with the end of his fingers. A few days afterwards the same difficulty occurred again but Victor was in his room and had no pencil-holder at hand to hold his chalk. I put it to the most industrious or the most inventive man to say, or rather do, what he did in order to procure one. He took an implement used in roasting, found in well-equipped kitchens but quite superfluous in one belonging to a poor creature such as he was, and which for that reason had remained forgotten and corroded with rust at the bottom of a little cupboard—namely a skewer. Such was the instrument which he took to replace the one he lacked and which by a further inspiration of really creative imagination he was clever enough to convert into a real pencil-holder by replacing the slide with a few turns of thread. Pardon, My Lord, the importance which I attach to this act. One must have experienced all the anguish of a course of instruction as painful as this had been; one must have followed and directed this man-plant in his laborious developments from the first act of attention up to this first spark of imagination before one can have any idea of the joy that I felt, and can pardon me for introducing at this moment, and with something of a flourish, so ordinary and so simple a fact. What also added to the importance of this result when considered as a proof of actual progress and as a guarantee of future improvement is that, instead of occurring as an isolated incident which might have made it appear accidental, it was one among many incidents, doubtless less striking, but which, coming at the same period and evidently emanating from the same source, appeared in the eyes of an attentive observer to be diverse results of a general impulse. It is, indeed, worthy of notice that from this moment many routine habits which the pupil had contracted when applying himself to the little occupations prescribed for him, spontaneously disappeared. While rigidly refraining from making forced comparisons or drawing remote conclusions, one may, I think, at least suspect that this new way of looking at familiar things which gave birth to the idea of making new applications of them, might be expected to have precisely the result of forcing the pupil out of the unvarying round of, so to speak, automatic habits.

XXXI. Thoroughly convinced at last that I had completely established in Victor's mind the connection of the objects with their signs, it only remained for me to increase the number gradually. If the procedure by which I established the meaning of the first signs has been thoroughly grasped it will be seen that it could be applied only to a limited number of objects and to things small in size, and that a bed, a room, a tree, or a person, as well as the constituent and inseparable parts of a whole, could not be labeled in the same way. I did not find any difficulty in making the sense of these new words understood, although I could not, as in the preceding experiments bind them visibly to the things they represented. In order to be understood it was sufficient for me to point to the new word with a finger and with the other hand to show the object to which the word belonged. I had little more trouble in making him understand the names of the parts which enter into the composition of the whole object. Thus for a long time the words fingers, hands, forearms could not offer any distinct meaning to the pupil. This confusion in attaching the signs was evidently due to the fact that he had not yet understood that the parts of a body considered separately formed in their turn distinct objects which had their particular names. In order to give him the idea I took a bound book, tore off its covers, and detached several of its leaves. As I gave Victor each of these separate parts I wrote its name upon the blackboard. Then taking from his hands the various pieces, I made him in turn indicate their names to me. When they were thoroughly engraved on his memory, I replaced the separated parts and when I again asked their names he indicated them as before; then showing him the whole book without indicating any part in particular, I asked him the name. He pointed to the word book.

XXXII. This is all that was necessary to render him familiar with the names of the various parts of compound bodies; and to avoid confusion between the names of the separate parts and the general name of the object, I was careful in my demonstrations to touch each part directly and, when applying the general name, to content myself with indicating the thing vaguely without touching it.

XXXIII. From this lesson I passed on to the qualities of the bodies. Here I entered into the field of abstractions and I entered it with the fear of not being able to penetrate or finding myself soon halted by insurmountable difficulties. None showed themselves, and my first lesson was grasped instantly although it bore upon one of the most abstract qualities, that of extension. I took two books of similar bindings but of different sizes, the one an octodecimo, the other an octavo. I touched the first. Victor opened his book and pointed to the word *book*. I touched the second. The pupil indicated the same word. I began again several times and always with the same result. Next I took the little book, and giving it to Victor, made him put his hand flat upon the cover which it hid almost entirely. I then made him do the same thing with the octavo volume; his hand covered scarcely half of it. So that he could not mistake my intention I showed him the part which remained uncovered, and induced him to stretch out his fingers towards this part which he could not do without uncovering a part equal to that which he covered. After this experiment which demonstrated in such a tangible manner to my pupil the difference in size of these two objects, I again asked him the name. Victor hesitated. He felt that the same name could no longer be applied indiscriminately to two things which he had just found so unequal. This was what I was waiting for. I wrote the word *book* upon two cards and placed one upon each book. I next wrote upon a third the word *big*, and the word *little* upon a fourth. I placed them beside the others, the one on the octavo and the other upon the small volume. Having made Victor notice this arrangement I took the labels again, mixed them several times, and then gave them to him to be replaced. This was done correctly.

XXXIV. Had I been understood? Had the respective sense of the words *big* and *little* been grasped? In order to be certain and to have complete proof, this is what I did. I got two nails of unequal length. I compared them in almost the same way as I had done with the books. Then having written upon two cards the word *nail* I gave them to him without adding the two adjectives big and little, hoping that if my preceding lesson had been thoroughly grasped he would apply to the nails the same signs of relative size as he had served to mark the difference of dimension of the two books. He did this with a promptness that rendered the proof still more conclusive. Such was the procedure by which I gave him the idea of size. I used it with the same success to render intelligible the signs which represent the other sensible qualities of bodies such as color, weight, resistance, etc.

XXXV. After the explanation of the adjective, came the verb. To make this understood by the pupil I had only to submit to several kinds of action an object of which he knew the name. These actions I designated as soon as executed, by the infinitive of the verb in question. For example I took a key and wrote its name upon the blackboard. Then *touching* it, *throwing* it, *picking* it up, *kissing* it, *putting* it back in its place, and so on, I simultaneously wrote in a column at the side of the word *key*, the verbs *to touch, to throw, to pick up, to kiss, to replace*, etc. For the word *key* I then substituted the name of another object which I submitted to the same functions, pointing at the same time to the verbs already written. It often happened that in thus replacing at random one object by another in order to have it governed by the same verbs, there was such an inconsistency between them and the nature of the object that the action asked for became odd or impossible. The embarrassment in which the pupil found himself generally turned out to his advantage as much as to my own satisfaction; for it gave him the chance to exercise his discernment and me the opportunity of gathering proofs of his intelligence. For example, when I found myself one day, after successive changes of the objects of the verbs, with such strange association of words as *to tear stone, to cut cup, to eat broom*, he evaded the difficulty very well by changing the two actions indicated by the first two verbs into others less incompatible with the nature of their objects. Thus he took a hammer to break the stone and dropped the cup to break it. Coming to the third verb (eat) and not being able to find any word to replace it, he looked for something else to serve as the object of the verb. He took a piece of bread and ate it.

In our study of these grammatical difficulties we were obliged to creep painfully and by endless detours, and so we simultaneously practised writing both as an auxiliary means of instruction and as a necessary diversion. As I had anticipated, the beginning of this work offered innumerable difficulties. Writing is an exercise in imitation, and imitation was yet to be born in our savage. Thus when for the first time I gave him a bit of chalk and arranged it conveniently in his fingers, I could obtain from him no line or stroke which might lead me to suspect any intention on the pupil's part to imitate what he had seen me do. Here then it was necessary once more to retrace our steps and to try and rouse from their inertia the imitative faculties by submitting them, as we had the others, to a kind of gradual education. I proceeded to the execution of this plan by practising Victor in the performance of acts when imitation is crude, such as lifting his arms, putting forward his foot, sitting down and getting up at the same time as myself; then opening his hand, shutting it, and repeating with his fingers many movements, first simple, then combined, that I performed in front of him. I next put into his hand, as in my own, a long rod sharpened to a point, and made him hold it as if it were a quill for writing, with the double intention of giving more strength and poise to his fingers through the difficulty of holding this imitation pen in equilibrium, and of making visible, and consequently capable of imitation, even the slightest movement of the rod.

XXXVII. Thus prepared by preliminary exercises we placed ourselves before the blackboard, each furnished with a piece of chalk, and placing our two hands at the same height I began by making a slow vertical movement towards the bottom of the board. The pupil did just the same, following exactly the same direction and dividing his attention between his line and mine, looking without intermission from the one to the other as if he wished to compare them successively at all points.

The result of our actions was two lines exactly parallel. My subsequent lessons were merely a development of the same procedure. I will not describe them. I will only say that the result was such that at the end of some months Victor could copy the words of which he already knew the meaning. Soon after he could reproduce them from memory, and finally make use of his writing, entirely unformed though it was and has remained, to express his wants, to solicit the means to satisfy them and to grasp by the same method of expression the needs or the will of others.

XXXVIII. In considering my experiments as a real course in imitation, I believed that the actions should not be limited to manual activity. I introduced several procedures which had no connection with the mechanism of writing but which were much more conducive to the exercise of intelligence. Such among others is the following. I drew upon a blackboard two circles almost equal, one opposite myself and the other in front of Victor. I arranged upon six or eight points of the circumference of these circles six or eight letters of the alphabet and wrote the same letters within the circles but disposed them differently. Next I drew several lines in one of the circles leading to the letters placed in the circumference. Victor did the same thing on the other circle. But because of the different arrangement of the letters, the most exact imitation nevertheless gave an entirely different figure from the one I had just offered as a model. Thence was to come the idea of a special kind of imitation which was not a matter of slavishly copying a given form but one of reproducing its spirit and manner without being held up by the apparent difference in the result. Here was no longer a routine repetition of what the pupil saw being done, such as can be obtained up to a certain point from certain imitative animals, but an intelligent and reasoned imitation, as variable in its method as in its applications, and in a word, such as one has a right to expect from a man endowed with the free use of all his intellectual faculties.

XXXIX. Of all the phenomena observable during the first developments of a child perhaps the most astonishing is the facility with which he learns to speak. When one thinks that speech, which is without question the most marvelous act of imitation, is also its first result, admiration is redoubled for that Supreme Intelligence whose masterpiece is man, and Who, wishing to make speech the principal promoter of education, could not let imitation, like the other faculties, develop progressively, and therefore necessarily made it fruitful as well as active from its beginning. But this imitative faculty, the influence of which extends throughout the whole of life, varies in its application according to age. It is used in learning to speak only during earliest childhood. Later other functions come under its influence and it abandons, so to speak, the vocal instrument, so that a young child, even an adolescent, after leaving his native country, promptly loses its manners, etiquette and language, but never loses those intonations of voice which constitute what is called accent. It follows from this physiological truth that in awakening the faculty of imitation in this young savage, now an adolescent, I ought not to have expected to find any disposition in the vocal organ to profit by this development of the imitative faculties, even supposing that I had not found a second obstacle in the obstinate lethargy of the sense of hearing. With respect to hearing, Victor could be considered as a deaf mute although he was certainly much inferior to this class of unfortunates since they are essentially observers and imitators.

XL. Nevertheless, I did not believe that I should allow this difference to bring me to a standstill or to let it deprive me of the hope of making him speak, with all the resulting advantages which I promised myself. I felt I should try a last resource, which was to lead him to the use of speech through the sense of sight, since it was out of the question to do so through the sense of hearing. Here the problem was to practise his eye in observing the mechanism of the articulation of sounds, and to practise his voice in the reproduction of the sounds by the use of a happy combination of attention and imitation. For more than a year all my work and all our exercises were directed towards this end. In order to follow the previous methods of insensible gradation, I preceded the study of the visible articulation of sounds by the slightly easier imitation of movements of the face muscles, beginning with those which were most easily seen. Thus we have instructor and pupil facing each other and grimacing their hardest; that is to say, putting the muscles of the eyes, forehead, mouth and jaw into all varieties of motion, little by little concentrating upon the muscles of the lips. Then after persisting for a long time with the movements of the fleshy part of the organ of speech, namely the tongue, we submitted it also to the same exercises, but varied them much more and continued them for a longer time.

XLI. Prepared in this way, it seemed to me that the organ of speech ought to lend itself without further trouble to the imitation of articulate sounds and I considered this result both near and inevitable. I was entirely mistaken. This long preparation resulted in nothing but the emission of unformed monosyllables sometimes shrill, sometimes deep and still far less clear than those which I had obtained in my first experiments. Nevertheless, I persisted, and still struggled for a long time against the obstinacy of the organ. Finally, however, seeing that the continuation of my efforts and the passing of time brought about no change, I resigned myself to the necessity of giving up any attempt to produce speech, and abandoned my pupil to incurable dumbness.

3. Organic Brain Syndromes

These disorders are caused by or associated with impairment of brain tissue function and are manifested by the following symptoms: impairment of orientation; impairment of memory; impairment of all intellectual functions such as comprehension, calculation, knowledge, learning, etc.; impairment of judgment; lability and shallowness of affect. The syndrome may be the only disturbance present or may be associated with psychotic symptoms and behavioral disturbances. The severity of the associated symptoms is affected by and related to not only the precipitating organic disorder but also the patient's inherent personality patterns, present emotional conflicts, his environmental situation, and interpersonal relations. Psychoses associated with syndromes such as senile and pre-senile dementia, alcohol poisoning, intracranial infection such as general paralysis or epidemic encephalitis, or other cerebral or physical conditions are categorized separately from psychoses not caused by physical conditions (see Section 4). However, it is important to note that patients may have an organic brain syndrome but not be psychotic.

3. Treatment of the Psychosis of General Paresis with Combined Sodium Amytal and Psychotherapy: Report of a Case*

Robert S. Wallerstein

The determination of a relationship between syphilitic infection and general paralysis (also general paresis, dementia paralytica) has been an outstanding accomplishment in the field of clinical psychopathology. Esquirol made observations concerning this relationship as early as 1805, but confirmation waited more than a century for the discovery that a minute organism, theponema pallidum, was the cause of syphilis and responsible for the destruction of nerve tissue in the brain.

In this case study of a 53-year-old man with a psychotic general paralysis, Wallerstein aims to demonstrate that the patient's psychotic behavior results not only from the organic condition (post-mortem examination of paretic patients typically shows atrophy of the frontal and temporal lobes), but also from pre-morbid personality factors that are significant in the mental functioning. The author suggests that the organic condition triggers the psychotic behavior, and supports this contention by presenting evidence to show that the mental picture frequently does not improve with serologic and neurologic improvement. He utilizes a psychoanalytic explanation of regression to early stages to account for the psy-

*This paper is sponsored by the Veterans Administration and is published with the approval of the Chief Medical Director. The statements and conclusions published by the author are results of his own study and do not necessarily reflect the opinion or policy of the Veterans Administration. Reprinted by special permission of the author and The William Alanson White Psychiatric Foundation, Inc., from *Psychiatry*, 1951, **14**, 307-317. Copyright © 1951, The William Alanson White Psychiatric Foundation, Inc.

*chotic development and offers the hypothesis that narcosis induced by
sodium amytal would render the patient more accessible to psychotherapy.*

*Sodium amytal, administered orally or by injection, is a barbiturate
hypnotic of intermediate duration of action and has been a widely used
drug for narcotherapy. The author notes that the effectiveness of sodium
amytal stems from a reduction in the patient's vulnerability to the pain
of psychological disclosure. Although Wallerstein's patient showed improvement in treatment, little appears to be known of the way in which
sodium amytal induces biochemical effects in behavior change.*

This communication discusses the extent of the potential reversibility
of so-called organic deterioration and dementia as illustrated in the
treatment of a patient with general paresis. Within this framework the
following aspects of this problem are dealt with: (1) the effects of drugs
and the peculiar effectiveness of sodium amytal in distinguishing the "functional" and reversible elements in "organic" mental syndromes with apparent deterioration; (2) the utilization of the transitory pharmacologically
induced remission as a lever to permit contact on a sustained psychotherapeutic basis; (3) a description of the psychotherapeutic process to
date, involving the question of the limitations of personal capacities imposed by the brain damage; and (4) some theoretical considerations as
to the nature and dynamics of the psychotic regression in the organic
brain syndromes.

General paresis has long been the prototype of the organic psychosis
and has been held as the classic demonstration of organic pathology
determining psychotic symptomatology. In 1902, Nissl was able to state
of this disorder, "Nothing is known to me of psychological explanations.
Here [in the mental symptoms of the paretic psychosis] one accepts the
same thing over which one is completely puzzled in other diseases as
something self-evident and necessary which is founded in the very nature
of the paretic process."[1] Since then, however, a continued search for these
"psychological explanations" has occurred. And as observations have mul-
tiplied, there has been an increasing awareness that the mental phenomena
manifested by patients with this organic psychosis are susceptible of psychologic explanation and their genesis can be dynamically understood just

---

[1]Nissl, "Hysterische Symptoms bei einfachen Seelenstorungen," *Zentralbl. f. Ner-
venh. u. Psychiat.* (1902) 13:2. Quoted in: Stefan Hollós and Sandor Ferenczi,
Psychoanalysis and the Psychic Disorder of General Paresis; New York, N. and M.
Disease Publishing Co., 1925; p. 1.

as those of the so-called functional psychoses. The significance of a person's premorbid personality structure and of his characteristic ego defenses for the psychologic make-up of this psychosis has been especially emphasized.[2] Hollós and Ferenczi in their monograph on *Psychoanalysis and the Psychic Disorder of General Paresis*,[3] published in 1925, elaborated a psychoanalytic explanation of the phenomenology of the disorder. Kenyon, Rapaport, and Lozoff in 1941 reviewed the literature to that date on the psychological investigations of the symptoms of general paresis. They summed up the main theses of Hollós and Ferenczi:

> General paresis is a pathopsychosis. The general impairment of mental functions is responded to by withdrawal of libido from the functions concerned. Thus regression to earlier stages of psychic development in which the damaged functions were not yet existent, occurs, permitting maintenance of self-esteem, since the damaged functions do not have any significance in those stages of development to which the patients regressed. No specific differentiation of this regression from others is given.
>
> The organic damage only initiates the psychosis. It has a limited role in the makeup of the psychosis which follows the psychological laws of regression. The dementia as a special problem is not discussed by the authors.
>
> The psychosis commences with a neurasthenic and depressive phase. While, according to Freud, the loss of love-object is the cause of melancholia, it is maintained that in paresis the losses of the ego inflicted by the organic damage (narcissistic loss) are equated with the loss of object and effect the depression and its compensation, the mania.[4]

If regression is the basic psychologic phenomenon of the paretic psychosis, then its occasional reversibility can be readily understood. Since the inception of specific somatic therapies—hyperpyrexia, tryparsamide, and now penicillin—physicians have continued to be puzzled by the lack of correlation between the degrees of serologic and neurologic improvement affected under treatment, on the one hand, and remissions in the mental picture, on the other. Frequently, despite vigorous therapy and

---

[2]Lawrence F. Woolley, "Personality Factors in the Psychosis of General Paresis," *Urol. & Cutan. Rev.* (1945) 49:3-6.

Vivian Bishop Kenyon, Milton Lozoff, and David Rapaport, "Metrazol Convulsions in the Treatment of the Psychosis of Dementia Paralytica," *Arch. Neurol. and Psychiat.* (1941) 46:884-896.

Vivian Bishop Kenyon, David Rapaport, and Milton Lozoff, "Notes on Metrazol in General Paresis: A Psychosomatic Study," *Psychiatry* (1941) 4:165-176.

[3]Reference footnote 1.

[4]Kenyon *et al.*, "Notes on Metrazol in General Paresis: A Psychosomatic Study," reference footnote 2; p. 167.

adequate serologic and neurologic restitution, no remission of the psychosis has followed. In addition, it has been repeatedly shown that there is no correlation between the anatomic degenerative and inflammatory processes seen at post-mortem examination and the clinical psychotic picture. These observations may be explained if we think of the somatic therapies as directed in some manner, as yet not completely elucidated, against only the initial inciting and function-damaging cause, presumably the spirochete itself. These somatic therapies, if successful, would therefore be able to arrest and possibly even partially reverse the organic component of the total loss of functioning—that is, the neurologic stigmata and, mentally, the dementia. But they would affect only in an accidental and uncontrolled manner the psychotic picture caused by the regression in ego functioning under the onslaught of the organic impairment of the ego's higher integrative faculties.

According to this reasoning, the same therapies, both somatic and psychologic, that have helped in the management of the so-called functional psychoses might well be indicated as concomitants to specific somatic antisyphilitic therapy. This would seem particularly applicable to those patients who have shown no improvement in mental functioning upon the use of fever therapy, arsenicals, and penicillin. Using this rationale, Kenyon, Rapaport, and Lozoff[5] treated 16 paretic patients with metrazol, the somatic agent then in use in the treatment of schizophrenia. Of these, 12 had been previously treated with fever and/or hyperpyrexia without substantial improvement of the psychotic symptomatology. In the remaining 4 of this group, metrazol was administered to patients who had had no prior somatic therapy of any kind to determine whether this agent alone could effect significant improvement. Of the 16, 5 showed good improvement both clinically and in their objective psychological testing results, leading to release from the hospital of 4 out of the 5; 5 showed slight improvement sustained over a short time only; and 6 showed no essential change. The improvement noted with metrazol would support the theory that the psychosis of dementia paralytica is not a simple consequence of the organic damage usually present in this disease, but is rather a potentially reversible psychologic response (regression) on the part of the ego to the weakening of its cardinal functions of reality-testing and control over the instinctual impulses,[6] which is a consequence of the syphilitic damage. Metrazol appeared to act upon this regressive process in the same manner as in the functional psychoses, and seemed therefore

---

[5]Vivian Bishop Kenyon and David Rapaport, "The Etiology of the Psychosis of Dementia Paralytica with a Preliminary Report of the Treatment of a Case of This Psychosis with Metrazol," *J. N. and M. Disease* (1941) 94:147-159. Also reference footnote 2.

[6]Isador H. Coriat, "A Psychoanalytic Interpretation of the Mental Symptoms of Paresis," *Psychoanalytic Rev.* (1945) 32:253-262.

of practical therapeutic benefit, as well as of theoretical interest, in those cases of the psychosis of dementia paralytica which were unresponsive to standard antisyphilitic therapy.

Since this first work with metrazol, numerous authors have utilized the same rationale and the same therapeutic approach with metrazol,[7] insulin coma,[8] insulin subcoma,[9] electroconvulsive therapy,[10] nonconvulsive electric (faradic) shock,[11] and combined ECT and insulin subcoma.[12] All but one[13] reported good results. Several of these investigators[14] pointed out that the efficacy of the therapy seemed related to the type of psychotic symptomatology and the nature of the underlying personality structure much as it does in the functional psychoses. Thus Tomlinson found that of his paretic patients, all those who showed predominant affective (manic) or catatonic coloring did well. Of those primarily paranoid, only one improved, and of those who showed what he called a predominant picture of organic deterioration, none did well. He concluded that "the sphere of greatest use would appear to be in catatonic and manic reactions which continue after adequate specific therapy has been given."[15] Solomon *et al.* concurred that "in schizophrenic-like pictures, it [ECT] . . .

---

[7]Eldo Broggi, "Weitere Ergebnisse mit der Krampfbehandlung (mit Cardiazol oder Elektro-schock) der Progresiven Paralyse," *Psychiat.-Neurol. Wchnschr.* (1942) 44:65-67.

[8]D. V. Conwell, personal communication; quoted in Kenyon *et al.,* "Notes on Metrazol in General Paresis: A Psychosomatic Study," reference footnote 2; p. 165.

F. Marco Merenciano, "Paralisis General Progresiva, Notas Clínicas y Primeros Essayos con Tratamiento Insulínico," *Med. Españ.* (1942) 8:468-481.

A. Puca, "Paralisi Progresiva e Terapia da Shock," *Riforma Med.* (1947) 61:209-212.

[9]Paul J. Tomlinson, "Insulin and Electric Therapy in General Paresis," *Psychiatric Quart.* (1944) 18:413-421.

[10]Reference footnote 7. Reference footnote 9.

Thomas J. Heldt and Nicholas P. Dallis, "Electroshock in Therapeutically Refractory General Paresis," *Urol. & Cutan. Rev.* (1945) 49:40-42.

M. C. Petersen, "Electric Shock Therapy for Psychosis with Special Reference to Dementia Paralytica," *Proc. Staff Meet. Mayo Clinic* (1944) 19:278-283.

M. C. Petersen, "Electric Shock in the Treatment of Dementia Paralytica," *Proc. Staff Meet. Mayo Clinic* (1945) 20: 107-112.

Harry C. Solomon, Augustus S. Rose, and Robert E. Arnot, "Electric Shock Therapy in General Paresis." *J. N. and M. Disease* (1948) 107:377-381.

Gert Heilbrunn and Paul Feldman, "Electric Shock Treatment in General Paresis," *Amer. J. Psychiatry* (1943) 99:702-705.

[11]Nathaniel J. Berkwitz, "Non-Convulsive Electric (Faradic) Shock Therapy of Psychoses Associated with Alcoholism, Drug Intoxication and Syphilis: A Psychosomatic Approach in the Treatment of 'Reaction of Delirium,' " *Amer. J. Psychiatry* (1942) 99:364-373.

[12]Reference footnote 9.

[13]Heilbrunn and Feldman, reference footnote 10.

[14]Reference footnote 9. Solomon *et al.,* reference footnote 10. Reference footnote 11.

[15]Reference footnote 9; p. 420.

is of little value," but that "cases of general paresis with predominant affective components in the psychosis respond well to electric shock even though signs and symptoms of organic brain disease may be present. Since the improvement is almost immediate it is hardly possible that tissue repair plays any role in the result."[16]

Since the introduction of the barbiturate drugs and especially sodium amytal in the treatment of psychiatric disorders, these drugs have been explored in a wide variety of ways against the entire gamut of psychiatric nosology. Bleckwenn's[17] original concept was that a prolonged period of narcosis would permit some sort of psychic reconstitution leading to a normal lucid interval following awakening. He used this rationale in treating manic behavior, depressed patients, involutional agitated depressions, and catatonic excitements. He felt that amytal narcosis definitely shortened the course of affective illnesses and resulted in brief lucid intervals in the schizophrenic. It was soon found that smaller, nonnarcotic doses of amytal likewise arouse the catatonic patient, reverse (temporarily) his withdrawal, and for a few hours at least make him verbally accessible.[18] A period of emotional rapport ensues, giving access to thought content ordinarily well guarded by repressive defenses, and "shifts the emotional state along the depression-elation scale in the direction of elation."[19] This effect occurs to greater or lesser degree in both 'normal' people and patients in catatonic stupor. The transient ameliorating effect of intravenous amytal on the catatonic symptomatology has been used by some workers[20] as a fairly reliable sign of ultimate prognosis of the current schizophrenic episode whether treated with or without somatic therapies. The dynamics

---

[16]Solomon *et al.*, reference footnote 10; p. 380.

[17]W. J. Bleckwenn, "Narcosis as Therapy in Neuropsychiatric Conditions," *J. A. M. A.* (1930) 95:1168-1171.

[18]Erich Lindemann, "The Psychopathological Effect of Sodium Amytal," *Proc. Soc. Exper. Biol. Med.* (1931) 28:864-866.

Erich Lindemann, "Psychological Changes in Normal and Abnormal Individuals under the Influence of Sodium Amytal," *Amer. J. Psychiatry* (1932) 88:1083-1091.

Meyer M. Harris and Siegfried E. Katz, "The Effect of the Administration of Sodium Amytal and Sodium Rhodonate on Mental Patients," *Amer J. Psychiatry* (1933) 89:1065-1083.

Erich Lindemann and William Malamud, "Experimental Analysis of the Psychopathological Effects of Intoxicating Drugs," *Amer. J. Psychiatry* (1934) 90:853-881.

Lother B. Kalinowsky and Paul H. Hoch, *Shock Treatments and Other Somatic Procedures in Psychiatry;* New York, Grune and Stratton, 1946; p. 202.

[19]Erich Lindemann, "Psychological Changes in Normal and Abnormal Individuals under the Influence of Sodium Amytal," reference footnote 18; p. 1088.

[20]M. M. Harris, William A. Horwitz, and E. A. Milch, "Regarding Sodium Amytal as a Prognostic Aid in Insulin and Metrazol Shock Therapy of Mental Patients (Dementia Praecox)," *Amer. J. Psychiatry* (1939) 96:327-333.

Jacques S. Gottlieb and Justin M. Hope, "Prognostic Value of Intravenous Administration of Sodium Amytal in Cases of Schizophrenia," *Arch. Neurol. and Psychiat.* (1941) 46:86-100.

of the effect of the drug on a person's psychologic functioning has been discussed by Kubie and Margolin. They state that "the drug lowers the intensity of the reaction to such unpleasant emotions as rage, anxiety and guilt, allows a patient to explore painful areas of experience without immediate psychic withdrawal at the first warnings of discomfort."[21] The personality is therefore less vulnerable to the psychic pain of exposure to material that would be otherwise intolerable.

In the light of the foregoing review, the application of sodium amytal to the management of the patient with an organic psychosis, such as general paresis, should offer like prospects of heightened accessibility to psychotherapy. For the psychosis of general paresis may be potentially reversible by the application of the same agents sometimes effective in the therapeutic management of the functional psychoses. Very few such attempts have been recorded, however. It is the purpose of this paper to present in detail one such use of sodium amytal in a patient with general paresis to demonstrate (1) the pharmacologic reversibility of a picture of apparent irreversible organic dementia and deterioration, and (2) the utilization of the transitory pharmacologically induced remission as a lever to permit contact on a sustained psychotherapeutic basis.

Case Report

The patient is a 53-year-old, white, World War I veteran, admitted to Winter VA Hospital for the first time in December, 1947, because of irritability, moroseness, seclusiveness, restless aimless overactivity, neglect of his business, and deterioration of personal habits—all of which had increased over a period of several months. Just prior to admission he had collapsed while downtown shopping. Five years before, in 1942, a positive blood Wasserman had been discovered, and he had been treated with arsenic and bismuth for over two years. Lumbar puncture was not done at that time.

The patient was born in 1897, the third of four sons of a hard-working German immigrant family in rural Kansas. The father was a diligent, thrifty farmer, economically successful, and a serious-minded, moralistic person who stressed decorum and industriousness. The mother was likewise cold, rigid, and moralistic, and was overly ambitious for the academic advancement of her children. The father's word was law at home. Discipline and obedience were rigidly enforced. Little companionship was offered the children, and only rarely were visitors entertained in the home or social evenings enjoyed. When the patient was 12, the

---

[21]Lawrence S. Kubie and Sydney G. Margolin, "The Therapeutic Role of Drugs in the Process of Repression, Dissociation, and Synthesis," *Psychosomatic Med.* (1945) 7:147-151; p. 147.

father was killed in a hunting accident. This resulted in the breakup of the home, the children moving in with the maternal grandparents, the mother going to California. From then to the time of her death years later, contacts between mother and children were minimal, consisting only of occasional letters and rare visits. When the mother was dying of carcinoma, the patient did nothing to help her and seemed quite indifferent to her death.

The patient was a compliant, controlled, passive youngster. He disliked school and was only a mediocre student. He enjoyed spending time by himself doing woodwork and "tinkering with mechanics." After he finished high school, he took a special trades course in mechanics at which he was apparently adept. He was at all times lonely and alone, had no close friends, and showed no particular interest in girls.

Following a two-year period of farming and an interval of service in World War I, the patient settled down to a lifetime of single-minded absorption in business in a small Kansas town. In succession, he built up several enterprises: a bus line, an automobile sales agency, a Delco equipment and repair shop. He operated these with tenacity, business acumen, single-minded concentration, and a willingness to engage in dubious, conniving practices designed to squeeze out competitors. Financially he became one of the leading citizens of the town, but he had no real friends, only business associates, and he led a constricted, lonely, schizoid existence which he shared with a dog or cat.

Outside his business, his only other real concern seemed to be a hypochondriacal absorption with his various bodily organ systems. He frequently consulted doctors, was addicted to numerous patent medicine preparations and was constantly absorbed in his somatic complaints. At 40, he suddenly married. This was both a surprise to his associates, who wondered when he could have had the time for courtship, and a joke to them that such a "fussy, old, confirmed bachelor" would marry. The courtship had apparently been of 12 years' duration, the patient having had to satisfy himself over that period that he was not making a mistake. His marriage introduced little change in his lonely existence. He and his wife seldom went out and usually stayed at home listening to the radio. He continually complained and nagged at his wife, largely about his various ailments. They had no children. His wife had a daughter by a previous marriage.

In 1942, when he was 45, the positive serology was discovered. A doctor assured the patient that this illness could have been contracted from a toilet seat. Despite two years of intensive antisyphilitic therapy, the mental symptoms already described became evident in 1947 and led to his first admission to Winter Hospital in December of that year. On admission he was restless, overactive, confused, and given to sporadic temper outbursts. He showed a mixture of euphoria and hypochondriasis. He had somatic complaints referable to every organ system. Memory and judgment were grossly impaired, and insight almost totally lacking. He had Argyll-Robertson pupils, mild optic atrophy, diminished deep tendon reflexes, impaired coordination and vibratory sense, and a cord bladder. Both blood and spinal fluid serology were positive. A diagnosis of taboparesis was made.

Following treatment with malaria and penicillin, the patient showed considerable improvement with good contact and accessibility, improved judgment, and diminution of his hypochondriacal complaints. Blood serology had become negative, and the spinal fluid cell count and protein fell to normal limits. The gold curve and the spinal fluid serology were unchanged. In July, 1948, he was adjudged well enough to go home on a trial visit and in October, 1948, ten months after admission, was discharged from the hospital rolls. At home both the townspeople and his wife seemed to have written him off permanently. His difficulties in attempting to re-establish himself in the community culminated in his wife's leaving him and securing a divorce.

Four months after discharge, in February, 1949, the patient returned to the hospital for a checkup because of recurrence of his hypochondriacal complaints in practically every organ system. Physical and neurological examination showed no evidence of relapse or progression of the disease process, and the improvement in his blood and spinal fluid was maintained unchanged: blood Kahn and complement fixation, negative; spinal fluid, no cells; 26 mg. percent protein; 4+ serology; and gold curve 5554320000. He was sent home where he continued on a gradual downhill course, became more hypochondriacal, depressed, confused, disoriented, and combative. He was sent to the County Farm where he was mute and semistuporous, refused food, and was incontinent of urine. In this state he was returned to Winter Hospital in May, 1949, about three months after his checkup. Again physical and neurologic examination showed no change from his initial admission and no evidence of progression. Further, the improvement originally noted in the laboratory examinations was still sustained with no sign of a relapse. Blood Kahn and complement fixation were negative, and spinal fluid cell count (3 lymphocytes) and protein (32 mg. percent) remained within normal limits. Spinal fluid Wasserman continued 4+, there were 4 Kolmer units, and gold curve was 5554320000. Despite the lack of evidence of progression of the organic syphilitic process, the patient was treated again with penicillin but with no perceptible effect on his psychological state.

During this time, the patient continued to be tense, apprehensive, mute, semistuporous. He was fearful and tremulous and would occasionally whimper and mumble. Sometimes he was hyperactive and ran moaning up and down the ward. He was negativistic; only with persistent coaxing could he be induced to eat. He was incontinent of urine. He was, above all, intensely resistive and fearful, and interpreted every attention or manipulation—such as being shaved, having his wet pants changed, and so on—as an attack, threatening immediate doom, which he must fight off at all costs. His fearful resistiveness to all ministrations resulted in repeated minor injuries to the patient and much difficulty to the personnel. In order to facilitate the performance of certain necessary procedures—such as a shave or an occasional enema—with as little trauma as possible, it was decided to attempt sedation of the patient with oral amytal just prior to the performance of these tasks. He was given two 3-grain capsules by mouth.

Under the influence of the amytal there was a startling transformation of the patient's appearance and behavior. After a half hour or so, he became suddenly talkative, even boisterous, active, and alert. In a sudden burst of activity, he wrote letters, started cleaning the ward, polished his shoes, changed his clothes, washed himself, and paid considerable attention to his grooming. He became loquacious, expansive, and cheerful. He was very importunate, made limitless, insistent small demands, and at times became quite irritable when these were denied. This effect lasted the better part of the day. The following day, the patient was again his more usual mute, fearful, incontinent, dilapidated self. The sodium amytal was repeated on numerous occasions, always with days in between, and the same sequence invariably ensued.

Various modifications in this regimen were attempted. Oral amytal in smaller doses and intramuscular amytal in the same dose both led to a similar reaction but of lesser intensity and of shorter duration, lasting only a few hours at most. Other barbiturates were tried in varying doses and administered in varying ways. Seconal made the patient somewhat alert and responsive, but the effect of the drug was less constant, lasted a much shorter time, and often led to marked drowsiness. Phenobarbital likewise made the patient only sparingly communicative for brief periods. Other nonbarbiturate sedatives, such as chloral hydrate or paraldehyde, no matter how administered or in what dose, had no demonstrable effect. The physiologically opposed, analeptic drugs, such as benzedrine or caffeine sodium benzoate, likewise evoked no discernible response. The unique efficacy of oral sodium amytal in bringing the patient from a mute, semistuporous, dilapidated state to a level of fairly good reality contact and personal tidiness seemed well established. This effect was produced repeatedly and unfailingly with amytal, and generally lasted through the day.

During these accessible intervals, the patient was seen in frequent interviews. The mental content was actively psychotic and delusional. The patient constantly voiced nihilistic and bizarre somatic delusions: "The ward's too small. It's shrunk down. There's not enough room. Not enough air or ventilation. I can't get any place competing with all these big guys. I'm so small. They crowd me out. They're all breathers. They use up all the ventilation. This place is too crowded with big fellows who take up all the room. I'm just a little fellow. I used to weigh 180. I used to be taller. I shrunk. I don't even weigh 100 pounds. I'm not even five foot. My blood is gone. My face is shriveling." He voiced pessimism about his own prospects for recovery and made numerous demands: "I'll never get better around here. I'll die here. I can't build myself up. The food's no good. . . . I need exercise. I need medicine. I want my kidney pills. My kidneys are bad. . . . I want to go to the library. I want to leave the hospital for a few days." There was always important business requiring immediate attention outside the hospital, but he was never able to specify what this might be. All unpleasant elements in his reality situation were denied. He was *not* divorced. He still loved his wife. She would come back. She had no reasons for divorce. She left temporarily because her hay fever bothered her. With apparent indifference he revealed his recent sexual impotence. He continually stressed how *well* he did under *previous* doctors—"not that I'm complaining about you." Whenever asked to account for his fluctuating levels of awareness and accessibility, he countered with denial and evasion or by explaining that on certain days he didn't feel good, listing various somatic complaints.

After experimentation with various dosages and drugs, it was decided to maintain the patient on a daily maintenance dose of amytal—two 3-grain tablets an hour apart at 7:30 and 8:30 a.m.—and to use that as a lever to make him accessible to an attempt at a prolonged, intensive, ego-supportive, psychotherapeutic relationship. Once the amytal was regularly given as part of the patient's routine therapeutic regimen, its effect was no longer as constant or as striking. Some days the patient was up, alert, and active; on other days he was withdrawn, incontinent, lay on his bed, and refused food. At no time, however, was he as completely withdrawn and unapproachable as he had been before the maintenance amytal regimen was instituted. When withdrawn and seclusive he could nonetheless with difficulty and patience be reached. Regular psychotherapeutic hours were scheduled twice weekly. Previously actual interviews had been held only when the patient was in good contact. Under the new schedule, interviews were held both at times when the patient was active and at times when he was withdrawn and seclusive. When up and alert, he greeted the therapist warmly, and eagerly came to the office for sessions up to an hour in length. When withdrawn and semistuporous he lay on his bed, moaned constantly, insisted that he felt unable to get up, and verbalized his sense of impending doom and destruction. At these times he often became both self-accusatory and accusatory of important figures in his environment—primarily his one surviving brother and the therapist —for abandoning him. On these occasions interviews were shorter and consisted, on the patient's part, largely of mumbled monosyllabic responses.

For months the patient continued to weave the same themes into his productions. He often and loudly voiced numerous somatic complaints and nihilistic delusions of the kind already described. He projected all of his difficulties onto numerous external factors, both persons and inanimate objects in his environment: "That damned radio. Playing all the time. How can a fellow get well in here?" He constantly accused the other patients of conspiring to harm him and prevent his recovery. Both the therapist and the patient's brother were accused of neglect: "Why don't you come *every* day? I'll never get well this way."

At other times, however, all complaints and bizarre delusions dropped away and the patient confidently voiced his belief in his rapid and complete recovery. On these occasions he pressed demands to be moved to a "better" ward, to be given passes, to be allowed to go home for a few days. He would point out that he was now "ready." When the therapist indicated that this state of "readiness" usually lasted only a few days and that he would then relapse into a semistupor and that transfer to another ward would be effected when he was truly ready as indicated by sustained improvement, the patient would counter in one of two ways. One would be a defiant "I'll show you"; the other a more despondent "I'll never get off the ward. If you don't let me go now, I'll never be ready. I'll get worse."

The therapist continued to pursue the role of aggressively, persistently, and painstakingly confronting the patient with reality, together with support to help the patient bear the awareness of the often intolerable nature of that reality. Doubt was cast on the veracity of the patient's repeatedly voiced somatic delusions. The reality core was seized and the rest ignored. The patient was faced over and over again with the facts of his fluctuating level of ego organization and their implications for him as an attempt through self-destructive withdrawal to cope with intolerable psychic distress. Little by little he accepted bits of reality that at first he had tried to deny—like the reality of his divorce—and reintegrated this awareness into his psychic functioning. Throughout these interview situations the patient continued in a clinging, passive-dependent, almost devouring attitude towards the therapist. He clung constantly to every available moment, often making it extremely difficult to terminate interviews. He made repeated demands of incredible variety; and the gratification of any of these led to the further extension of these demands so that they became impossible of fulfillment, and he could then turn on the object of his demands with feelings of rejection and deprivation. This pattern he attempted to re-enact constantly with both his brother—who visited him occasionally at the hospital—and the therapist.

Gradually the relationship with the therapist appeared to become strengthened. The patient at times shook hands spontaneously at the end of interviews and finally on one occasion verbalized, "I knew you'd come. You always keep your promise." Concomitantly, he showed a slow but definite clinical improvement evidenced in the increased amount of time during which he was up and alert and in the degree of reality contact and absence of delusional material during those periods. Periods of withdrawal as they occurred were interpreted to him as retreats before a too painful reality, and the therapist would relate each such withdrawal to specific disappointment or frustration in the reality situation. This the patient would deny and follow by projection of the difficulty and distress onto various externals. But over a period of time he developed an increased capacity to handle that particular kind of trauma without as much regression. As the improvement became more sustained, the patient was moved to a ward with more privileges, and was allowed to attend off-hospital events in town. After about six months, the patient was able to work through to the verbalization about the amytal, "I don't need the pills any more." At that point the amytal was stopped. At present writing the patient has been without amytal for seven months and receives no medication other than an occasional aspirin for headaches. He is alert and active on most days. On other days when he again tends to withdraw, this can usually be reversed by a visit from the therapist or by a determined show of interest on the part of the ward personnel. His mental content is not delusional or deviative. He needs the constant and firm support that he obtains within the relationship with the therapist. The psychotherapy is being continued. A further report of progress with this patient is anticipated.

DISCUSSION

In this patient with taboparesis and the mental picture of an organic psychosis in an apparent advanced stage of deterioration and dementia, a partial remission has thus far been induced by a combination of sodium amytal medication and intensive psychotherapeutic interviews. Previous intensive antisyphilitic therapy with malaria and penicillin had arrested the progress of the organic damage but had failed to halt the developing psychotic picture. Though at first the amytal was essential to make the psychotherapeutic contact possible, after some six months it was possible to dispense with the amytal without deterioration in psychic functioning. At present the psychotherapy continues.

The use of sodium amytal in this case played a unique and withal still inadequately understood role, deserving of discussion from several aspects. Certainly it demonstrates that so-called organic dementia is not necessarily to be dismissed as such. Under the impact of the awareness both of the functional impairment and of the loss of painfully acquired ego-integrative functions, the patient experiences a psychotic regression. It is not clearly established how amytal acts pharmacologically—and on what integrative levels in the central nervous system—to permit a reversal of this psychologic regressive process and a re-establishment of reality contact on the highest level of ego functioning possible to the organically damaged organism. Kubie and Margolin[22] have outlined the psychologic dynamics of this process. They state that the use of amytal reduces tremendously the "psychic pain" that awareness of the painful reality—that is, the organic process at work in the brain—would cause in the ordinary waking state. This would explain how amytal facilitates the abreaction of repressed battle trauma in the therapy of the war neuroses, how it brings a mute catatonic patient out of his withdrawal from an unacceptable reality back into contact with it, and similarly how it effects the same result in this paretic patient who in the face of *his* reality (the paresis) had to resort to a psychotic regression until amytal made it possible to partially reverse this process, temporarily.

This same effect of amytal has been noted in depressed patients where "diminution of anxiety and tension . . . with sodium amytal . . . has had a temporary ameliorating effect upon the symptoms of depression. It is an effective antidepressant." The patients feel more "comfortable, pleasant, and alert."[23] Whether the nature of the withdrawal in the patient presented here is depressive or catatonic is a matter of dynamic speculation. Whatever its nature, the need for it, in this patient, could be lessened under amytal.

One similar case was described in considerable detail by Fellows in 1932. His patient was a 32-year-old general paretic who did poorly on antisyphilitic therapy and six weeks after admission presented a picture described as: ". . . deteriorated rather rapidly, would no longer speak at

---

22Reference footnote 21.
23Jacques S. Gottlieb, "The Use of Sodium Amytal and Benzedrine Sulfate in the Symptomatic Treatment of Depressions," *Dis. Nerv. System* (1949) 10:50-52; p. 50. See also:
Jacques S. Gottlieb and Frank E. Coburn, "Psychopharmacologic Study of Schizophrenia and Depressions: Intravenous Administration of Sodium Amytal and Amphetamine Sulfate Separately and in Various Combinations," *Arch. Neurol. and Psychiat.* (1944) 51:260-263.
Jacques S. Gottlieb, Howard Krouse, and Arthur W. Freidinger, "Psychopharmacologic Study of Schizophrenia and Depressions: Comparison of Tolerance to Sodium Amytal and Amphetamine Sulfate," *Arch. Neurol. and Psychiat.* (1945) 54:372-377.

all, stood by the window naked, gazing out with an expressionless face for hours at a time. . . . He defecated and urinated upon the floor without moving or changing his position. He refused all nourishment; when fluids were put into his mouth he would not swallow them but let the fluid run out of his mouth, necessitating daily tube feedings." With oral amytal a remarkable change ensued. The patient "spoke intelligibly, ate unassisted, read newspapers, discussed his friends, etc."[24] This phenomenon lasted for about three hours and was repeated almost daily. The patient went on to improve and after about six weeks was taken off amytal. Kenyon *et al.*[25] reported a followup on Fellows' case. The patient was shortly paroled from the hospital, following which he soon relapsed, was admitted to another hospital and died. No attempt at formal psychotherapy had been made. Apparently referring to the same case, Karl Menninger in *Man Against Himself* states, "The whole question of just how different drugs affect the different instinctual strivings and the different structural and functional faculties of the psyche is almost entirely unexplored. In this connection, one of my colleagues was particularly struck some years ago by the modification of the super-ego effected by sodium amytal in a case of general paresis. It is an impressive thing when the administration of a drug suddenly makes a man responsive to the demands of civilization who, only a few hours before that time, was acting like a wild beast or an imbecile, the more startling because the response is lost as the effects of the drug wear off."[26] Solomon *et al.* refer briefly to a similar experience: "A patient who had recently been treated for general paresis was admitted from a general hospital with catatonic mutism and refusal to eat." With amytal he "became tractable" and "ate ravenously."[27]

In addition to thus demonstrating the pharmacologic reversibility of the psychosis of general paresis, amytal also poses a psychotherapeutic challenge, in that, theoretically at least, psychologic reversal on a sustained basis is therefore also possible. The capacity of the patient under discussion in this paper to respond to intensive psychotherapeutic contact and even ultimately to dispense voluntarily with the amytal demonstrates the validity of this hypothesis. The amytal, of course, not only served to demonstrate the reversible nature of the psychotic regressive process in this patient but greatly facilitated the psychotherapeutic contact itself.

---

[24]Ralph M. Fellows, "Sodium Amytal in the Treatment of Paresis: Preliminary Report," *J. Missouri State Med. Assn.* (1932) 29:194-196; p. 194.

[25]Kenyon *et al.*, "Notes on Metrazol in General Paresis: A Psychosomatic Study," reference footnote 2.

[26]Karl A. Menninger, *Man Against Himself;* New York, Harcourt, Brace, 1938; pp. 431-432.

[27]Solomon *et al.*, reference footnote 10; p. 377.

Pertinent to these observations is a report of a similar kind of work dealing with the use of psychotherapy in organically brain-damaged patients who were aphasic as a result of wartime craniocerebral injuries. This report, by Linn and Stein,[28] postulated that the functional impairment in these aphasic patients was due not only to the actual structural damage but also to the awareness of loss of the original mastery over the environment. The patients responded to this awareness with enormous anxiety and feelings of inadequacy, and reacted to new situations with verbal withdrawal in order to avoid the anxiety engendered by recurrent failure. Under amytal, anxiety lessened, and their vocabulary and sentence structure increased in breadth and complexity. This improvement of performance could then be worked with in helping the patient again to face reality and perform maximally within the limitations imposed by the actual structural damage.

---

[28]Louis Linn and Martin H. Stein, "Sodium Amytal in Treatment of Aphasia," *Bull. U. S. Army Med. Dept.* (1946) 5:705-708.

4. "Model Psychosis" Produced by Inhalation of Gasoline Fumes*

Eliere J. Tolan and Friedrich A. Lingl

The "model psychosis," or artificially-induced psychotic-like state, offers psychology both a research tool and a therapeutic adjunct. "Model psychotic" states, also called experimental or artificial psychoses, are alterations in psychic and body functioning resembling the actual morbid states. "Model psychoses" are induced by a number of agents, mainly lysergic acid diethylamide (LSD – 25), mescaline, and psilocybin. These drugs are considered among the hallucinogenic (producing hallucinations) and psychotomimetic (producing states mimicking psychosis) substances. The three drugs are rather closely related in chemical structure, and physiological theorists believe that when these drugs are introduced into the body they become even more closely related through interaction with body chemicals and may all cause their effects through the same mechanism.

In the following article, Tolan and Lingl describe two case studies of adolescents who experienced states akin to the "model psychosis" brought about by the hallucinogens. However, in both cases the states were induced by the inhalation of gasoline fumes which are not related to the psychotomimetic drugs in chemical structure.

Recent research with the psychotomimetics, consisting almost entirely of work with LSD – 25 (the most powerful of the drugs), has been approached from two sides. Physiological psychologists have utilized "model psychoses" in an attempt to discover the neurophysiological basis of

*Reprinted by permission of the authors and the American Psychiatric Association from the *American Journal of Psychiatry*, 1964, **120**, 757-761. Copyright 1964, the American Psychiatric Association.

their action, hoping that this discovery might lead to a physiological theory of psychosis. Clinicians, on the other hand, have observed subjects who are experiencing "model psychoses" in attempts to better understand psychotic mental functioning and thereby improve therapeutic techniques. In addition, some therapists use the drugs as a part of their therapy.

Since the mid-1950s, the dominant neurophysiological theory of the psychotomimetic agents has considered LSD – 25 and the other hallucinogens as somehow affecting the normal action of the neurohumor serotonin, a chemical which some physiologists believe may play a major part in synaptic impulse conduction in the central nervous system. The authors ask how the "model psychosis" produced by gasoline fumes can be related to current theory and, in addition, note that the hallucinations and delusions of these patients were often quite significant on a personal level. They also point out that the patients' initial experiences were compelling enough to prompt several more episodes. This problem is shared with the hallucinogens, the unauthorized use of which has prompted federal control.

The practice of inhaling gasoline fumes has recently led to the hospitalization of two adolescent boys with clinical syndromes resembling the "model psychoses" produced by many hallucinogenic and psychotomimetic drugs. One patient was a member of a group of 6 boys in Clark County, Ohio, who had engaged in the practice for several months. The other patient, from Marion County, claims he adopted the practice by accident. The seriousness of the practice is evident from the reports of 23 cases of inhalation of fumes from gasoline or wood glue in Columbus, Ohio, with two deaths caused by exploding gasoline.

Case 1. A single white male of 15 was admitted 2/21/63 with a history of smelling gasoline fumes for 6 months and having periods of amnesia after intoxication culminating in an episode in which he broke furniture and a glass door, and attacked his mother's dog. The parents had divorced during the mother's pregnancy. The mother married 4 times and the second step-father dealt in dope. The patient was reared by grandparents and resented his mother. He was doing average work in the 8th grade at the time of admission. He had been arrested 4 times for stealing and twice had been intoxicated. In social situations he was nervous, afraid to make new friends, and preferred older boys. He had had both heterosexual and homosexual experiences since the age of 12. Physical, neurological and laboratory findings were in normal limits. Two EEG's were normal. The psychological report indicated that the patient was severely anxious and indecisive. His explosive aggressiveness reflected the struggle against his childish reactions in the effort to become a "man." The tests showed neither organicity nor psychosis. Mental examination disclosed a tall, mature-looking youth of 15, who was restless but cooperative and friendly. He talked freely despite some uneasy defensiveness, and readily recalled his symptoms and hallucinations. Verbatim excerpts follow from his description of his experiences:

My first experience with the gasoline fume inhalations was in Dayton, Ohio, where I was visiting friends, 6 months ago. When I found them they were acting like crazy, jumping around and shouting. I wondered how they felt and I tried it. At first, I felt nauseated, real stuporous, light, like floating away. We were swinging our arms. Some of the boys were getting on the top of the garage and jumping off. Then I started to hear a constant buzzing as if someone was talking real fast. It sounded like echoes pretty far away. When talking to each other I could understand and I could see, but seeing a little bit more than usual. Then everything went back to normal, I guess I didn't take too much.

The second time I tried it was in Midway with 3 other boys. At first I barely felt it, then I felt like getting drunk. I was getting pretty ,high, higher than from drinking whiskey. I felt this kind of lightheadedness every time I inhaled the fumes. I started seeing little ants like crawling all over the ground real fast. There were billions. I felt like I was in a dream, like in another world. It does not seem like you're in reality. It gets to the point that you don't want to go back to reality. Then I saw walls change colors from real light blue to a real dark purple, then to a light red. Our clothes changed colors. One of the boys looked like a sailor with a blue suit, tie and hat all in colors. Then I felt I was floating again in the air; everything and everyone was smaller than normal size and in color.

I was dreaming like I was in hell, lying in a fire pit and the flames were rolling out. I got scared and stopped smelling and everything stopped. The next morning I had a headache, but I felt like doing it again.

The third time I tried it was in New Carlisle, Ohio, in a garage with a group of 6 boys. I went through the same experiences. First I felt very light, then I started seeing colors. They glittered like, and I saw peoples' clothes changing color. I felt like I was up and looking down. I could see clear through the garage floor. I looked like I was swinging up there and things below were swinging. The floor was moving back and forth. Then I felt that the whole garage was picked up and the earth looked smaller and smaller and things were flying in the air real fast, then they slowed down to a real slow pace, and then speeded up again. People were small and looked like elves or something, only 3 inches tall. Then I heard this buzzing noise again. The cars and the airplanes sounded like a real high shrill buzz, and the garage floor was covered all over with small tools and I saw colored patterns on the garage walls. If I would imagine purple, the whole wall would turn purple. Then I saw little animals like deer and an indian carrying a big torch, and the flame looked real, but it was cold. I could feel it.

The next thing I felt was that something was pulling me up against the wall like a magnet. Then I started seeing genii all of different colors moving out of a box like. I felt I was right in with these genii. They talked to me but I couldn't understand them, and they would motion at me or they would type things out on the walls, but I could never read it or understand it. I wanted somebody to talk to. I just wanted somebody who I could be with because I couldn't be with anyone. I felt like I was taking part in all these activities.

After awhile I felt like I was out in the open and there were clouds floating around with different shapes like Lone Ranger or Robin Hood running through the trees and that buzzing noise was with me all the time hurting my ears.

Then I saw people: half-cow, half-woman, half-horse and half people, all kinds of people. One of the small people was shoveling salt and as soon as he would shovel it the next one would shovel it and the next and so on.

I saw rock and roll pictures all over the place moving very fast, colored pictures clashing together. Then they started to get smaller. Things will get lighter and fade away and pretty soon you barely see these things anymore except for a little movement. The colors disappeared; there were only lines left, until they all disappear and everything is normal again.

If I would stare at the window and then look away, all I would see is that window pattern. Walking out on the streets I would see the peoples' faces, the houses and trees, all green and then turned blue, and the sky would turn a real dark red and pink and yellow. The tree leaves would merge together like a picture making the shape of an ape or a giant. Or I would see things like in a movie—the Statue of Liberty all over the walls, and then it will change and I would see a captain of the Civil War with a little cap on.

Then all of a sudden time would stop and I felt just like I was froze in space. I couldn't move. Then slowly I would move around and looking down I could see that the floor had disappeared and a great big dark hole was there and people were trying to push me in it. Looking up I would see angels floating and it seemed like every angel had a burnt spot on his back. At one time I heard girls' voices saying, "yes, yes."

I feel that most of the things you see are in your mind. It's all what you imagine. It's like you'd see something you didn't want to see, and it will come in your imagination. Or you would try to think of a different thing, but you would see something else, or at other times whatever you want to see you will see.

For days I lost my appetite, food didn't have a taste, cigarettes tasted like straw. I would be nauseated and vomit. Everything would taste like gasoline, even coughing or spitting. After days you still smell gasoline. Your clothes and your body perspiration and your breath; nothing will get rid of it.

Case 2. A single white male of 19 was admitted 3/7/63 because of unusual behavior after smelling gasoline for one and a half months. He mewed like a cat, saying, "I am having kittens." He slept in a pen with a pregnant sow, tried to choke his older brother, threatened to kill his sister, cut his clothing with a knife and acted as if drunk. He was easily angered, with periods of amnesia. His mother reported that at the age of one he began putting things into his ears and continued this behavior until the sixth grade. His mother taped his ears. At 10 he had an appendectomy and put things into the incision to get attention. In 1959 epilepsy was diagnosed. Since 1962 he had been having nightmares. He had been put in a special class in the sixth grade. Since stopping school he worked at odd jobs. He mixed easily and had sexual relations with an older woman. He had done some drinking, even trying rubbing alcohol. Physical, neurological and laboratory findings were within normal limits. The EEG was abnormal, with diffuse slowing in frontal area and spiking during hyperventilation. Psychological tests indicated dull normal intelligence. Projective tests suggested emotional repression and impoverishment, immaturity, suggestibility and impulsiveness. Psychosis was suspected. During examination the patient was cooperative and oriented but displayed some memory defects. He was ambivalent toward his parents but not delusional. He readily reported his abnormal experiences.

His first experience with gasoline inhalation occurred 2/7/63. The patient gave the following account: I was putting gasoline in the lawnmower. The fumes smelled good. I always liked to smell gas, so I got down by the tank and was sniffing it about 4 or 5 times.

The first sensation I had was that it seemed to me that I was in some big beautiful place, like a big city or something, and all I could see or hear were people and their voices. I couldn't make out what they were saying, just heard their voices. The voices were not clear, like little old honeybees buzzing. I felt like I was supposed to be dead or something, and I told a lie or I had done something. I don't know what it was. It was like a dream, and I started spinning around in circles real fast and all I could hear was a little bee buzzing. Then I saw a little honeybee. It was buzzing around and it kept saying, "Tell the truth, tell the truth." It seems like I said something. I sat down and I felt very dizzy and spinning. Then in a few minutes everything was over. I passed out and my brother found me by the mower.

After I done it once I had the urge to do it again and again. The second time I used the lawnmower I tried it again. My mother caught me in time and whipped me, but I guess I didn't feel it—just like my whole body was numbed.

It was like an urge or impulse to do it again, and I did it about 5 times at least. After the first two times I took gasoline cans and inhaled the fumes all alone. Everytime this place or city-like would appear. It was like a big town, all lit up with beautiful lights and forms all in colors, all kinds of colors, just all over, on everything. It was like a Walt Disney world in colors and everything was colorful and bright including the houses, but it couldn't have been a city because a city isn't decorated like that. It was like a dream, something out of this world.

There were people in this city, but when they talked you couldn't make out what they said. It sounded like a "Hoooo," and there were flowers there of all the colors. The houses looked like pretty rocks in all colors, and the windows were in colors, and every house was in different colors, and they were shining, just like you would take a brick and paint it red or blue or green, and you put a lightbulb in it so the whole house will be shining in different shades of color. The whole place was like that— all different colors. Every building was different from the others in its own colors. One building would be red with different shades of red, the next one blue with all the shades of blue in it, the next one yellow and so on.

At another time it seemed that it wasn't a city. It was just like a huge sheet of something all colored and pretty or like colored pictures. I don't know for sure what it was. Another time I saw a field just like you would look out there at that field, and it was all colored, no trees or nothing, just a colorful field, and I was standing out in that field and then at the end I saw that bee again. It seemed like that bee came back everytime. Then I felt I was going around in circles, and I'd be dizzy. I could see the blurry figure of a man saying something, and I would answer him, and that's when I'd see the bee, and I would be spinning around inside or something. The sky would go around in circles and everything around me was going around in circles fast, then stop real quick. Then I was able to get up, but I was still dizzy. For days afterward walking down the streets I would hear a man's voice calling my name and I'd turn around and there wouldn't be anyone. Or when I was out in the yard I would hear mother's voice calling me. When I would go in the house and ask her, she said she didn't call.

The next time I was inhaling the gas, beside seeing this beautiful place in colors, I would see little stones and square rocks in all colors and shapes and they were moving very fast. They would be there for a couple of seconds, then they'd go. I felt weak and didn't feel like doing anything. It felt like you're floating away loose and keep going up, just like you are weightless, like an astronaut. After I came out of it, I had to drive the tractor back home. I felt like something snapped in my ears for a couple of seconds and I found myself driving in the ditch. I was confused, and days after I felt confused-like a little, but I could think and do things. But food and cigarettes wouldn't taste the same. It would taste different—funny—like gas, and my whole body smelled like gas, and I was afraid that they would smell it on me.

Another time I was under the gas, I felt I was ten feet tall, like walking on the air, and I felt like I was taller than anyone else and stronger than anybody and that they couldn't do anything to you. Then I would hear an airplane or a car going and it would sound like a humming noise for a long time, very loud, and it would keep getting louder and keep that loud until it got further and further away. I couldn't tell if it was a car or an airplane until I looked. Things around look the same but they were all going around in circles like a merry-go-round, and I was going around with them, and the old honeybee would go around and she would pull me like a magnet and I would go around in circles with her. It seemed like that bee was after me for something, like I told a lie or something. Then it seemed like an innertube just kind of hunched all around me and pulled me up, made me go up like a little ball and that beautiful place in colors appeared again. A place that could be no place like it; I never saw nor heard of anything like it, and I could see people and automobiles and everything else in it, but I couldn't make out what they would be saying, and they looked blue, everything looked light blue. At times I couldn't see the city, it was just like a huge sign in colors or like bricks all in colors, I could always see the bricks, the stones, but in different places and arranged different, just like a pattern or a picture in colors. It was something to look at and it made me feel good and I often thought that if something like that could come true it would be wonderful.

Table 1 permits comparison of the findings in our cases with those reported in the psychotic syndromes produced by mescaline, LSD – 25, and psilocybin (1-3).

Our data were obtained from the subjective recollections of the patients. Neither patient was examined during the acute toxic phase. This fact may account for the absence of motor and certain autonomic findings from our symptom list.

It is apparent that substances of very different chemical structure are capable of eliciting similar toxic reactions. Solubility in liquid tissues may be a common factor. It is also noteworthy that each patient reported

TABLE 1

	"Model Psychosis"	Gasoline Inhalation
Autonomic-somatic	Flushing, pallor Dilated pupils Altered salivation Nausea Sweating Diuresis Palpitation Drowsiness Dizziness Weakness Headache Malaise Blurred vision Change of appetite	Unpleasant taste Nausea Loss of appetite Excessive salivation Drowsiness Weakness Lightheadedness
Motor	Restlessness Tremor Ataxia Dysarthria	
Perceptual	Altered shapes and colors Hyperacusis Distortion of space and time Distortion of proprioception and body image Depersonalization Hallucinations Illusions Synesthesias Dreamlike state	Sense of physical lightness Sense of spinning, moving, floating, and magnetic pull Distorted space perception Altered shapes and colors Micropsia Amnesia Hyperacusis Visual, auditory and tactile hallucinations Dreamlike state
Affective	Lability Euphoria Anxiety Irritability Suspicion Depression	Euphoria Fear Guilt Loneliness
Ideational	Delusional misinterpretations Impaired concentration Thinking disorders Symbolic distortions	Grandiosity Temporary misinterpretations

personally significant symbolic visions and distortions (hell fire, angels, semi-human creatures, feeling pushed into a dark hole, feelings of exaggerated size and strength, *etc.*) evidently related to the patient's life experiences and emotional difficulties.

REFERENCES

1. Hoch, P. H., *et al.: Am. J. Psychiat.* 108:579, 1952.
2. Hollister, L. E., and Hartman, A. M.: *Compr. Psychiat.* 3:235, 1962.
3. Silva, F., *et al.:* Recent Advances Biol., *Psychiat.* 3: 1960.

4. Functional Psychoses

This major category is for patients whose psychosis is not caused by such physical conditions as noted in Section 3. Patients are described as psychotic when their mental functioning is sufficiently impaired to interfere grossly with their capacity to meet the ordinary demands of life. The impairment may result from a serious distortion in their capacity to recognize reality. Hallucinations and delusions, for example, may distort their perceptions. Alternations of mood may be so profound that the patient's capacity to respond appropriately is grossly impaired. Deficits in perception, language, and memory may be so severe that the patient's capacity for mental grasp of his situation is effectively lost. Categories include schizophrenia, affective disorders, paranoid states, and psychotic depressive reactions.

The category of schizophrenia includes a group of disorders manifested by characteristic disturbances of thinking, mood, and behavior. Disturbances in thinking are marked by alternations of concept formation which may lead to misinterpretation of reality and sometimes to delusions and hallucinations, which frequently appear psychologically self-protective. Mood changes include ambivalent, constricted, and inappropriate emotional responsiveness and loss of empathy with others. Behavior may be withdrawn, regressive, and bizarre. The schizophrenias, in which the mental status is attributable primarily to a *thought* disorder, are distinguished from the major affective illnesses which are dominated by a *mood* disorder. Types of schizophrenia include hebephrenic, catatonic, and paranoid.

The major affective disorders are characterized by a single disorder of mood, either extreme depression or elation, that dominates the mental life of the patient and is responsible for whatever loss of contact he has with his environment. The onset of the mood does not seem to be related directly to a precipitating life experience. Affective psychoses include involutional melancholia, and various types of manic-depressive illness.

Paranoid states are psychotic disorders in which a delusion, generally persecutory or grandiose, is the essential abnormality. Disturbances in mood, behavior, and thinking (including hallucinations) are derived from this delusion. Psychotic depressive reactions are distinguished by a depressive mood attributable to some experience.

5. Volition and Value: A Study Based on Catatonic Schizophrenia*

Silvano Arieti

In this paper, the author is concerned primarily with the role of volition (will) as it affects catatonic behavior. He sees the immobility of the catatonic, and the compliance of the state called waxy flexibility, primarily as a disturbance of volitionary functioning and not as a disorder of motor apparatus. Volition develops early in childhood as an inhibitory reaction to a reflex movement. According to Arieti, toilet training and the inhibitory control of the anal sphincter appear to form the earliest model of volitional behavior. The explanation for the acculturation of the elimination process is found in Sullivan's theory of interpersonal relations, namely, that security is to be gained by socialization and approval. Normal development allows for freedom of action and decision but the patient who becomes catatonic develops extreme anxiety when carrying out acts of decision.

John, the patient discussed by Arieti, illustrates severe disturbance in volition with a resultant schizophrenic behavior. When in a situation which had stimulated intolerable homosexual thoughts, the patient avoided them by translating them into doubting and symbolic acts. These acts and thoughts were obsessive and compulsive, and their main purpose was to guard against the possibility of carrying out a dreaded behavior. The regression to obsessions and compulsions is assumed to be an abnormal safety factor in response to forbidden sexual thoughts, while the catatonic stupor represents the last refuge.

*Read at the mid-winter meeting of the Academy of Psychoanalysis, New York, December .11, 1960. Reprinted by permission of the author and Grune & Stratton, Inc., from *Comprehensive Psychiatry*, 1961, **2,** 74-82.

I hope I shall be permitted to begin my presentation with a personal memory, which goes back to more than twenty years ago, when I first arrived in this country.

Among the many things that came to my attention was the fact that undoubtedly Dante's *Divine Comedy* was the best known work of Italian literature in America. For the second place, however, two books were actively competing: one was *Decameron* by Boccaccio; the other *Pinocchio*, a little book for children, written by an otherwise obscure author named Collodi.

That *Decameron* should enjoy such popularity in America I was not surprised, being not completely unaware of the universal appeal of its subject matter. But that Pinocchio should be so well known, that was amazing!

What was so fascinating about the story of this wooden puppet? Pinocchio was a puppet, but unlike his sibling puppets, did not need a puppeteer to move his strings. He was capable of motions on his own, of willed acts. But what was the result? From the very first moment that his father, carpenter Geppetto, finishes making him, he gets into trouble. As soon as Geppetto gives the last touch to his legs, the legs start to move and kick Geppetto. And from that moment on it is one naughty thing after another. Pinocchio is a real psychopath.

In a leap of artistic imagination Collodi overlooked the great evolutionary process of billions of years, which first gives autonomous movement to organic matter, then coordinated motion, finally voluntary acts and moral deeds.

Collodi's intuition created a paradoxical situation; while Pinocchio must act as a moral human being, he cannot. As the story evolves in the book he becomes tamed, socialized, industrious and acquires a conscience. When this gradual transformation is completed, he has miraculously changed into a child of flesh and blood, a regular member of the human race.

I do not have the time to go into the many fascinating allegorical implications of Pinocchio, nor do I have the time to give even a succinct summary of that evolutionary process, which starting with the most elementary movement ends with those highest moral deeds that Western man exemplifies in accordance with the paradigms of the various roots of our civilization: as *areté*, or the harmonious action of the Greeks; as *mitzva*, or the good deed of the Jews; as *virtus*, or the way of man, according to the Romans.

In the first part of this paper I shall present some of the highlights of this phylogenetic and ontogenetic process, and some of the psychopathological arrests and deviations. Lest I am misunderstood, my references to phylogenetic mechanisms are not attempts to explain, in Jungian fashion, the dynamics of psychopathological conditions occurring today. Phylogenetic studies are important in studying the structural or formal mechanisms, but not content or motivation. In the second part of this paper I shall make an attempt to show how catatonic schizophrenia represents the most dramatic disintegration of this development. This will be illustrated with a case report.

The first movements that we must study in relation to motor actions are no longer the reflexes, as we did until a few years ago, but the so-called autorhythmic movements (12, 16), spontaneous movements of the organism from which eventually reflexes or fixed patterns of responses emerge in evolution. But neither autorhythmic movements nor reflexes can be called real volitional acts.

The first real volitional act is an inhibition, or at least an inhibition of a reflex response. For instance, during toilet training, the baby has the impulse to defecate when the rectum is distended by the passage of feces. The child, however, learns not to yield to the impulse and to postpone defecation in spite of the fact that it would be more pleasant to do so. He learns to control his sphincters because his ability to do so will affect his relation with mother. Obviously he has the neurophysiologic potentiality for sphincter control, but such control, inasmuch as it affects the people in his environment, is not purely a physiological act; it is also a social one. Furthermore in order to control himself, he must inhibit the still available simpler and more pleasant physiological mechanisms of immediate defecation.

His first act of will is thus at the same time an inhibition and a compliance to the will of others. It seems almost a paradoxical contradiction, just as paradoxical as negativism is a little later as an assertion of the emerging will (Arieti, 5). But will is a very complicated and portentous function, and like many other complicated functions appears to originate from what at first seems its opposite, just as logical thought originates from what at first seems its opposite: irrational thought. But somebody could object: Are acts of inhibition and compliance, as they occur, for instance, in toilet training, really the first voluntary acts? What about those actions of the baby, who toward the fifth or sixth month of life grabs rattles and other objects? Certainly these acts of the baby, like grabbing a rattle, must be included under the large category of conative acts, but actually they are not volitional in a mature sense; they are protovolitional. The baby responds to the stimulus rattle and enjoys the pleasure of the response which later on he seeks again. But there is no choice, not even a minimum of conflict, as there is between pleasing mother and defecating. If the action is a reflex response or, though conative, has the purpose only of maintaining the homeostasis or of producing immediate pleasure, without alternative possibilities, we do not yet have volition, but protovolition.

Inasmuch as these alternative possibilities are at first created by the exposure to the interpersonal situation, the act of will becomes, so to say, socialized. The action loses its primitive characteristic of a purely motor or physiologic mechanism because its outcome is anticipated in relation to the interpersonal world. As Parsons (13, 14) writes, action is not concerned only with the internal structure or processes of the organism, but with the organism in a sort of relationship. Action has additional dimensions, which may be called at the same time the social and the moral dimensions.

At this early ontogenetic level, volition is not only inhibition but also, as I said before, extreme submission. It is more than submission: it is enormous receptivity to the interpersonal world. This enormous receptivity is necessary for the development of the social self, or, as Erikson (8) would say, for the epigenesis of the ego. It has some hypnotic qualities and may be related to the phenomenon of hypnosis. Hypnosis may be a more acute artificial reproduction of this stage of life when the child is extremely receptive to the will of others and does not remember who gave the instructions or suggestions. Later on he may rationalize his unconsciously introjected attitudes. The transference is also a repetition of attitudes generally acquired during this period of high receptivity. The origin of the transference is repressed and the phenomenon is rationalized. We have thus that triad of characteristics that Spiegel (15) considers inherent in the hypnotic situation.

This transient period of suggestibility has more manifest sequels in primitive cultures, where mass hypnosis, voodoo phenomena, and latah are relatively common (Arieti and Meth, 6). It is perhaps not too difficult to understand the importance of suggestibility in primitive society. As Kelsen (10) has described, in primitive societies *to do* and *to be guilty* are approximately the same thing. To do is at least potentially to be guilty because often one does not know the event that will follow one's action. The event might even have an effect on the whole tribe, such as an epidemic or drought. When the prevailing way of thinking is ruled not by deterministic or scientific causality, but by what is considered the will of animate things, the will becomes a portentous and frightening weapon. Its possession is liable to make one feel very guilty. But one will not feel very guilty if one accepts the will of others, of the gods, or the collective will of the tribe in a form of almost automatic obedience.

Automatic obedience is not the only way primitive men free themselves from guilt and fear. They also refrain from acting freely; they perform only those acts which are sanctioned by the tribe. For any desired effect, the tribe teaches the individual what act to perform. The life of primitive man is completely regulated by a tremendous number of norms and restrictions. The individual has to follow the ritual for practically everything he does. By performing the act according to the ritual, the primitive believes that he will avoid guilt for the act. These rituals are found again at an ontogenetic level as compulsive acts. The individual, who has not been able to develop his potentiality of acting freely without anxiety or guilt may resort to obsessive-compulsive mechanisms to obviate this anxiety and guilt.

In normal development we find a minimal quantity of compulsive behavior, just as we find traces of autism and of automatic obedience, etc. But in persons whose development was accompanied by excessive anxiety, obsessive-compulsive behavior may remain more pronounced than normal, and later on, when the individual is confronted by difficulties, obsessive-compulsive patterns may be resorted to again.

The psychopathic person does not resort to obsessive behavior. His attempt to remove anxiety will consist in allowing his actions to follow his desires without consideration of the interpersonal world, or of the rightness or wrongness of the act.

The patient who is to become catatonic is generally a person given to fits of overpowering anxiety, especially anxiety connected with the carrying out of some action. He generally does not resort to hypnotic or autohypnotic mechanisms, nor to psychopathic denial of responsibility. When in his life he is confronted with an important challenge or decision which causes him excessive anxiety, he fabricates many obsessive-compulsive mechanisms. But the anxiety may overpower him acutely, and he may not have time to manufacture compulsions. The anxiety will then be experienced as fear and guilt connected with any action and will be generalized to every action, to every movement determined by the will. He has a last resort to avoid these feelings: to fall into catatonic immobility. In stupor the immobility is complete, but in other less pronounced catatonic conditions it is not. The patient follows orders given by others not because he is in a state of automatic obedience or hypnosis, but because these orders are willed by others, and therefore he does not have the responsibility for them. In the state called waxy flexibility he retains the positions imposed by others, even if uncomfortable, because he cannot will to change position.

Most of these acute catatonic episodes are forgotten by the patient when he recovers, so that there is a scarity of reports in the literature about these experiences and their interpretation. I have been able to collect a few rare cases in which full memory was retained, and I have reported some of them elsewhere (3, 5).

I am now going to report the case of John, which bears striking similarities to others reported by me, but which also bears some important differences that, in my opinion, may increase our understanding somewhat of the pathology of volition and value.

CASE REPORT

John is an intelligent professional man in his thirties, Catholic, who was referred to me because of his rapidly increasing anxiety—anxiety which reminded him of the one he experienced about ten years previously, when he developed a full catatonic episode. Wanting to prevent a recurrence of the event, he sought treatment.

The following is not a complete report but only a brief history of the patient and a description and interpretation of his catatonic episode as it was reconstructed and analyzed during the treatment.

The patient is one of four children. The father is described as a bad husband, an adventurer who, although a good provider, always caused trouble and home instability. The mother is a somewhat inadequate person, distant from the patient. John was raised more or less by a maternal aunt who lived in the family and acted as a housekeeper.

Early childhood memories are mostly unpleasant for John. He recollects attacks of anxiety going back to his early childhood. He also remembers how he needed to cling to his aunt; how painful it always was to separate from her. The aunt also had the habit of undressing in his presence, causing him mixed feelings of sexual excitement and guilt. Between 9 and 10 there was an attempted homosexual relation with his best friend. During his prepuberal period he remembers his desire to look at pictures of naked women, and how occasionally he would surreptitiously borrow some pornographic books or magazines from his father's collection and look at them. Fleeting homosexual desires would also occur occasionally. He masturbated with fantasies of women, but he had to stimulate his rectum with his fingers in order to experience, he says, "a greater pleasure." Among the things that he remembers from his early life are also obsessive preoccupations with feces of animals and excretions in general of human beings. He had a special admiration for horses, because "They excreted such beautiful feces coming from such statuesque bodies."

In spite of all these circumstances, John managed to grow more or less adequately, was not too disturbed by the death of his aunt, and did well in school. There were practically no dates with girls until much later in life. After puberty he became very interested in religion, especially in order to find a method to control his sexual impulses. Anything connected with sex was evil and had to be eliminated. This attitude was in a certain way the opposite of that of one of his sisters who was leading a very promiscuous life. John considered the possibility of becoming a monk several times; however, he was discouraged from doing so by a priest he had consulted. When he finished college at the age of 20, he decided to make a complete attempt to remove sex from his life. He also decided to go for a rest and summer vacation at a farm for young men where he would cut trees, enjoy the country, and be far away from the temptations of the city. On this farm, however, he soon became anxious and depressed. He found out that he resented the other fellows more and more. They were rough guys. They used profane language. He felt as if he were going to pieces progressively. He remembers that one night he was saying to himself, "I cannot stand it any more. Why am I in this way, so anxious for no reason? I have done no wrong in my whole life. Perhaps I should become a priest or get married." When he was feeling very badly he would console himself by thinking that perhaps what he was experiencing was in accordance with the will of God.

Obsessions and compulsions acquired more and more prominence. The campers had to go chopping wood. This practice became an ordeal for John because he was possessed by doubts. He would think, for instance: "Maybe I should not cut this tree because it is too small. Next year it will be bigger. But if I don't cut this tree another fellow will. Maybe it is better if he cuts it, or maybe that I do so." As he expressed himself, he found himself "doubting and doubting his doubts, and doubting the doubting of his doubts." It was an overwhelming, spreading anxiety. The anxiety gradually extended to every act he had to perform. He was literally possessed by intense terror. One day, while he was in this predicament, he observed another phenomenon which he could not understand. There was a discrepancy between the act he wanted to perform and the action that he really carried out. For instance, when he was undressing he wanted to drop a shoe, and instead he dropped a big log; he wanted to put something in a drawer and instead he threw a stone away. However, there was a similarity between the act that he had wanted and anticipated and the act he actually performed. The same phenomenon appeared in talking. He would utter words, which were not the ones he meant to say, but related to them. Later, however, his actions became more and more disconnected. He was mentally lucid and able to perceive what was happening but he realized he had no control over his actions. He thought he could commit crimes, even kill somebody and became even more afraid. He was saying to himself: "I don't want to be damned in this world as well as in the other. I am trying to be good and I can't. It is not fair. I may kill somebody when I want a piece of bread." At other times he had different feelings. He felt as if some movement or action he would make could produce disaster not only to himself but to the whole camp. By not acting or moving he was protecting the whole group. He felt that he had become his brothers' keeper.

Fear soon became connected with any possible movement. The fear was so intense as to actually inhibit any movement. He was almost literally petrified. To use his own words, he "saw himself solidifying, assuming statuesque positions." However, he was not always in this condition. As a matter of fact, the following day he could move again and go to chop wood. He had one purpose in mind: to kill himself. He remembers that he was very capable of observing himself, and of deciding that it would be better for him to die than to commit crimes. He climbed a big tree and jumped down in an attempt to kill himself but received only minor contusions. The other men, who ran to help him, realized that he was mentally ill, and he was soon sent to a psychiatric hospital. He remembers understanding that he was taken to the hospital and being happy about it; at least he was considered sick and not a criminal. But in the hospjtal he found that he could not move at all. He was like a statue of stone.

There were some actions, however, which could escape this otherwise complete immobility: the actions needed for the purpose of committing suicide. In fact he was sure that he had to die to avoid the terror of becoming a murderer. He had to kill himself before that could happen.

During his hospitalization, John made 71 suicidal attempts. Although he was generally in a state of catatonia he would occasionally make impulsive acts such as tearing his strait jacket to pieces and making a rope of it to hang himself. Another time he broke a dish in order to cut the veins of his wrist. Other times he swallowed stones. He was always put under restraint after a suicidal attempt. He remembers, however, understanding everything that was going on. As a matter of fact, his acuity in devising methods for committing suicide seemed sharpened.

When I questioned him further about this long series of suicidal attempts, John added that the most drastic attempts were actually the first ten or twelve. Only these could really have killed him. Later, the suicidal attempts were not very dangerous. He performed such acts as swallowing a small object or inflicting a small injury on himself with a sharp object. When I asked him whether he knew why he had to repeat these token suicidal attempts, he gave me two reasons. The first was to relieve his feeling of guilt and fulfill his duty of preventing himself from committing crimes. But the second reason, which he discovered during the present treatment, is even stranger. To commit suicide was the only act which he could perform, the only act which would go beyond the barrier of immobility. Thus, to commit suicide was to live; the only act of life left to him.

The patient was given a course of electric shock treatment. The exact number could not be ascertained. He improved for about two weeks, but then he relapsed into catatonic stupor interrupted only by additional suicidal attempts. While he was in stupor he remembered a young psychiatrist saying to a nurse, "Poor fellow, so young and so sick. He will continue to deteriorate for the rest of his life." After five or six months of hospitalization his catatonic state became somewhat less rigid and he was able to walk and to utter a few words. At this time he had noticed that a new doctor seemed to take some interest in him. One day this doctor told him, "You want to kill yourself. Isn't there anything at all in life that you want?" With great effort the patient mumbled, "Eat, to eat." In fact, he really was hungry as his immobility prevented him from eating properly, and he was inefficiently spoon fed. The doctor took him to the patients' cafeteria and told him, "You may eat anything you want." John immediately grabbed a large quantity of food and ate in a ravenous manner. The doctor noticed that John liked soup and told him to take even more soup. From that day on John lived only for the sake of eating. He gained about sixty pounds in a few weeks. When I asked him if he ate so much because he was really hungry, he said, "No, that was only at the beginning. The pleasure in eating consisted partially in grabbing food and putting it into my mouth." Later it was discovered by the attendants that John would not only eat a lot but he would also hoard food in his drawers and under his mattress.

I cannot go into detail about many other interesting episodes which occurred in the course of his illness. John continued to improve and in a few months he was able to leave the hospital. He was able to make a satisfactory adjustment, to work, and later to go to a professional school and obtain his Ph.D. degree. On the whole he has managed fairly well until shortly before he decided to come for psychoanalytic treatment.

I shall now attempt an interpretation of these phenomena. It is obvious that John underwent an overpowering increase in anxiety when he went to the camp and was exposed to close homosexual stimulation. His early interpersonal relations had subjected him to great instability and insecurity and had made him very vulnerable to many sources of anxiety. This anxiety, however, retained a propensity to be aroused by or be channeled in the pattern of sexual stimulation and inhibition. His personality defenses and cultural background made the situation worse. John was not like Pinocchio, i.e., deprived of that part of the self called social self, conscience or superego; nor could he go against his cultural-religious background as his philandering father and promiscuous sister. Sex was evil for him, and homosexuality much more so. As a matter of fact, homosexual desires were not even permitted to become fully conscious.

When he was about to be overwhelmed by the anxiety, he at first resorted to some of the defenses commonly found in precatatonics. He found refuge in religious feelings. God or religion gave him the order of eliminating sex from his life and of becoming a monk. This may be considered a form of autohypnosis, but as we have already mentioned at the beginning of this paper, hypnosis and autohypnosis do not work well with catatonics. He resorted, then, to obsessive-compulsive mechanisms. The anxiety which presumably was at first connected with any action that had something to do with sexual feelings became extended to practically every action. Incidentally, Ferenczi (9) has reported similar feelings in one patient. Every action became loaded with a sense of responsibility. Every willed movement came to be seen not as a function but as a moral issue. Every motion was not considered as a fact but as a value. This primitive generalization of his responsibility extended to what he could cause to the whole community. By moving he could produce havoc not only to himself but to the whole camp. His feelings were reminiscent of the feelings of cosmic power or negative omnipotence experienced by other catatonics who believe that by acting they may cause the destruction of the universe (Arieti, 5).

To protect himself at first, John resorted to obsessive thinking and compulsions, as, for instance, when he was cutting trees. But even this defense was not sufficient to dam his anxiety; as a matter of fact, it made the situation worse and gave rise to other symptoms. The first one was the unrelatedness between the act, as anticipated and willed, and the action which followed. But, and this is a point of great importance, at first the actions were not completely unrelated from their anticipation. They were analogic. In other words, two actions, like dropping a shoe and dropping a log, had become psychologically equivalent, i.e., they were identified just because they were similar or had something in common. This fact is, in my opinion, of theoretical importance because it extends to the area of volition or of willed mobility those characteristics which have already been described in paleologic or analogic thinking of schizophrenics (Arieti, 4). It would seem to indicate that the same basic formal psychopathological mechanisms apply to every area of the psyche. It may also be connected with neurological studies of motor integration, as recently outlined by Denny-Brown (7). The analogic movement may be viewed as a "release" or "dedifferentation or loss of restriction to specific attributes of adequate stimulus."

The reason why this phenomenon of generalized analogic movement escapes notice and has not been reported in the literature so far, is to be found in the fact that it is of very transient occurrence. In most patients the symptomatology proceeds rapidly to following stages, e.g., the stage where the actions are completely unrelated to the will, as in catatonic excitement, or the stage in which the actions are all eliminated, as in catatonic stupor. The catatonic excitement may be the result of two facts. In some cases the patient senses that he is sinking into stupor because he is afraid to act and tries to prevent this occurrence by becoming overactive and submerging himself in a rapid sequence of aimless acts. In other instances the opposite is true and the patient acts, but his actions are so unrelated to the conceived or willed actions as to result in a real movement-salad, the motor equivalent of word-salad. The patient then has no other resort but to sink into the immobility of the stupor.

In many cases the barrier of immobility is not completely closed. In a very selective way it may allow passage to actions of obedience to the will of others or to some special actions of the patient himself.

In the case of John the actions necessary for the suicidal attempts were allowed to go through. Incidentally, these suicidal attempts in catatonics, accompanied by religious feelings and eventually by stupor, have often led to the wrong diagnosis of the depressed form of manic-depressive psychosis. Kraepelin (11) himself described suicidal attempts and ideas of sin in catatonics, but did not give to them any psychodynamic significance. What is of particular interest in our case is the fact that the suicidal act eventually became for John the only act of living. It is not possible here to examine in greater detail the therapeutic effect of the encounter of John with the doctor in the hospital. Important is the fact that the doctor gave John permission to eat as much as he wanted. Thus the only previously possible act (of killing oneself) was replaced with one of the most primitive acts of life, nourishing oneself. I have described the placing-into-mouth habit in very regressed schizophrenics (1). In slightly less regressed patients we find the hoarding habit (2), a stage John went through in his progress toward recovery. In acute cases of catatonia we often find, in very acute form, symptoms appearing in other types of schizophrenia after many years of regression.

Many other aspects of the interesting case of John cannot be examined for lack of space. However, I feel that adding what we have learned from John to what has been reported about other cases (3, 4, 5), some conclusions may be drawn:

1) Catatonia is predominantly a disorder of the will. It is not a disorder of the motor apparatus.

2) Contrary to appearance, the state of catatonia is not that of an ivory tower. It is a state where volition is connected with a pathologically intensified sense of value, so that torturing responsibility spreads like fire to every possible act. Such pathological sense of responsibility reaches the acme of intensity when a little movement of the patient is considered capable of destroying the world. Alas! This conception of the psychotic mind reminds us of its possible actuality today, when the pushing of a button may have such cosmic effects! Only the oceanic responsibility of the catatonic could include this up-to-now unconceived possibility.

3) The passivity to the suggestion of others found in some catatonics is not an acceptance of power from others, as in hypnosis, but a relief from responsibility.

4) Only those actions may go through the catatonic barrier which may compensate or atone for the intensified responsibility. This selectivity is dramatically exemplified in our case report, where only the movements necessary for self-inflicted death penalty could be carried out, but even more than that—where self-inflicted death penalty became the only voluntary movement, thus life itself.

5) Catatonia may present certain phenomena such as the analogic movement which may be related to the general pathological functioning of the psyche as well as to principles of neurological disorganization.

6) The recognition that the catatonic patient is not an ivory tower but, on the contrary, a volcano of not at all petrified feelings, lends itself to possible therapeutic maneuvers, already in course in other cases, which will be reported elsewhere.

REFERENCES

1. Arieti, S.: The "placing-into-mouth" and coprophagic habits. *J. Nerv. & Ment. Dis.* 102:307, 1945.

2. ———: Primitive habits in the preterminal stage of schizophrenia. *J. Nerv. & Ment. Dis.* 102:367, 1945.

3. ———: *Interpretation of Schizophrenia.* New York, Brunner, 1955, pp. 109-129.

4. ———: *Interpretation of Schizophrenia.* New York, Brunner, 1955, pp. 194-209.

5. ———: *Interpretation of Schizophrenia.* New York, Brunner, 1955, pp. 219-238.

6. ———, and Meth, J.: Rare, unclassifiable, collective and exotic psychotic syndromes, *in* Arieti, S. (Ed.) *American Handbook of Psychiatry.* Vol. 1, chapter 27, p. 546. New York, Basic Books, 1959.

7. Denny-Brown, D.: Motor mechanisms—introduction: The general principles of motor integration, *in* Field, J. (Ed.) *Handbook of Physiology.* Washington, American Physiological Society 2:781, 1960.

8. Erikson, E. H.: *Identity and the life cycle. Psychological Issues.* New York, International University Press, 1959, Vol. 2.

9. Ferenczi, S.: Some clinical observations on paranoia and paraphrenia, *in Sex in Psychoanalysis.* New York, Basic Books, 1950.

10. Kelsen, H.: *Society and Nature—A Sociological Inquiry.* Chicago, University of Chicago Press, 1943.

11. Kraepelin, E.: *Dementia Praecox and Paraphrenia.* Edinburgh, Livingston, 1925.

12. Lorenz, K. Z.: Comparative behaviorology in *Discussions on Child Development.* New York, International University Press, 1954, Vol. 1.

13. Parsons, I.: *The Social System*. Glencoe, The Free Press, 1951.

14. ———, and Shies, E. A.: *Toward a General Theory of Action*. Cambridge, Harvard University Press, 1951.

15. Spiegel, H.: Hypnosis and transference: A theoretical formulation. *A.M.A. Arch of General Psychiatry* 1:634, 1959.

16. Von Holst, E.: Von Dualismus der motorischen und der automatisch-rhythmischen Funktion im Ruckenmark und von Wesen des automatischen Rhythmus Pflug. *Arch. ges. Physiol.* 237:356, 1936.

6. The Analytic Treatment of a Psychotic*

Reuben Fine

In this paper, the author uses the term "analytic" rather than "psycho-analytic." Although Jung preferred the term "analysis" as opposed to "psychoanalysis" the interpretations and diagnosis presented here are seen in terms of Freudian psychology.

The patient is a 44-year-old woman diagnosed as paranoid schizophrenic. She had been through marked psychotic episodes and hospitalization and had been in treatment with a psychiatrist who had to leave the case. The former therapist had managed most of the patient's affairs, a procedure considered antithetical to psychoanalysis. Because of her dependency on the previous therapist, the author felt that in the transfer of therapists some support should be given to the patient in order to make a transition possible. Because of this support, and the need to deal with the practical affairs of the patient, Fine anticipated that his treatment might be questioned as to its being truly psychoanalytic. He indicated that it was, since the process included the working through of transference and resistance, interpretation of unconscious material, and strengthening of the ego. Fine relinquished another feature ordinarily considered basic to psychoanalysis: the emphasis on free association and dream interpretation. The reduction of emphasis on these features seemed necessary because the frail ego of the patient could not have dealt with the abundance of primitive material released by free association in certain aspects of dream analysis (material which usually poses a problem in the psychoanalysis of

*Reprinted by permission of the author and publisher from *Psychotherapy: Theory, Research & Practice*, 1964, **1**, 166-177.

psychotics). However, alleviation of this psychotic disorder was obtained by relating faulty reality testing to psychosexual development and disturbances at the anal, oral, and phallic levels. The patient was helped to gain functioning independence through successful analysis of her (oral) primary infantile dependency on her mother, and her (anal) inadequacy in early achievement. Oedipal conflicts are seen as resistant to change, and mature psychosocial and psychosexual functioning (which Freudian psychology ascribes to a full genital psychosexual state) were not achieved in this case.

The patient, a 44-year-old woman who looked much older than her age, was referred to me by the psychiatrist who had been treating her for several years. He had to leave town, and the referral was made on a few days notice. The patient had no opportunity to work through the separation.

The patient appeared somewhat agitated but in adequate control of herself. She called for an appointment (arranged for the next day). An hour later she called again and asked to see me the same day. I agreed. When she came, she explained that she was frightened by the change and wanted to "nail her fear" down as soon as possible. Initially, I saw her three times a week.

Her history had been most traumatic. Her mother died when the patient was a year-and-a-half old. The father took her to live with his parents. When she was three he went to Puerto Rico for five years, and she lived with her maternal grandparents. There were no other children present. The grandfather was deaf and used an ear trumpet.

When she was six, she developed some sickness of unclear origin and was kept out of school for a year.

When she was eight her father returned home, but did not take her to live with him. Just before her tenth birthday, he remarried and brought the girl to his home. By his second marriage he had four children, all of whom are alive and well.

When the patient was about fourteen, the father again left. He took along his wife and four children but not the patient. Consciously, the patient had never experienced any resentment toward her father for this continued rejection, nor did she ever really grasp how serious it had been in the course of her therapy. She was left with an aunt for a while, then sent to boarding school.

In adolescence, the patient became an active homosexual, and had a number of violent affairs with other girls. In these she was usually the passive partner who admired and looked up to the other girl. After a while, whipping fantasies became prominent, which culminated in inducing another girl to whip her with a tree twig when she was about eighteen. She was unable to finish high school.

When she was twenty she made up her mind to give up homosexuality, and carried out her resolution.

When she was 26 she was married to a man with similar interests, and for a number of years the marriage seemed to be a very happy one.

Shortly after the birth of her children, she began to go to psychiatrists. The first symptom was the fear that she was a homosexual. No one, however, seemed to be able to help her, and she grew steadily worse. For reasons which she could not fully clarify, she switched therapists some eight or ten times.

During this period, her husband came back from an assignment in Europe and told her he had fallen in love with a European woman. He said nothing would come of it, and he never expected to see her again. Not long after, the patient's symptoms worsened. She was in poor contact with people and developed the strong conviction that nobody wanted her. When she was hospitalized, she was sure that the hospital would not accept her because harm would befall them. She had delusions that people were after her. At one point, she got a gun, determined to kill herself. Later she did attempt suicide with sleeping tablets. She presented a typical picture of paranoid schizophrenia.

Before coming to see me, she had been hospitalized three times. She had been given ECT the first time and insulin the last.

During the last hospitalization, she was treated by Dr. A., the psychiatrist who referred her to me. He was a dashing, handsome man to whom the patient, for the first time, made a strong transference. After some nine months in the hospital, she was discharged, considerably improved. The psychotic symptoms had disappeared, although she was still extremely frightened and dependent. Dr. A. continued to see her three times a week.

Unfortunately, Dr. A. also managed the patient's affairs *in toto*. While she was in the hospital, recovering from insulin shock, he approached her with the advice to divorce her husband. Since he recommended it, she went along. This had made the dependency on the psychiatrist much stronger, so that his sudden departure was even more of a blow than it would otherwise have been.

The husband agreed to support her, so that she could get along on a very modest scale without working, and could still manage to pay for the therapy.

Because of the way in which she had been handled by Dr. A., the treatment with me began on a completely supportive level. She would bring me letters she had written to her husband, or the children, or part of a manuscript she was writing about the hospital experience, and ask for my opinion. Naturally, the weaning away from her dependency had to be gradual, and in the initial period I referred her to a lawyer and a doctor, and made various other decisions for her.

About five weeks after the therapy with me began, she received a note from her husband telling her of his remarriage; the note came before she had been officially notified that the divorce decree was final.

This incident naturally caused some regression, but the full effects were not immediately apparent. She denied any feeling about the remarriage: it was one of those things, and she fully accepted it.

The whipping fantasies became stronger. Her homosexual wishes also increased. Her attitude towards therapy became markedly ambivalent. One week she would not even think of work, but would concentrate entirely on treatment; the next week she did not feel that treatment was really so essential, she was all right, and it would be better to spend the money for a home with the children.

Around this time she had a dream:

> I'm talking to D.E. (a cousin). He's laughing and full of high
> spirits. I touch him; he shrivels up.

The dream was used only to try to help her to see how angry she was, but she completely denied any such feelings.

A few days later she came out with the idea that she was doing people harm. This was the beginning of the recurrence of the psychosis.

On the next appointment she was quite disturbed, and could not talk too clearly. She had to move that very day. She had arranged to take another room which was far beyond her means. I forbade any change, and took a much more active role. I explained to her that the sickness was breaking out again, and that she would have to come in every day for treatment. From this point on, for the next two months, I saw her seven days a week, and encouraged her to come twice a day if she felt the need for it; this did happen several times.

From here on, more and more of the psychotic material came out. This can be grouped under several headings:

(1) *Auditory Hallucinations:* Voices said a number of things. One said, "That B.— woman," referring to Dr. B., a female physician who had treated her over a period of years. Voices shouted the names of other

people whom she had known in the past. The radio talked about her, mentioning names of people she knew.

At other times she heard: "You're a bathroom woman." "You're a bedroom woman." "You're a Commie."

(2) *Delusions of Harm:* She became convinced that she was doing harm. She felt marked out and peculiar. "I riffle people," she said. She felt that she could do me no harm only because I was an analyst.

After a few weeks she began to visit Fountain House, a rehabilitation center for discharged psychotics. She soon came to believe that she caused "consternation" there, and stopped going.

(3) *Bizarre Ideas:* For a while she told of police cars driving up to her and the policeman saying, "Clink you." Once she reported that when the hotel clerk gave her the *New York Times* a razor blade was hidden in the paper. An especially persistent conviction was that someone came into her room and disarranged her things. Particularly, the marking up of library books by this unknown stranger was awfully frightening to her, and for a long time she was advised to stay away from libraries.

She thought that she was "dripping information," and that she was a "public woman." One night she was "boiling," and everybody outside in the hall where she lived was "boiling."

The intensity of the psychotic material varied from day to day. At times the voices would be almost continuous. At other times they would come over her in what she called "flurries" and then disappear for a while.

The therapeutic approach: She was encouraged to call on the telephone whenever she felt the need to do so. The analyst adopted an air of absolute certainty, and repeatedly assured her that he knew exactly what she was going through. He would also comment that she acted better or worse on certain days. The analyst made direct suggestions about handling environmental problems, and kept himself fully informed about every aspect of her life. These suggestions were usually followed, though they did not always work out.

Within this framework, the material produced was treated analytically. Hallucinations were explained as inability to distinguish between what was going on inside her and what was going on outside, and related to her wishes. The difference between a wish and an action was emphasized. Peculiar words were traced to their sources via associations, in exactly the same way that dream-language is analyzed in the ordinary analysand. Her confusion of some words, and their double usage, was worked out. The transference was handled as an oral regression, which she talked about but did not really grasp; she once said, "You're a very strange-looking mother to me." Wherever feasible, her present symptoms were linked up with the past.

Some examples of the therapeutic approach may be cited from the daily notes written at the end of each day. The daily sessions began in March, 1952, her fifty-second session with me.

Session 56: She's still worried; begins every session this way. She must move from the hotel because she is hurting the people there. I explained that she was not hurting anybody; it was a fear inside her, and a fear differs from an act.

Session 58: She repeated almost incessantly that she must move to another apartment before she could continue treatment. She is "wide open," "dripping" information. The radio is talking about her, mentioning the names of people she knew. I explained these as her thoughts, and again told her not to move.

Session 59: She was feeling much better, though the radio was still talking about her. Her need to attach herself to me, and make me the only person in the world, was interpreted to her. Would I know if she did anybody any harm, she wanted to know? I assured her that I would.

Session 60: When my telephone rang she heard a voice say: "That B. woman." I explained to her how she develops hateful feelings when I stop paying attention to her, just like a child, and turns these against herself. This was tied up with her early deprivations.

Session 61: She can't read the *New York Times* because if she does she will hurt the people on the *Times*. She can't get over the feeling that in the past few months she has made some horrible mistake. She thought that analysis would rip the children wide open. These fears were explained as the outcome of her own hostile feelings.

Session 63: She saw the children today briefly, and everything went fine. She thinks that if she doesn't stay with them too long she won't do them any harm.

I suggested that the radio announcements might be an idea in her mind—she looked very startled. Then I asked whether it is frightening to think that all these ideas might be in her mind—she said no, on the contrary, it would be a great relief.

At the end she asked whether she was getting any better. I asked her what she thought; she said, "I'm feeling better." I agreed.

Session 65: Today she confided that last week she had become angry when I said that she wanted to be a baby, but did not feel it at the time. As she came in the building today, there was a "flurry" because the people in the house were going to protect me from her. I interpreted that I am to be protected against her hostile wishes, and again explained the difference between a wish and an action.

Session 70: I explained the voices to her as reproaches; she is bawling herself out all the time. I went into the mechanism of how such a reproach becomes a voice. She has been working in her room. A voice says, "You can't work in your room." I explained this as a reproach.

Session 74: During the night one of the women in the place opened the door around 2 or 3 o'clock, evidently discovered it was the wrong room, and went away. She feels bad about living there. I interpreted this as a fear of her homosexual wishes.

After leaving here yesterday, there was a great commotion, voices talking all over the place. It lasted so long it couldn't be a hallucination. I showed her that it was.

Session 75: Yesterday she went to Fountain House; it was all right. She spoke a little, did some lace work. Some people looked worried.

Last night she had a strange experience—a ringing in the ears. She seemed fogged, in the process of closing up. I interpreted this as an exaggeration of bodily sensations.

She thinks I don't understand the seriousness of her situation fully. (What makes you feel that?) She may be doing harm, particularly to children, without me knowing about it. She went into the fact that she does have an effect on other people—if she looks distracted or worried, they notice it. I said that she exaggerates their normal reactions in her hypersensitive state. We discussed her friendly feelings, and the difficulties she has with them in this state, which makes her want to do harm.

She is wondering about the cause of the relapse. She thinks it is because she was coming to grips with living alone.

Session 77: I suggested we get at this relapse by comparing it with what happened three years ago: Then she did not hear voices, nor did she have such terrible tension, but was strained by fantasies, sexual and whipping. Now these have disappeared. She thinks maybe subconsciously she was affected by her husband's remarriage. After all, she had a sex life for 20 years and now she had to give it up. I explained how this led to feelings of unworthiness and ideas of doing harm.

Lately she's been experiencing some smells—coffee is especially strong, and laundry. Voices say, "You stink." I explained the difference between fear and reality.

Occasional voices and fears remain. She now realizes that she was much sicker than she thought.

Session 78: She went to the Met. yesterday, and felt that people were talking about her. Her fears are greater than yesterday, which I tied up with her coming back to life and going to the movies and the Met.

She hears voices calling her "clinker" and "that B. woman." For the first time she revealed that her mother's first name was the same as Dr. B.'s. She has tremendous admiration for Dr. B. I pointed out that Dr. B. is like a mother.

This session she produced a dream for the first time since the relapse. It occurred last night:

> I'm in an office with an oblong desk; I go in and out a number of times. The children are mixed up in it somehow or other. Then my father comes in and he is perfectly all right.

The dream was merely used to get whatever associations she cared to make. She remembered that three years ago she was overcome once by the fear that her father had died.

Session 81: On the way here she heard, "She is a clinker," and, "Look at that B. woman." People looked at her and saw that she was a peculiar person, but she is able to force herself through these fears and do things now. . . .

Session 83: At the end she wanted to take an empty cigarette box along; I laughingly urged her to leave it.

Session 84: Today she came in terribly frightened. These voices are not hallucinations, she insisted; there's some reality to them. Last night there were musicians in the courtyard who were there just to mock her. Army planes fly over and clink her. That incident with the police that time was real—they did call her a clinker.

I inquired what had happened to frighten her so. Yesterday when she left, she said, there was a silly grin on my face, and she knew that she had upset me. If even an analyst cannot get along with her, what was the use? I reminded her of the cigarette box incident—she said yes, she was afraid that she had done me harm.

I reminded her that a week ago she realized that all these things were hallucinations. That, she said, was because she hadn't been around so much. Now she's been around, and knows that they're real.

I pointed out the cigarette box incident, that the day was Sunday, and Fountain House was closed—all this made her so terribly afraid.

She was not convinced; there is an element of reality, she kept on repeating.

Session 85: Much better than yesterday. In spite of everything yesterday, she went down to Fountain House.

The voices were again discussed, particularly clinker and clinking. Today she associated drinking to it, but there is still no great clarification.

The highlights of the next few months can be briefly indicated. The hallucinations and delusions were treated as experiences of anxiety so far as possible. Where she could not grasp the explanations no matter how often they were repeated, the subject was either dropped or environmental manipulation resorted to.

Session 87: She revealed that when she was sick she had the fear that she was a radio antenna, and that her head was made of ravioli; no associations could be obtained. Now she thinks that there's cotton wool in her head and feels closed up.

Session 89: The present-day material could be related to her childhood for the first time. She had heard a voice say "apple-tree." When asked for her associations, she recalled that when she was 4 or 5 years old she ate a crabapple and it was sour, added that an apple a day keeps the doctor away, and that she is a sour patient. The voices could thus be seen as stemming from the childhood feeling that she was a bad or "sour" girl.

Session 91: She reported a dream:

> There is a girl at a lecture. The lecturer looks like my Uncle C. They move from room to room. The lecturer is talking. The girl gets up to say something; he waves her down. Finally, she gets up and says, "I'm leaving." She leaves with 7 or 8 people. I watch all this and become angry with her, but repress it.

The dream was used to help her to see her anger at me, caused by a previous interpretation. The difference between her angry wish to destroy and events in the outside world was again emphasized; *e.g.*, the day before she had reported that there was a tremendous explosion in the subway, for which she thought she was responsible. . . .

Session 115: She spoke of some sexual feelings. The next session she reported a dream:

> I entered a boat at the invitation of a strange middle-aged man. It was a small, open boat, and we both stood in it. It was night, and I was talking to him, relating a strange occurrence in the sky that had happened in the previous part of the dream. Suddenly the moon shone, abnormally clear and bright, seeming very close— almost frighteningly close, and I pointed to it and said, "Like that." In a moment or two it changed to resemble a globe of the world, still retaining a brilliant light around it in the dark sky. Then another boat, open at the stern end which was toward our craft, came toward us very rapidly. I was frightened and jumped overboard. The men in the other boat seemed menacing, and I jumped from fear.

The luminosity and fear were tied up with her sexual feelings. However, any efforts at sexual interpretations and any attempt to let her talk more directly about her sexual feelings met with such violent resistance that I did not persist. Earlier, in the sixty-second session, she had once spoken of a feeling in her breasts—they rose occasionally. When I asked her more about it, she said, "Do you want to drive me completely crazy? Do you want the radio broadcasting such things?"

Session 118: She came out more directly with some hostile feelings toward me. She said that the children (who had met me once for a few moments) did not like me as much as they had the previous therapist; I was not as warm.

After this release of feeling, she had a sexual dream:

> I'm in an old house; there are children outside playing and laughing. A man is there, he is joking and talking. He lies down on the bed and invites me to lie down too.

She denied anything sexual about this dream. The man she recognized as an old bachelor from her home town; he looked somewhat like the therapist.

Around this time I had already decided on my summer vacation plans. Although it was still six weeks off, preparations were made to transfer her to another therapist while I was away, and her reactions to the vacation and shift were discussed. I was going to be away for six weeks. In order to make the separation easier, the frequency of sessions was cut down to five, then four, then three a week. After I left, a social worker was also retained to see her three times a week socially, because of the continued shakiness of her reality adjustment.

Session 132: She was again noticeably upset. She thought she was marked out, knew that these things were real, heard a voice say, "We'll tweak you in the vagina," wanted to know if I was familiar with her entire history, if I had been in touch with her previous therapist, etc. I interpreted her anxiety in terms of my vacation, which she vigorously denied. . . .

Session 135: She brought another dream:

> Three trees stood on a sandy plain and not much life around. Suddenly all three trees fall as if in an explosion, though there was no sound and no signs of such.

To the three trees she associated herself and the children. To the explosion she associated one which had occurred at a friend's house when she was in her teens, and for which she thought herself responsible. The explosion was interpreted as her anger, and the dream as a fear of what her anger might do.

In a sense, this dream was quite similar to the one which had preceded the recurrence of the psychosis, in which she touched her cousin and shriveled him up. In the meantime, the fear of doing harm had assumed delusional forms, and then diminished gradually, though a number of the delusions were still present at this stage.

During the session I burped. She expressed the feeling that she gave me indigestion and caused me to burp.

Session 137: She said that she wanted to get a radio for her room. She still heard names she knew on the radio, and said that she heard my name a lot. I said I thought it best that she should not have a radio, and she complied.

There was some increase in anxiety shortly before I left. At one point, she even expressed the thought that she should go back to the hospital. I discouraged that idea, and interpreted her fears in terms of her reaction to my vacation.

The switch to the vacation therapist occurred without incident. When she arrived at his office, his electric clock had temporarily stopped, and she felt responsible; she also told him that she withers flowers. However, she established a satisfactory relationship with him, and weathered the summer without any noticeable storm.

Psychodynamically, the hallucinations generally lent themselves to analysis, though the degree to which she grasped the explanations remained an open question. Eventually, the cries of *dink-tink-rink* were related to stink, and a feeling of slight loss of bowel control. One sequence, which was worked out much later, related to the idea that when she came into a room there was a "flurry" of people talking. It came out that she thought she created an odor, and people were too polite to tell her, so they talked more loudly to cover it up. The cries of "That B. woman" embodied both a reproach for sexuality (Dr. B. was a gynecologist) and a wish for her mother (Dr. B. had the same name as her mother). The feeling that children especially laughed at her and saw her as marked and peculiar was tied up with memories of her own childhood, and reproaches felt because of her inability to take care of her children.

Although she seemed to have improved considerably as a result of the intensive analysis, the amount of insight acquired was small. When she did not hear voices, her explanation was that the outside world had changed, so that there were no voices to be heard. The idea that her fears could lead to hearing voices remained totally incomprehensible; she said, quite logically, how can fears inside me produce voices outside? Yet, there were some glimmers of understanding, and several times an insight jelled after many years of intensive denial on her part.

Upon my return from vacation, I found the patient in substantially the same condition as when I had left.

The analysis was resumed three sessions per week. The social worker continued to see her on alternate days, three times per week, so that some therapeutic contact was available six days per week. Naturally, this also helped me to get a first-hand version of her behavior away from therapy.

An attempt was made to enlist the aid of friends or relatives to give her more of a social life, since she was extremely isolated. A number of possible contacts turned out to be either psychotic (hospitalized) or to have been psychotic at some time in the past. One interested relative was found, an unmarried woman in her fifties. She allowed the patient to share her apartment. After six months, the relative had to be rehospitalized. Thus no real emotional help from the family was ever available.

In this period her therapeutic time was dominated by two particularly strong fears: that others knew what is happening in her, and that she forces others to conduct conversations. These fears did not lend themselves either to clarification or to a ready therapeutic resolution, and remained prominent for a number of years.

The extreme fear and clinging dependency on me which she had displayed at the time of the acute psychosis from March through June now began to give way to a variety of negative transference manifestations. She had always compared me unfavorably with the previous therapist, Dr. A., to whom she had felt much closer. At one time she even expressed the thought that maybe the relapse was my fault.

After the vacation she also began to compare me with the substitute therapist. She also found him much warmer and much more understanding. Curiously, this led to a strengthening of her tie to me. Now that she knew one of my friends, and he was so nice, I could not be so bad, and she could place much more faith in me.

For a long time, the negative transference centered around three questions which were repeated over and over again: (1) What objective reasons did she have for placing confidence in me? (2) Was I taking care of her properly? (3) Why didn't I provide her with a third person to talk to and handle her affairs, one who was closer to her family? This last demand, of course, was for the restoration of her family.

The transference phenomena were handled by a combination of release, reassurance, and interpretation. Naturally, here she had a chance to release hostility towards me without suffering the consequences, and every effort was made to help her to see that.

Apart from the transference, the major focus of the analysis in this year was placed on the life history, and its connection with her illness. No hostility could ever be elicited against any of the major figures in her life, however. Even the idea that her father could have taken better care of her was vigorously denied. He was a poor man, he had to work, if his work carried him to Puerto Rico that was unavoidable. Of course, at this point in the therapy she was greatly preoccupied with her own adequacy as a mother, and to blame her father would have meant to invite blame for her own conduct, which was too much for her to handle. Thus, the denial mechanism served to reinforce the crushing superego formation, and erected a formidable barrier against the therapeutic effort to lighten superego pressure.

A good deal of time was devoted to her father's remarriage, which occurred when she was nine.

The therapeutic attempt to understand her life met with increasing resistance as time went on. She would harp repetitively on certain fears or preoccupations, such as whether we could not arrange for a third person to handle her affairs, what she could do about the children, or money, which were extraordinarily difficult to handle therapeutically. The situation was unduly complicated by the all-encompassing solicitude of the previous therapist. I felt that it would be wisest to urge her to seek more real life contacts.

The relative who has been mentioned (the woman who shared her apartment with the patient) arranged for an interview with an employment agency, and then contributed a small sum to allow an educational institution to employ the patient, who, of course, did not know that her employment was subsidized.

Though she felt very peculiar, she managed to go to work regularly and to do what was assigned to her. The main symptom that appeared at work was the feeling that she created a peculiar impression on others. Some of this was an obvious, disguised expression of homosexual wishes, but no interpretation at that level was ventured.

She had now progressed sufficiently to get along without a substitute therapist during my vacation, which lasted three weeks.

In the fall she struck out for a job on her own, and succeeded in obtaining employment a level below her pre-war employment, but still using many of her abilities.

The social worker was discharged. Roughly 15 months after the acute psychosis had subsided, she was able to work and manage her affairs. Naturally, she was still quite disturbed and in need of much intensive therapy.

She stayed two-and-a-half years at her new job. A new problem now dominated the therapy for most of the period of her employment. Her new boss was a woman, Susan, in her late twenties. The patient developed a strong crush on Susan.

At first she was quite certain that Susan had some homosexual leanings, and thought about the possibility of an affair with her. Susan was married, mother of one child, and a short time later became pregnant again. The patient reported nothing that pointed to lesbian tendencies in Susan, but the patient could not be shaken from her conviction. As she (in a sense quite reasonably) argued, how could I know that Susan was not homosexual; I did not know the woman.

No attempt was made to act out the homosexual side of her transference to Susan, but she did try to make a mother of her. She wrote her letters, asking for an opportunity to discuss personal problems with her. In Susan she saw the possible "third person" whom she had dreamed about so long. Since Susan was also a mother, she wanted particularly to discuss the children with her, since she was so troubled by the thought of being a bad mother.

Susan insisted on keeping the relationship on a purely business level. Eventually, Susan's continued rejection, my persistent interpretation of the whole fantasy as search for a mother, and her own slow but gradual growth, served to keep the crush within reasonable bounds. Characteristically, however, she never really gave up the conviction that Susan would respond to her, given the proper circumstances.

Most of the earlier complex of symptoms, particularly the hallucinations and delusions, disappeared in the course of time. More exactly, whenever they appeared, they were systematically analyzed in the manner indicated above, and yielded to the analysis.

One triad of symptoms, however, persisted many years after all the others had vanished. When she became anxious, she could not recognize the feeling but complained (1) that somebody had entered her room and disarranged objects there; (2) library books were marked up by some unknown person; (3) people, usually children, were laughing at her.

No amount of interpretation could convince her that this triad was not part of reality. After all, I wasn't there, how did I know that people did not enter her room?

In view of her obduracy, these symptoms, when they occurred, were encapsulated by the analyst, and separated for her from the rest of her functioning. I explained to her that whenever she became upset these symptoms would appear, and that it was important to bear that in mind even though she could not see the connection. By this method the symptoms would come and go, and she learned to handle them, even though she could not grasp what was happening.

By the spring of 1954 (330 sessions), some two years after the acute psychotic attack, we reached an impasse. The patient complained bitterly that she was overworked, always tired (her physician found her in satisfactory health), and could not manage to come to therapy three times a week. I felt that we had gone about as far as we could, and allowed her to cut down to two sessions a week. From here on, the treatment became almost completely supportive. She had come a long way for a woman with her history, and I did not want to risk another outbreak. By the fall of that year she had cut down to one session per week and in the next spring once every two weeks. Up to that time she had had 384 sessions.

The treatment has not been terminated completely; she has been encouraged to come back and see me whenever she felt the need to. I have functioned mainly as an advisor, although on rare occasions it has been possible to offer her some usable interpretation.

In this supportive period, I have found it possible to handle symptoms by merely ignoring them. Once she said that 6-year-old children were laughing at her at 11 o'clock at night outside her window, at another time she complained that somebody had entered her room and cut a hole in her bathrobe. Both of these symptoms disappeared without further consequence. Evidently she can have hallucinatory or delusional experiences and simply get over them, just as the ordinary person has a blue spell and gets over it.

The follow-up period since then has occasionally necessitated more intensive therapy. In nine years she has had roughly eighty sessions.

Her capacity to tolerate rejection has been remarkably good. In these years she has passed through a number of experiences which could easily shake a so-called normal person. Her roommate broke down in her presence, and had to be removed to a mental hospital. Her father died. An old friend's son committed suicide shortly after she had seen him. She was fired from her job. She witnessed one man beating another to unconsciousness in the street. Her novel was rejected by a number of publishers. Her daughters have married and she acquired two grandchildren. Her family consistently refused to help her, in spite of numerous pleas; usually they blamed her for not taking care of herself.

As we know, any one of the above incidents might set off an acute episode in a schizophrenic personality. That none of them did shows that her ego was strengthened considerably by the therapeutic process.

An important source of ego gratification for the patient was the novel she wrote about her hospital experiences. A few chapters had been written before she started with me. When the acute episode broke out, she put it to one side, and I discouraged her from taking it up again for several years thereafter. Finally she did get back to it, and completed a manuscript of some 180 pages. The book is a starkly realistic account of one patient's reactions to a mental hospital. It brings out the fear, monotony and isolation she experienced as a patient. It is a moving document, but she has yet to find a publisher.

Anyone seeing her these past few years would have no inkling of the tremendous storms she has passed through. She lives the life of a normal spinster in her early fifties. Her basic financial needs are taken care of by the alimony from her ex-husband, but she obtains work occasionally and supplements it, although consciously her main source of worry is money.

She is a quiet, rather soft-spoken woman. Her clothes are unpretentious, but adequate. She prefers to dress in a business-like way; to some extent this is due to her lack of money. Much of her time is spent alone, reading or working on her novel, or more recently attempting other kinds of writing. Occasionally she visits with her ex-mother-in-law, now in her eighties, and some friends; at times her daughters come to see her. As time has gone on, she looks more and more cheerful, no doubt because the fear which was so dramatically stamped on her face for so many years has gone. Her health is good. It has been at least six years since any of the severe psychotic symptoms has bothered her.

THEORETICAL COMMENTS

In reflecting on my therapeutic techniques, I would stress three in particular:

(a) *Intensive contact:* As soon as the acute psychosis reappeared, the frequency of sessions was stepped up to one a day, on occasion two. This contact served to gratify the increased dependency needs, and helped the therapist get a more rounded picture of what was happening to her.

That intense contact is *per se* therapeutic has been noted by a number of observers (Fromm-Reichmann, 1948; Harlow, 1958; Knight, 1946; Sechehaye, 1951; Weininger, 1938). Even the most regressed schizophrenics may respond to prolonged human concern shown by another person.

The situation, however, is not as simple as: provide contact and the patient will improve. If too much love is given, the patient may regress further and become more inaccessible (Searles, 1955).

Had I offered to see my patient seven times a week when she first came to me, she would probably have protested and refused to cooperate. It was the recurrence of the illness which made her accessible to the offer of maternal care on my part. There is a timing factor: the therapist must gauge when the patient's psychic economy is prepared to accept the increased contact.

The signal here came as an overwhelming increase in anxiety, which I handled both theoretically and actually as a cry for the mother.

The idea that anxiety in general and schizophrenic panic in particular is dynamically a cry for the mother follows fairly directly from Freud's second theory of anxiety.

For some years now in Amsterdam, Holland, there has been an emergency service for psychotics, a psychiatrist on call twenty-four hours a day. Whenever a request comes in to hospitalize a person, the psychiatrist goes out to that person and makes a home visit immediately; it is in the same category as any medical emergency. One result reported is a reduction in the incidence of hospitalization and a shorter length of stay while the patient is in the hospital.

(b) *Alternation of gratification and interpretation of oral needs:* The patient's symptoms were explained to her as a regression to an oral level (naturally in language she would understand), particularly with regard to the longing for a mother and the loss of ability to distinguish between inner and outer reality.

Most of the symptoms make sense when looked at theoretically as the infant-mother relationship: both the previous therapist and her husband were mother-substitutes; when she lost them, it revived the memory of the loss of her own mother. She tried to restore the mother by magical means. But the mother rejected her; she told her, "You're a stinker." This enraged the patient, and she wished to destroy everybody. The wish was not recognized as such; she attributed magical destructive powers to herself.

The auditory hallucinations for the most part represented a wish for the mother, and the reproach that she is bad if she has such a wish; *i.e.,* the ambivalent mother, good and bad. Badness also took in much symbolism from the anal level. The hallucinations about "dink" "rink" "tink," all ending in "ink," seemed to be versions of "stink." *E.g.,* when the police car pulled up and said "clink," it was first a hallucinated wish that mother (the police) was coming to her and simultaneously the reproach from mother: "You stink." When she entered a restaurant (food = mother), she thought she stank; the patrons (mother) wanted to say, "You stink," but were polite and merely talked louder.

The most persistent of all symptoms was the idea that her library books were marked up; it lasted long after the other hallucinations and delusions were gone. Later, we did trace it to the fact that the previous therapist, Dr. A., had on several occasions loaned her some books from his own library; those books he had heavily marked up with red pencil. The delusion was thus a disguised longing for Dr. A. In addition, in view of her lifelong love of books, and preoccupation with them, books must always have been a mother-symbol to her.

As I have indicated, the therapy did not proceed on purely analytical lines; a parameter (Eissler, 1953b) of gratifying her dependency needs had to be introduced. This varied with her psychic state; at times, I made many decisions for her, at times, few. The shift from gratification to analysis and back, the determination of how much she could handle at any particular time, and of what had best be avoided, represented by far the most difficult part of the therapist's task, and yet the most important.

(c) *Persistence in interpretation in the face of denial and incomprehension by the patient:* This is one of the most puzzling and most trying features of the analysis. Throughout she verbalized almost no insight. When the hallucinations disappeared, it was because the outside world had changed. When the delusions of doing harm vanished, it was because she no longer had those powers. To the repeated explanations of the difference between a wish and an action, she usually countered with the statement that she could not see how her wishes could influence the outside world.

In the absence of confirmation from the patient, I relied on my own subjective conviction of correctness. Whenever I could fit together pieces of the puzzling mosaic, I tucked them away in my mind and presented them to her when a suitable occasion appeared.

Nevertheless, the fact remains that although in terms of her own verbalizations she grasped almost nothing, she continued to make progress. A skeptic might say that the interpretations were all a waste of time, and that she got better by accident (spontaneous remission), or because I paid attention to her. Neither of these explanations is particularly convincing.

Negative transference was probably at play here. Similar phenomena, though not on such an extensive scale, are often seen with neurotics. One sometimes sees the statement that in analysis an interpretation is not really effective unless the patient first denies it.

Thus, with one part of her mind she could accept the interpretation, at least in part, while with another she would push me away. This is the same kind of ambivalence displayed in her hallucinations. After all, the mother (analyst) whom she restitutes is always calling her a stinker, so she had better be wary of everything she says.

The discouragement of the therapist has been noted by many theoreticians as one of the primary counter-transference problems with schizophrenics. Even before the large-scale advent of psychoanalytically-oriented therapy, Bleuler (1950) set down as his principal rule that "No patient must ever be completely given up."

In terms of her ultimate adjustment, some comments are in order. In the course of the years, she eventually left her family, husband and children, and adopted a rather solitary mode of life. Her adaptation now is on a rather infantile level; she is the baby who is taken care of by the world, though as time has gone on, she has shown more signs of wanting to be independent.

We have mentioned that the limits of the therapy were reached when libidinal material began to come up. She can handle the oral phase, but object relations are too frightening. This would explain another baffling feature of her adjustment, the abandonment of homosexuality. Of course, in the period with Susan, the homosexual urges were strong, and were analyzed as a wish for a mother. Since then no trace of them has appeared. The maternal need involved in homosexuality has been analyzed. The bodily needs, like the heterosexual ones, are repressed. No doubt also age plays a part (she is now 55).

In view of the existence of spontaneous and physiologically-induced remissions, the question may be raised as to the nature of the effectiveness of this therapy. The answer, I think, lies in the way in which the patient gets over the illness. Since her treatment, as mentioned above, she has lived through a variety of traumatic experiences which frequently affect even fairly normal people adversely; yet she has shown no reaction. We can assume that, as a result of the therapy, the ego has been strengthened to tolerate more anxiety, and to handle it differently, while superego pressure has been considerably reduced.

The persistence in interpretation must have meant to her that there was a stable figure in her environment who would not change or leave, no matter what she did, even to the extent of accepting her hostility. No such figure had ever existed in this woman's life before: sooner or later she had been abandoned by everybody, including all her previous therapists. For this reason, the insistence by the therapist that he was available for the rest of her life was important. Any indication that the relationship was terminated once and for all might conceivably have precipitated another crisis. The whole experience makes any crisis situation less threatening to her.

If we put these facets together, we get to an inner-dynamic change which could not be duplicated by any other method currently at our disposal.

Some theoreticians have raised the question as to whether a procedure of the type adopted here should be called analysis. I believe that it should be, since there is a working through of transference and resistance, a release and interpretation of unconscious material, and a reorganization of the ego structure.

REFERENCES

1. Belak, L.: *Schizophrenia*. New York: Logos Press, 1958.
2. Bleuler, E.: *Dementia Praecox or the Group of Schizophrenias*. New York: International Universities Press, 1950.
3. Bychowski, G.: *Psychotherapy of Psychosis*. New York: Grune & Stratton, 1952.
4. Cohen, M. B.: The therapeutic community and therapy. *Psychiatry*, 1957, **20**, 173-175.
5. Eissler, K.: Notes upon the emotionality of a schizophrenic patient and

its relation to problems of technique. *Psychoanalytic Study of the Child,* 1953, **8**, 199-251.

6. Eissler, K.: The effect of the structure of the ego on psychoanalytic technique. *J. Amer. Psychoanal. Assoc.,* 1953b, **1**, 104-143.

7. Fenichel, O.: *The Psychoanalytic Theory of Neurosis.* New York: W. W. Norton & Co., 1945.

8. Fine, R.: The logic of psychology. *Psychoanal. & Psychoanal. Rev.,* 1959, **45**, 15-41.

9. Fromm-Reichmann, F.: Notes on the development of schizophrenics by psychoanalytic therapy. *Psychiatry,* 1948, **11**, 263-272.

10. Harlow, H.: The nature of love. *Amer. Psychol.,* 1958, **13**, 673-686.

11. Hill, L. B.: *Psychotherapeutic Intervention in Schizophrenia.* Chicago: University of Chicago Press, 1955.

12. Knight, R. P.: Psychotherapy of adolescent catatonic schizophrenia with mutism, study in empathy and establishing contact. *Psychiatry,* 1946, **9**, 323-339.

13. Kronhausen, E., and Kronhausen, P. C.: The therapeutic family—the family's role in emotional disturbance and rehabilitation. *Marriage & Family Living,* 1959, **21**, 29-35.

14. Rachlin, H. L.; Goldman, G. S.; Gurwitz, M.; Lurie, A.; and Rachlin, L.: Follow-up study of 317 patients discharged from Hillside Hospital in 1950. *J. Hillside Hosp.,* 1956, **5**, 17-40.

15. Roheim, G.: *Magic and Schizophrenia.* New York: International Universities Press, 1953.

16. Rosen, J.: *Direct Analysis.* New York: Grune & Stratton, 1953.

17. Rosenfeld, H.: Considerations regarding the psychoanalytic approach to acute and chronic schizophrenia. *Int. J. Psychoanal.,* 1954, **35**, 135-140.

18. Searles, H. F.: Dependency processes in the therapy of schizophrenia. *J. Amer. Psychoanal. Assoc.,* 1955, **3**, 19-66.

19. Sechehaye, M. A.: *Symbolic Realization.* New York: International Universities Press, 1951.

20. Sullivan, H. S.: The oral complex. *Psychoanal. Rev.,* 1925, **12**, 31-38.

21. Weininger, B.: Psychotherapy during convalescence from psychosis. *Psychiatry,* 1938, **1**, 257-264.

7.   An Electric Shock Patient Tells His Story*

Thelma G. Alper

Electric convulsive therapy is effected by placing electrodes on both sides of the patient's forehead and applying electric current of 70–130 volts for a period of 1/10 to 5/10 of a second. Anectin, a muscle relaxant, may be used to reduce chances of physical injury during the convulsive seizure which lasts about a minute. In some cases, sodium amytal is used to counteract postconvulsive excitation.

The nature of electric shock therapy, and its value as a treatment, has stirred much controversy among psychologists and psychiatrists. Some reports state that the patient has no pain or memory of the shock. Alper, however, reports that her subject experienced great pain and fear. For a number of psychiatrists, electric convulsive therapy is the chosen treatment for all recalcitrant depressions, while others feel it reasonable as a last resort and a means of reducing suicidal risks. Still others feel that its effects are both psychologically and physiologically detrimental, and that its use is never warranted. Certain psychoanalysts theorize that the experience of electric convulsive therapy is supported by a belief the patient accepts as part of a death-rebirth fantasy. The suggestion is conveyed to the patient that the sick person will be killed and the healthy one reborn. A more physiological position suggests that a cerebral anoxia may somehow be the basis for improvement. Electric convulsive therapy raises brain activity to such a high level that cerebral functioning cannot be sustained

---

by the oxygen and glucose coming to the brain in the blood. Cortical inhibition may follow, allowing the activation of subcortical areas and stronger emotional expression. The manic-depressive psychosis is one of the disorders which are said to respond well to electric convulsive therapy.

The case study presented here describes the course of a manic-depressive illness and a young male patient's response to a series of shocks. This case also provides a dramatic view of the symptomatology and the periodicity of the disorder, even though it does not offer a biochemical or psychodynamic explanation for either the psychosis or electric shock treatment. Alper's conclusion is similar to that of other empiricists who feel that electric convulsive therapy alone is insufficient treatment but will provide reasonably good results when used along with psychotherapy.

Although electric shock therapy has been widely used in the treatment of many types of psychotic and of psychoneurotic illnesses since 1938, very little case material is available for understanding the patient's subjective reactions to it. Yet without such material it is difficult, if not impossible, to evaluate some of the current theories of cure.[1] Judging from the patient's behavior, the trembling, the profuse sweating, and the impassioned verbal pleas for help and release, it would appear that most patients find at least the preparatory phase of the treatment very unpleasant. So marked are these overt anxiety reactions that they have been accepted by many investigators as basic to psychogenic theories of cure. It has been suggested, for example, that the treatment threatens the patient with death and offers him an opportunity of rebirth cleansed of previous fears, anxieties, and confusions; or, that the treatment is a form of punishment which absolves the patient from overwhelming guilt feelings. Evidence in support of such theories, however, is not very great and, to date, neither psychogenic nor organic theories of cure have been generally acceptable (7).

Only a few investigators have tried to test any of the psychogenic theories by soliciting pre- and post-treatment accounts from their patients [cf. Fraser and Sargant (3), Millet and Mosse (10), Mosse (11), and Silbermann (12)]. Unfortunately, however, most of the accounts published by these authors are fragmentary, and of only limited usefulness for understanding the psychological elements in the curative process.

---

[1]See Stainbrook (13) and Kalinowsky and Hoch (8) for summaries both of the empirical findings and the theoretical discussions in this area.

Typically, the patient is too ill, or too anxious, both before and after treatment, to cooperate with the therapist.[2] This may be one reason why so few studies in this field include accounts by patients. But another, and perhaps even more basic, reason for the dearth of published case material written by patients themselves may be that therapists have not been sufficiently aware of the potential usefulness of such personal documents for understanding the dynamics of the individual illness or for predicting the likelihood of a successful cure by electric shock therapy.

An unusual opportunity to procure a personal document from a former patient presented itself to the writer when a student in an elementary psychology course offered to write an account of his own manic-depressive episodes and reactions to electric shock therapy. His story, written in the summer of 1946 during a lucid interval between recurrent manic-depressive attacks, appears below. Some suggestions as to how such material could be used for prognostic purposes in the individual case, and a brief discussion of the relation of this material to current psychogenic theories of shock, follow the patient's story.[3]

MY ELECTRIC SHOCK TREATMENT

Introduction: the Course of the Illness. In 1940-41, I was a senior at college. I had already gone through mild episodes of both elation and depression but I had managed to get my work done and to stay in college. If I could stick to the end of the year I would graduate in June.

But the spring of 1941 was different. Before it was over things got out of hand. I took my divisionals but I was convinced that I had flunked them, that I would never graduate, that I would never be able to hold down a job, that I would be a continual burden upon my parents. I left college without taking a final course examination and without waiting to hear about my divisionals.

By the middle of that summer things had gotten much worse. I was severely depressed. Such tasks as getting out of bed in the morning had taken on the proportions of hard labor. Sitting in a deep chair looking at the pictures in old copies of *Life Magazine* was about all I was able to manage. My family accounted for my blues by the sudden death of

---

[2]Gillespie (5) and Wiedeking (14) have attempted to supplement studies of patients by investigating the reactions of normal Ss to shock treatment. Such studies have yielded material consistent with patient material though their usefulness for the interpretation of patient reactions is limited. The normal person, by definition, is typically neither anxiety ridden nor disoriented before "treatment" is instituted.

[3]Liberties have been taken only with the introductory portions of the document. These consist primarily of rearranging certain portions of the material in order to present a clearer chronology than the document originally afforded. The original document was written in the third person. For present purposes it was recast into the first person.

my father a month after my failure to graduate from college. I had also lost the job I had procured for myself that summer because the plant was closed down by a strike. And it remained shut down for three and one-half months.

But as the fall drew nearer my family thought things were going better and they decided that I should return to college for one semester. I *had* passed my divisionals. In fact, I had done surprisingly well on them. But since I had so sold myself on the idea that I had flunked and had not taken the final exam, I did not complete my course in Freshman Physics.

When September finally came around, and I was to return to college, I was out of control. For example, I had decided that the building material of the twentieth century should be diatomite, a rock made up of the skeletons of millions of microscopic organisms. Deposits of diatomite were known in every state of the union, with one source of supply in Lompac, California that extended over several counties and had a known thickness of almost three quarters of a mile. I worked on my plans diligently, frequently staying up without sleep for 48 hours at a time until I was able to work 64 hours straight without a break, except to drink several glasses of milk to keep myself going. I was making elaborate plans to prefabricate small houses from diatomite blocks. My family realized that hospitalization was required, and instead of returning to college that fall, I was committed to the State Hospital.

The Hospital Period. I was in the hospital for a large part of the next three years. During this time I had studied myself until I could catalogue every move. I was a textbook example of a manic-depressive. Perfect. I enjoyed reading about manic-depressives in elementary psychology books. It was as though the author was watching me, jotting down all of my thoughts and actions. I had learned all about my cycle, and how it affected me. I boasted that I could tell the day of the year, the time of the day, by asking myself how I felt. This was a joke, but it wasn't the exaggeration it sounds. My cycle was as regular as a chronometer: three months elation, six weeks normalcy, six months of depression, six weeks of normalcy, and another year had gone by, but the cycle continued, and it took exactly a year for it to make one revolution. I knew that for the three months of my elation I would be locked up in the hospital; when I was depressed I would be out on pass. In spite of this I always looked forward to the elation; it was the depression that scared me. On two different occasions I bet with my brother that by the fifteenth of the coming September I would be back at the hospital. In each case I won. The first time I missed the date by eleven days, but the second time I was off by only two days.

I knew the game, knew it cold, nothing could surprise me. But in March of 1944 at one of the Friday afternoon hospital dances I had a new experience. I began to "hear voices." There was a great deal of conversation, noise, and general confusion. But suddenly every noise, every word was aimed at *me*. Everything that was being said, was being said about me. Everything that was being done, was being done because of me. For a short time I did my best to cope with this unusual situation. I tried to answer every remark, I tried to meet action with its proper counteraction. But in a short time it overwhelmed me. I knew something was radically wrong, and I told the attendant, who had brought me to the dance that I must see the doctor immediately. We started back to the ward together. On the way it slowly dawned on me that it would be impossible to see the doctor in my present "disturbed condition." The only other rational thought I had was that this situation must be brought to an end. I must get myself knocked out. The simplest way of accomplishing this was to go after an attendant. As soon as I got to the ward I made a beeline for my old friend, Mac.[4]

I have no clear recollection of the following two weeks, my last memory of the incident was running down the long corridor to get Mac. He told me all about it afterwards, but this is the only period in the entire three years that still remains vague, confused, distorted.

The next thing I remember was lying in the tub with my head resting on a small straw-filled, canvas-covered pillow. I was not at all surprised to find myself in the tubs. I could vaguely remember going haywire, but I couldn't recall any of the subsequent details. I could remember the experience of hearing voices; I would never forget it. I could remember the beginning of it all, but nothing else. I wasn't surprised at being in the tubs but I was surprised that I wasn't strapped in a hammock. The tubs were rather pleasant when you aren't rolled up in canvas so that you can scarcely blink your eyes. You can loll around, read magazines, if you don't get them too wet, you can even smoke cigarettes if you can bum them from the attendants. The only thing is that you can't quite go to sleep. Eight hours is a long time, and sleep is the ideal way to pass time.

There were five tubs in the white-tiled room, and in the five tubs were the five worst patients of the one hundred and fifty in the Reception Building. At least one was always raising the roof. I wondered if I had been that bad, but obviously I hadn't, or else I wouldn't be splashing around so comfortably. I dreamed and dreamed, and the morning passed. I didn't dare think about myself, for the first time I was scared, really

---

[4]Mac was a former alcoholic patient, a great big jovial fine-looking Irishman, and all in all one of the finest attendants the hospital ever had. When Mac and I had been patients together we became good friends. In the violent ward there are only a few patients that you can talk to. Mac had a parole, and before long we were allowed to go for long walks together through the extensive, beautifully landscaped hospital grounds. We were even allowed to go to town. We were together continually and when Mac became an attendant our friendship was only strengthened.

scared. I thought of the autobiography I was writing. I had started it back in 1941 sometime after I first came to the hospital. Two hundred pages were already written but I decided now that at last I had written the final period. This was the end. I'd be spending my life here in the hospital. So I started to dream again, the wilder the dream the better.

At lunch time Hap, the little Irishman in charge, passed out sandwiches and eggnog. Hap brought me my sandwiches first and asked:

"What the hell's been the matter with you?"

"I don't know, Hap."

"You went after Mac."

"I know I did."

"Mac's your best friend. What the hell did you do that for?"

"I don't know, Hap. What else did I do?"

"Oh, you've been making a damn fool of yourself. You've got more sense than that. Well, take it easy for a while. You'll be all right, fella."

Take it easy for a while. Three years of taking it easy for a while. I'd be all right. I'd be just dandy. But don't think; dream.

About one-thirty in the afternoon Mac came in carrying a county bathrobe, yellow county pajamas, and black felt carpet slippers. This meant that I had come down to the tubs wrapped in a sheet, that I had spent the night naked in a seclusion room and not in my regular bed in the dormitory. But, then, I couldn't expect to spend the night in the bridal suite at the Waldorf.

Mac said, "What do you say, Pal? You're looking better."

"Hi, Mac."

"We've got to take a cardiograph. Dr. S—— is going to give you shock treatment."

No other attendant would have bothered with this explanation. Electric shock, this was another surprise. Electric shock treatment had been suggested before for me but it never was seriously discussed. It was "too severe," "too drastic," a "last resort." When all else fails, try electric shock and hope for the best. Well, here it was. What would they try after electric shock failed? It would be worse if they gave up entirely. But don't think about it.

I got out of the tub, dried myself in a clean sheet, put on the pajamas and slippers, and holding the bathrobe close about me, I went down the corridor with Mac. Mac didn't seem mad at me, and even went so far as to make conversation, being careful to avoid referring to the entire business.

One of the doctors whom I didn't know, and a nurse whom I knew only by sight, made the necessary preparations for taking a cardiograph. There were a few feeble jokes about being electrocuted, and it was over. I expected to go back to the tubs, but Mac took me up to the Ward.

We stopped in at the office where the charge was admiring his new teeth in a small hand mirror. The charge had been a sergeant in the cavalry in the first World War. Mac said, "Sarge, our old college chum looks better today."

"How are you feeling, Ted?"

"Oh, pretty good, Sarge."

But this was a lie; I felt lousy. They could have taken me out in the field and buried me for fertilizer and I'd have made no kick.

"Do you want to sit around in the Ward for a while?" Sarge asked.

"Yeah, that'd be fine."

"O.K., fella. Take it easy."

I went down the long polished linoleum corridor to the day room. Another attendant was sitting in a rocker in the hallway.

"Hi, Ted. Sit down. Take it easy."

I sat down beside the attendant but there wasn't much talk. In a few minutes Mac came down the ward, and the three of us sat together.

"I hear he'll be getting shock treatment," the other attendant said.

"Yeah," Mac said.

The other attendant started off, "I'd be damned if I'd let any doctor give a relation of mine shock treatment."

"Why not?" Mac asked.

The attendant answered, "I've studied electricity long enough to know that it develops heat when it meets resistance." This man had been an electrician and had studied at Princeton for a short time, so you couldn't entirely laugh him off.

Mac said, "Dr. S—— wouldn't use it if it did any harm."

The attendant said, "What the hell does Dr. S—— know about electricity?"

It doesn't take much to get Mac mad when Dr. S——'s judgment is being bandied about and he said, in a fighting voice, "Well, he knows plenty more about it than you do, and I'll tell it to your face. If you know so much about electricity why don't you go out and get a job as an electrician? It'll pay a lot more than this lousy job."

"Well, all I know is that it generates heat, and heat will burn, and you can't tell me it doesn't destroy some of the brain cells."

"I wouldn't tell you anything," Mac said, and the conversation stopped.

Well, this was good. Electricity equals heat, equals burn. I'd never heard of a burned brain, but I was learning a lot lately, just when I thought nothing new could happen to me.

The next morning at six o'clock I was told to stay in bed. There would be no breakfast this morning because I was getting shock treatment. I already knew quite a bit about shock treatment. I had helped them give it to other patients many times. I worked in the dormitory, helping to lift the unconscious patients into bed from the wagon, covering them up, checking that no one swallowed the bandage gag that prevented the patient from biting his tongue or chipping his teeth, tying a man in bed if necessary, and occasionally holding the patient down in bed when things got really rough. It wasn't easy work and in a way I was glad not to be doing it this morning.

At half past six Mac came on duty. He came right up to my bed.

"Good morning, Ted. How are you feeling?" Mac asked with a big grin. You couldn't help smiling when Mac was feeling good.

At nine o'clock the doctor came on the Ward. The doctor was a good friend of mine and it was a nice feeling to know that someone was doing his best to help me. But at this moment I was none too happy. I hoped that I'd be the first on the list to get treatment. Yet I was glad to see another patient wheeled out first. I was scared and there was no getting around it. I tried to tell myself that I was just hungry. But I wasn't hungry at all. I tried to tell myself that I had had a bad night. But I'd slept like a log, as I always did. I wondered if I was going to burn, and if I did burn, whether I'd smell. But by this time there was an awful cry down the hall and I knew that the first patient's shock treatment had begun.

Soon a man was pushed into the dormitory and lifted into bed while another man on another wagon was pushed into the visiting room where the shock was administered. They had a system. Fifteen patients could be given shock treatment in an hour, easily.

Now it was my turn. I climbed up on the high wagon and stretched out. Three sand bags in the form of a pyramid stuck into the small of my back to expand my chest. Many of the men squirmed and fidgeted and fooled with the sand bags trying to make themselves comfortable. But you were never on the wagon long. A counterpane was pulled up to my neck and a small straw pillow, though covered with a clean towel, was wet with the sweat of the men who had gone before. I was wheeled out into the hall to wait my turn. There was another scream and a gurgling coughing groan, and the patient ahead of me was moved out down the hall and into the dormitory, with arms and legs and head flopping around. Before I realized it I was zooming down the hall. Mac was pushing me, and Mac was in a hurry.

The wagon bumped over the thick rubber matting that formed a hollow rectangle for the wagon to fill. The doctor was looking down, smiling.

"Hello there, young fellow."

"Good morning, Sir."

Sarge was rubbing some sticky stuff on my head beside my ears. I had seen tubes of the stuff in the office, "electrode jelly." After all you had to make a good contact—to burn. I was mighty scared and there was no use kidding about it. Mac held my right arm and pressed hard with the elbow just inside my shoulder muscle. Sarge had the other arm. Another attendant climbed up on the wagon and lay across my knees gripping the side of the wagon with hands and toes. The three attendants would hold me down during my convulsion. The theory was: the more severe the convulsion, the better the results.

I heard the doctor give the pretty blonde nurse a set of numbers, and I knew that she was setting the dials.

"God, don't let her give me an overdose."

Mac's face was about eight inches above my own. I looked up into Mac's eyes. Mac wasn't smiling a bit. I stared up into Mac's eyes and slowly said over and over to myself, "Mac, you big Irish lug, take care of me now." Very deliberately, very slowly a black shade came up over my eyes.

I woke up sometime later feeling completely refreshed, not tired or logy, or drugged with sleep, just ready for a big day. I started thinking what I would do today but I could think of nothing. I began looking around. I was in a large cream colored room with fifteen or twenty beds neatly made, and covered with white counterpanes. It looked like a hospital, but why should I be in a hospital? There were large windows all along one wall. The room looked strangely familiar. I shut my eyes and tried to think. But nothing came.

"What is the date?" I asked myself.

"I haven't any idea."

"What day of the week is it?"

"Don't be silly."

"What month is it?"

"I don't know."

"What year is it?"

That shouldn't be hard. But I wasn't sure. It was later than 1941. I tried to outsmart myself by asking how old I was and then figuring one year. But I didn't know how old I was.

"What season of the year is it?"

I looked out the windows. I couldn't see much, but I realized I didn't have on my glasses. I must have lost them. I rubbed my eyes. I wasn't alarmed at all. What difference did it make? I went back to sleep.

Then someone was shaking me.

"Come on, Pud." Mac sometimes called me Pudd'n'head.

"Good morning, Mac."

Mac laughed.

"Well, you remember my name anyhow."

"Why shouldn't I remember your name?"

"What else do you remember, smart boy?"

"I remember everything."

Mac laughed again.

"Where are you now?"

"I'm with you, I must be at O——."

"That doesn't say much for me, Pud, does it?"

I didn't feel quite up to snappy sayings.

"It's time to get up, Ted."

Going down the corridor I looked at the clock. Ten-thirty. It must have stopped. The ward was almost empty, and it was quiet. I didn't try to think much, I just watched. The first meal of the day was lunch. I began to pick up some of the details of the ward. Lunch was over by twelve. I started to help clean up the dishes, but there was too much confusion, so I went down back to the day room.

At one almost everyone went off to Occupational Therapy. The ward was again empty and quiet. I found a few old copies of *Life*. I looked at the pictures. There was a war going on. The date was 1944 or later.

By that evening I had gained enough confidence to sit with the attendants out in the hall. This was one of my privileges. But I didn't talk much, and I didn't ask any questions. I mostly listened.

I had two more shock treatments in the following five days. They didn't bother me as much as the first one, but I never looked forward to them. I always looked up at Mac's eyes above mine and thought, "Stick with me, old side kick. Don't let me down now."

At six-thirty the morning of my fourth treatment, Mac came over to my bed and said: "You're not getting treatment this morning, Ted. Dr. S—— has taken you off the list."

"Why? I've only had three." There were six treatments to a series.

"You don't need any more. You're coming along fine."

"Shall I help give treatment this morning?"

"No. Take it easy for a while."

This was the first time in years that I hadn't resented "take it easy for a while."

After breakfast I got another piece of paper from Sarge and started the routine which had become daily since my first day of shock treatment: my chronology—

1919—born
1920—1 year old
1921—2 years old

Very shortly I worked my way up to 1944. So I was twenty-four years old. But I had a hard time believing it. It must be so, but I couldn't remember my last birthday. I knew I had been in the hospital at that time. My mother would have visited me. My sister would have baked me a delicious chocolate birthday cake with an orange filling. She always did. My mother would have a big basket of fruit and presents from the rest of the family. I couldn't remember the cake, I couldn't remember the presents, I couldn't even remember the fruit and my mother always brought me a big basket of fruit, every week, often two or three times a week. Fruit was good for me, non-fattening, and I always gave it away.

Slowly I began to work out the chronology again. Slowly I began to remember things. Some things I couldn't remember at all. But this didn't worry me. All things came in time.

One day I realized that I was normal. I wasn't depressed, but I sure wasn't elated. I checked with the calendar. I should be normal. Damn the cycle. In a week or two I found I was getting depressed. This was mighty discouraging.

Mac came down the hall.

"Dr. S—— wants to see you, Ted," Mac said. Mac looked pretty pleased.

I followed Mac into Dr. S.——'s office.

Dr. S—— said, "Sarge and I have been talking it over, and we've decided that you're ready to go to work. You can go to work as an attendant here and work right with Mac and Sarge. We all know you can swing it. You've been working in the Ward as an unofficial attendant for a good part of three years, only now you'll be paid for it. Think it over, talk it over with your mother and let me know what you decide."

I went back down the hall and thought. I didn't want the damned job, but they would have to discharge me before they hired me. I had never before been discharged, and this would certainly be a big step in the right direction. Always before, when I left the hospital, I had been on Pass.

Four days later I was working as an attendant, white coat and all. I was still depressed and it was getting worse, but I was beginning to hold my head up. I was legally sane. I was supporting myself. I was saving a little money.

Six weeks later I broke my leg in a scramble. A patient fell on me sidewise. I went up to 57, the infirmary ward. I realized my days of attending were over and I felt fine. I had known that sooner or later I would get hurt, then I'd never work as an attendant again, if for no other reason than that my mother wouldn't allow it. I laughed for the first time in some months. A broken leg. That's cheap. I had been afraid that my eyes would be injured. I had to wear glasses, and on a lively day those glasses would spin across the smooth linoleum floor at a great rate. I stretched out in bed and decided to be lazy for at least four weeks. I had made a habit of asking myself how I felt, checking up on myself. I felt great. This was strange, for according to the calendar I should still be depressed. But I was way off my cycle, there was no denying it. I had been depressed for only three months, not six months. I watched myself. No elation followed. My cycle was a thing of the past. Get Thee behind me.

What threw me off my cycle? Was it shock treatment? Probably. But I was depressed following the shock treatment, even if only for a short time. What had the shock treatment done for me? It had given me a new chance. I was able to start over fresh. With no memory, no delusions, no fears. Or at least I had no memory of them for that period of days before I could again remember the details of my life. In that time I had been reoriented. I was on the right track for the first time in some years. I had been offered a job on a silver platter. In fact it had been forced upon me. That was a very smart move on Dr. S——'s part. And I was discharged as sane.

When my leg healed I left the hospital and got a job as a laboratory assistant. After a year I got a better job as a chemist. In February 1946 I returned to college. On June 6, 1946, I graduated. Four days later I had my diploma framed.

Conclusion: My Understanding of Shock Treatment. Electric shock treatment was successful in my case because there existed a "love relationship," a relationship similar to that between father and son, between myself and Mac, a relationship such as is established between psychiatrist and patient in narcosynthesis. I believe that this lucky accident proved to be the focal point of the entire treatment. This relationship must be reaffirmed and strengthened during the short period of complete loss of memory, following the awakening from unconsciousness, if the treatment is to be used with best results.

The personal document ends at this insightful point. The subsequent history is based on brief interviews and letters.

After graduation, the patient returned home and resumed his old job as a chemist. During a lull at the plant when the men were laid off for a few days, the patient completed his personal document and sent it off to the writer. With it came a letter dated June 24, 1946. In the letter he spoke of "working leisurely on the book." His family was encouraging him in this and wanted him to finish it. He ended the letter with the remark, "So I guess I have no choice."

Nothing further was heard from him until September 18, 1946. Then a brief note came saying, "I am sorry to write that I am once again back at the hospital as a patient. I went haywire July 23. I have had six shock treatments, and, as before, they have done me a great deal of good."

In November, 1946 he left the hospital on Pass and went back to his old job as a chemist. "Normally" the excited phase of the cycle would have caught up with him by June, 1947. But in a letter dated late in July he reported that he had "safely passed the June date." He was certain that the shock treatments were responsible for this but he himself raised the question as to whether the cycle had merely been delayed by the treatments, as had occurred in the past, or whether a permanent cure had been effected.

In November, 1947 he visited briefly with the writer. He was still holding down his job as a chemist. He was "feeling fine." It had been a good summer—plenty of fun and relaxation on weekends spent lazily drifting down inland streams. Would he stay well? He wasn't sure, but he was hopeful.

It is not possible, of course, to predict with certainty what the outcome in this case will be. If one checks the facts with the prognostic signs listed by Gold and Chiarello (6) as portending a good prognosis, the outlook is not too happy. In the present case, though the youthfulness of the patient is in his favor, he already has had more than one series of attacks, and at least one series of unsuccessful shock treatments. Moreover, it is not clear that exogenic factors played a significant role in precipitating the illness. There is also evidence from interviews that the patient had been fairly restricted in his interpersonal relations even before the illness. According to the criteria set forth by Gold and Chiarello, this combination of factors would seem to mitigate against a permanent recovery.

These authors also mention that personality factors, in addition to the nature of the patient's interpersonal relations, mitigate against recovery. They suggest that the prognosis is poor if the patient has "personality defects." They do not make clear, however, what the nature of these defects might be. Nor have other investigators of shock therapy treated the role of personality factors in this form of therapy any more extensively. The evidence from the personal document alone, in the present case, is, of course, inadequate for estimating whether or not there are "personality defects" here. A much more intensive case record, including the results of projective techniques and interview material, would be required. On the basis of the personal document alone, however, certain tentative hypotheses can be formulated.

Perhaps the clearest needs of this personality are in the nature of strong passive, dependent needs. Others decide things for him and he considers it right that they should: the family decides that he is to go back to college, that he should finish the book, and he has "no choice"; the mother, not he, will decide whether he should go back to work after the accident in the hospital. All of this he takes for granted. He even takes the horrors of the treatment for granted, pinning his hopes on his good friend Mac who will take care of him. He learns that he may end up with a "burned brain." He knows that electric shock treatment is a "last resort," that other patients dread it. Yet he does not resist it. The pain and fear of treatment would seem to serve not so much as a death threat, or as punishment, but rather as inevitable and to be endured because the good parent can be trusted here, as well as with respect to other details of his life. Whether the psychosis in this case is basically a giving-in to these passive dependent needs, or not, cannot categorically be stated. On the other hand, recognizing the existence of these needs one must also recognize that electric shock therapy alone does nothing to alter this patient's psychogenic need-structure. If anything, one might expect it to *increase* his dependency and to increase the likelihood of subsequent episodes.

On the other hand, the fact that the two sets of shocks did "throw the cycle off," that the period of depression was shortened and the period of normalcy was lengthened, is a hopeful sign. Even if subsequent attacks should occur, it may be that the duration of each attack can be considerably shortened if treatments are instituted at the first signs of manic breakdown [cf. Geoghegen (4)]. Moreover, if, along with the electric shock treatment, psychotherapy which is more than mere supportive therapy can be given, as is recommended in the recent report (7) of the Committee on Therapy of the Group for the Advancement of Psychiatry, the prognosis may be reasonably good. Somehow the personality needs to be strengthened. It is not enough merely to be given a "new chance, to start over fresh," as he himself puts it, "with no memory, no delusions, no fears." Unfortunately, the amnesia, as is typical in these cases, wears off and, without psychotherapy, the inner and outer life-situation of the patient remains essentially unchanged.

One further point needs to be stressed here. In spite of the confusion and seeming disorientation of the patient, it cannot be assumed that he is unaware of the discomfitures of other patients and of the attitudes and conversations of staff members. Clifford Beers (2) called this to our attention many years ago. Kindwell and Kinder (9) have written more recently. Shock treatment, whether it is insulin (1) or electric shock, is a terrifying experience for the patient. It has not yet been conclusively shown that the results of the wholesale use of electric shock therapy warrant inflicting such terror on the patient.

REFERENCES

1. Anonymous: Insulin and I. *Amer. J. Orthopsychiat.,* 1940, **10,** 810-814.
2. Beers, C.: *A mind that found itself: An autobiography.* New York: Longmans Green, 1908.
3. Fraser, R., and Sargant, W.: The subjective experiences of a schizophrenic illness. *Character & Pers.,* 1940-41, **9,** 139-151.
4. Geoghegen, J. J.: Manic depressive psychosis and electroshock. *Canadian Med. Ass. J.,* 1946, **55,** 54-55.

5. Gillespie, J. E. O. N.: Cardiazol convulsions, the subjective aspect. *London Lancet*, 1939, **1**, 391-392.

6. Gold, L., and Chiarello, C. J.: The prognostic value of clinical findings in cases treated with electric shock. *J. Nerv. Ment. Dis.*, 1944, **100**, 577-583.

7. Group for the Advancement of Psychiatry. Report #1. Formulated by Committee on Therapy. Sept. 15, 1947.

8. Kalinowsky, L. B., and Hoch, P. H.: *Shock treatments and other somatic procedures in psychiatry.* New York: Grune & Stratton, 1946.

9. Kindwell, J. A., and Kinder, E. F.: Postscript on a benign psychosis. *Psychiatry*, 1940, **3**, 527-534.

10. Millet, J. A. P., and Mosse, E. P.: On certain psychological aspects of electroshock therapy. *Psychosom. Med.*, 1944, **6**, 226-236.

11. Mosse, E. P.: Electroshock and personality structure. *J. Nerv. Ment. Dis.*, 1946, **104**, 296-302.

12. Silbermann, I.: The psychical experiences during the shocks in shock therapy. *Int. J. Psychoanal.*, 1940, **21**, 179-200.

13. Stainbrook, E.: Shock therapy: Psychologic theory and research. *Psychol. Bull.*, 1946, **43**, 21-60.

14. Wiedeking, I.: Selbstbeobachtungen in hypoglykämischen Zustand. *Z. Ges. Neurol. Psychiat.*, 1937, **159**, 417.

8. A Case of Paranoia Running Counter to the Psycho-analytical Theory of the Disease*

Sigmund Freud

Paranoia in which the delusion is encapsulated, leaving the rest of the personality free to function in a nonpsychotic fashion, has been described as a rare disorder. The psychoanalytic literature generally has not been as concerned as psychiatric texts with discriminating between paranoia and paranoid schizophrenia, and one may see the dynamics of paranoia and paranoid schizophrenia given the same nucleus of explanation by psychoanalysts. Freud, in fact, believed that paranoia and schizophrenia, for which he suggested the name paraphrenia, could coexist, and also that the schizophrenic fixation occurs earlier in development than paranoia. The psychoanalytic explanation of paranoia requires three basic ingredients: denial; homosexuality; and projection. The delusion, it is theorized, is constructed to protect the individual against threatening feelings of homosexuality resulting from the negative Oedipal complex (in which the child has identified with a person of the opposite sex and is attracted to a person of the same sex). The patient Freud studied for most of his formulations on paranoia protected himself from his homosexual tendencies in the following way: his first unconscious reaction to the homosexual attraction was, "I do not love him, I hate him." This, according to Freud, was changed, through projection, to "He hates me," and rationalized to "I hate him because he persecutes me." According to Freudian

*First published in *Zeitschrift*, Bd. III., 1915. Reprinted from the Standard Edition of the *Complete Psychological Works of Sigmund Freud* (vol. 14, pp. 263-272), revised and edited by James Strachey, by permission of Sigmund Freud Copyrights Ltd., The Institute of Psycho-Analysis, The Hogarth Press, Ltd., and Basic Books, Inc., Publishers, New York.

theory, the persecutor should be of the same sex to bear out the hypothe-
sized projected homosexual position.

This case study presents notes on a young woman who, following a
love affair, consulted a lawyer to ask for protection from the persecution
of her ex-lover. The lawyer, not convinced by her story, had her inter-
viewed by Freud. Freud's observations led him to believe that the woman
was delusional and a paranoiac. He stated that her delusion was some-
what different from the usual paranoiac delusion which remains fixated
on a person of the same sex. He explained, however, that progression
from female to male as the object of the delusion was possible on a
paranoiac basis since the man was merely a screen figure for a woman
(mother).

Some years ago a well-known lawyer consulted me about a case
which had raised some doubts in his mind. A young woman had asked
him to protect her from the molestations of a man who had drawn her
into a love-affair. She declared that this man had abused her confidence by
getting unseen witnesses to photograph them while they were making love,
and that by exhibiting these pictures it was now in his power to bring dis-
grace on her and force her to resign the post she occupied. Her legal
adviser was experienced enough to recognize the pathological stamp of
this accusation; he remarked, however, that, as what appears to be incredible often actually happens, he would appreciate the opinion of a
psychiatrist in the matter. He promised to call on me again, accompanied
by the plaintiff.

(Before I continue the account, I must confess that I have altered
the *milieu* of the case in order to preserve the incognito of the people
concerned, but that I have altered nothing else. I consider it a wrong practice, however excellent the motive may be, to alter any detail in the presentation of a case. One can never tell what aspect of a case may be
picked out by a reader of independent judgement, and one runs the risk of
leading him astray.)[1]

Shortly afterwards I met the patient in person. She was thirty years
old, a most attractive and handsome girl, who looked much younger than
her age and was of a distinctly feminine type. She obviously resented the
interference of a doctor and took no trouble to hide her distrust. It

---

[1]Cf. a footnote to the same effect added in 1924 at the end of Freud's case
history of 'Katharina' in Breuer and Freud, *Studies on Hysteria* (1895), *Standard Ed.,*
2, 134, and some remarks in the Introduction to the 'Rat Man' case history (1909*d*),
Standard Ed., **10**, 155-6.

was clear that only the influence of her legal adviser, who was present, induced her to tell me the story which follows and which set me a problem that will be mentioned later. Neither in her manner nor by any kind of expression of emotion did she betray the slightest shame or shyness, such as one would have expected her to feel in the presence of a stranger. She was completely under the spell of the apprehension brought on by her experience.

For many years she had been on the staff of a big business concern, in which she held a responsible post. Her work had given her satisfaction and had been appreciated by her superiors. She had never sought any love-affairs with men, but had lived quietly with her old mother, of whom she was the sole support. She had no brothers or sisters; her father had died many years before. Recently an employee in her office, a highly cultivated and attractive man, had paid her attentions and she in turn had been drawn towards him. For external reasons, marriage was out of the question, but the man would not hear of giving up their relationship on that account. He had pleaded that it was senseless to sacrifice to social convention all that they both longed for and had an indisputable right to enjoy, something that could enrich their life as nothing else could. As he had promised not to expose her to any risk, she had at last consented to visit him in his bachelor rooms in the daytime. There they kissed and embraced as they lay side by side, and he began to admire the charms which were now partly revealed. In the midst of this idyllic scene she was suddenly frightened by a noise, a kind of knock or click. It came from the direction of the writing-desk, which was standing across the window; the space between desk and window was partly taken up by a heavy curtain. She had at once asked her friend what this noise meant, and was told, so she said, that it probably came from the small clock on the writing-desk. I shall venture, however, to make a comment presently on this part of her narrative.

As she was leaving the house she had met two men on the staircase, who whispered something to each other when they saw her. One of the strangers was carrying something which was wrapped up and looked like a small box. She was much exercised over this meeting, and on her way home she had already put together the following notions: the box might easily have been a camera, and the man a photographer who had been hidden behind the curtain while she was in the room; the click had been the noise of the shutter; the photograph had been taken as soon as he saw her in a particularly compromising position which he wished to record. From that moment nothing could abate her suspicion of her lover. She pursued him with reproaches and pestered him for explanations and reassurances, not only when they met but also by letter. But it was in vain that he tried to convince her that his feelings were sincere and that her suspicions were entirely without foundation. At last she called on the lawyer, told him of her experience and handed over the letters which the suspect had written to her about the incident. Later I had an opportunity of seeing some of these letters. They made a very favourable impression on me, and consisted mainly in expressions of regret that such a beautiful and tender relationship should have been destroyed by this 'unfortunate morbid idea'.

I need hardly justify my agreement with this judgement. But the case had a special interest for me other than a merely diagnostic one. The view had already been put forward in psycho-analytic literature that patients suffering from paranoia are struggling against an intensification of their homosexual trends—a fact pointing back to a narcissistic object-choice. And a further interpretation had been made: that the persecutor is at bottom someone whom the patient loves or has loved in the past.[2] A synthesis of the two propositions would lead us to the necessary conclusion that the persecutor must be of the same sex as the person persecuted. We did not maintain, it is true, as universally and without exception valid the thesis that paranoia is determined by homosexuality; but this was only because our observations were not sufficiently numerous; the thesis was one of those which in view of certain considerations become important only when universal application can be claimed for them. In psychiatric literature there is certainly no lack of cases in which the patient imagines himself persecuted by a person of the opposite sex. It is one thing, however, to read of such cases, and quite a different thing to come into personal contact with one of them. My own observations and analyses and those of my friends had so far confirmed the relation between paranoia and homosexuality without any difficulty. But the present case emphatically contradicted it. The girl seemed to be defending herself against love for a man by directly transforming the lover into a persecutor: there was no sign of the influence of a woman, no trace of a struggle against a homosexual attachment.

In these circumstances the simplest thing would have been to abandon the theory that the delusion of persecution invariably depends on homosexuality, and at the same time to abandon everything that followed from that theory. Either the theory must be given up or else, in view of this departure from our expectations, we must side with the lawyer and assume that this was no paranoic combination but an actual experience which had been correctly interpreted. But I saw another way out, by which a final verdict could for the moment be postponed. I recollected how often wrong views have been taken about people who are ill psychically, simply because the physician has not studied them thoroughly

---

[2]See Part III of Freud's Schreber analysis (1911*c*).

enough and has thus not learnt enough about them. I therefore said that I could not form an immediate opinion, and asked the patient to call on me a second time, when she could relate her story again at greater length and add any subsidiary details that might have been omitted. Thanks to the lawyer's influence I secured this promise from the reluctant patient; and he helped me in another way by saying that at our second meeting his presence would be unnecessary.

The story told me by the patient on this second occasion did not conflict with the previous one, but the additional details she supplied resolved all doubts and difficulties. To begin with, she had visited the young man in his rooms not once but twice. It was on the second occasion that she had been disturbed by the suspicious noise: in her original story she had suppressed, or omitted to mention, the first visit because it had no longer seemed of importance to her. Nothing noteworthy had happened during this first visit, but something did happen on the day after it. Her department in the business was under the direction of an elderly lady whom she described as follows: 'She has white hair like my mother.' This elderly superior had a great liking for her and treated her with affection, though sometimes she teased her; the girl regarded herself as her particular favourite. On the day after her first visit to the young man's rooms he appeared in the office to discuss some business matter with this elderly lady. While they were talking in low voices the patient suddenly felt convinced that he was telling her about their adventure of the previous day—indeed, that the two of them had for some time been having a love-affair, which she had hitherto overlooked. The white-haired motherly old lady now knew everything, and her speech and conduct in the course of the day confirmed the patient's suspicion. At the first opportunity she took her lover to task about his betrayal. He naturally protested vigorously against what he called a senseless accusation. For the time being, in fact, he succeeded in freeing her from her delusion, and she regained enough confidence to repeat her visit to his rooms a short time—I believe it was a few weeks—afterwards. The rest we know already from her first narrative.

In the first place, this new information removes any doubts as to the pathological nature of her suspicion. It is easy to see that the white-haired elderly superior was a substitute for her mother, that in spite of his youth her lover had been put in the place of her father, and that it was the strength of her mother-complex which had driven the patient to suspect a love-relationship between these ill-matched partners, however unlikely such a relation might be. Moreover, this disposes of the apparent contradiction to the expectation, based on psycho-analytic theory, that the development of a delusion of persecution will turn out to be determined by an over-powerful homosexual attachment. The *original* persecutor—the agency whose influence the patient wishes to escape—is here again not a man but a woman. The superior knew about the girl's love affairs, disapproved of them, and showed her disapproval by mysterious hints. The patient's attachment to her own sex opposed her attempts to adopt a person of the other sex as a love-object. Her love for her mother had become the spokesman of all those tendencies which, playing the part of a 'conscience', seek to arrest a girl's first step along the new road to normal sexual satisfaction—in many respects a dangerous one; and indeed it succeeded in disturbing her relation with men.

When a mother hinders or arrests a daughter's sexual activity, she is fulfilling a normal function whose lines are laid down by events in childhood, which has powerful, unconscious motives, and has received the sanction of society. It is the daughter's business to emancipate herself from this influence and to decide for herself on broad and rational grounds what her share of enjoyment or denial of sexual pleasure shall be. If in the attempt to emancipate herself she falls a victim to a neurosis it implies the presence of a mother-complex which is as a rule overpowerful, and is certainly unmastered. The conflict between this complex and the new direction taken by the libido is dealt with in the form of one neurosis or another, according to the subject's disposition. The manifestation of the neurotic reaction will always be determined, however, not by her present-day relation to her actual mother but by her infantile relations to her earliest image of her mother.

We know that our patient had been fatherless for many years: we may also assume that she would not have kept away from men up to the age of thirty if she had not been supported by a powerful emotional attachment to her mother. This support became a heavy yoke when her libido began to turn to a man in response to his insistent wooing. She tried to free herself, to throw off her homosexual attachment; and her disposition, which need not be discussed here, enabled this to occur in the form of a paranoic delusion. The mother thus became the hostile and malevolent watcher and persecutor. As such she could have been overcome, had it not been that the mother-complex retained power enough to carry out its purpose of keeping the patient at a distance from men. Thus, at the end of the first phase of the conflict the patient had become estranged from her mother without having definitely gone over to the man. Indeed, both of them were plotting against her. Then the man's vigorous efforts succeeded in drawing her decisively to him. She conquered her mother's opposition in her mind and was willing to grant her lover a second meeting. In the later developments the mother did not reappear, but we may safely insist that in this [first] phase the lover had not become the persecutor directly but *via* the mother and in virtue of his relationship to the mother, who had played the leading part in the first delusion.

One would think that the resistance was now definitely overcome, that the girl who until now had been bound to her mother had succeeded in coming to love a man. But after the second visit a new delusion appeared, which, by making ingenious use of some accidental circumstances, destroyed this love and thus successfully carried through the purpose of the mother-complex. It still seems strange that a woman should protect herself against loving a man by means of a paranoic delusion; but before examining this state of things more closely, let us glance at the accidental circumstances that formed the basis of this second delusion, the one aimed exclusively against the man.

Lying partly undressed on the sofa beside her lover, she heard a noise like a click or beat. She did not know its cause, but she arrived at an interpretation of it after meeting two men on the staircase, one of whom was carrying something that looked like a covered box. She became convinced that someone acting on instructions from her lover had watched and photographed her during their intimate *tête-à-tête*. I do not for a moment imagine, of course, that if the unlucky noise had not occurred the delusion would not have been formed; on the contrary, something inevitable is to be seen behind this accidental circumstance, something which was bound to assert itself compulsively in the patient, just as when she supposed that there was a *liaison* between her lover and the elderly superior, her mother-substitute. Among the store of unconscious phantasies of all neurotics, and probably of all human beings, there is one which is seldom absent and which can be disclosed by analysis: this is the phantasy of watching sexual intercourse between the parents. I call such phantasies—of the observation of sexual intercourse between the parents, of seduction, of castration, and others—'primal phantasies'; and I shall discuss in detail elsewhere their origin and their relation to individual experience.[3] The accidental noise was thus merely playing the part of a provoking factor which activated the typical phantasy of overhearing which is a component of the parental complex. Indeed, it is doubtful whether we can rightly call the noise 'accidental'. As Otto Rank has remarked to me, such noises are on the contrary an indispensible part of the phantasy of listening, and they reproduce either the sounds which betray parental intercourse or those by which the listening child fears to betray itself. But now we know at once where we stand. The patient's

---

[3]The subject of 'primal phantasies' is discussed at length in Lecture XXIII of Freud's *Introductory Lectures* (1916-17) and in his case history of the 'Wolf Man' (1918*b*), *Standard Ed.*, **17**, 59-60 and 97.

lover was still her father, but she herself had taken her mother's place. The part of the listener had then to be allotted to a third person. We can see by what means the girl had freed herself from her homosexual dependence on her mother. It was by means of a small piece of regression: instead of choosing her mother as a love-object, she identified herself with her—she herself *became* her mother. The possibility of this regression points to the narcissistic origin of her homosexual object-choice and thus to the paranoic disposition in her.[4] One might sketch a train of thought which would bring about the same result as this identification: 'If my mother does it, I may do it too; I've just as good a right as she has.'

One can go a step further in disproving the accidental nature of the noise. We do not, however, ask our readers to follow us, since the absence of any deeper analytic investigation makes it impossible in this case to go beyond a certain degree of probability. The patient mentioned in her first interview with me that she had immediately demanded an explanation of the noise, and had been told that it was probably the ticking of the small clock on the writing-desk. I venture, however, to explain what she told me as a mistaken memory. It seems to me much more likely that at first she did not react to the noise at all, and that it became significant only after she met the two men on the staircase. Her lover, who had probably not even heard the noise, may have tried, perhaps on some later occasion when she assailed him with her suspicions, to account for it in this way: 'I don't know what noise you can have heard. Perhaps it was the small clock; it sometimes ticks like that.' This deferred use of impressions and this displacement of recollections often occur precisely in paranoia and are characteristic of it. But as I never met the man and could not continue the analysis of the woman, my hypothesis cannot be proved.

I might go still further in the analysis of this ostensibly real 'accident'. I do not believe that the clock ever ticked or that there was any noise to be heard at all. The woman's situation justified a sensation of a knock or beat in her clitoris. And it was this that she subsequently projected as a perception of an external object. Just the same sort of thing can occur in dreams. A hysterical woman patient of mine once related to me a short arousal dream to which she could bring no spontaneous associations. She dreamt simply that someone knocked and then she awoke. Nobody had knocked at the door, but during the previous nights she had been awakened by distressing sensations of pollutions: she thus had a motive for awakening as soon as she felt the first sign of genital excitation.

---

[4] Cf. the similar regression from object-love to identification described in 'Mourning and Melancholia' (1917*e*).

There had been a 'knock' in her clitoris.[5] In the case of our paranoic patient, I should substitute for the accidental noise a similar process of projection. I certainly cannot guarantee that in the course of our short acquaintance the patient, who was reluctantly yielding to compulsion, gave me a truthful account of all that had taken place during the two meetings of the lovers. But an isolated contraction of the clitoris would be in keeping with her statement that no contact of the genitals had taken place. In her subsequent rejection of the man, lack of satisfaction undoubtedly played a part as well as 'conscience'.

Let us consider again the outstanding fact that the patient protected herself against her love for a man by means of a paranoic delusion. The key to the understanding of this is to be found in the history of the development of the delusion. As we might have expected, the latter was at first aimed against the woman. But now, *on this paranoic basis, the advance from a female to a male object was accomplished.* Such an advance is unusual in paranoia; as a rule we find that the victim of persecution remains fixated to the same persons, and therefore to the same sex to which his love-objects belonged before the paranoic transformation took place. But neurotic disorder does not preclude an advance of this kind, and our observation may be typical of many others. There are many similar processes occurring outside paranoia which have not yet been looked at from this point of view, amongst them some which are very familiar. For instance, the so-called neurasthenic's unconscious attachment to incestuous love-objects prevents him from choosing a strange woman as his object and restricts his sexual activity to phantasy. But within the limits of phantasy he achieves the progress which is denied him, and he succeeds in replacing mother and sister by extraneous objects. Since the veto of the censorship does not come into action with these objects, he can become conscious in his phantasies of his choice of these substitute-figures.

These then are phenomena of an attempted advance from the new ground which has as a rule been regressively acquired; and we may set alongside them the efforts made in some neuroses to regain a position of the libido which was once held and subsequently lost. Indeed we can hardly draw any conceptual distinction between these two classes of phenomena. We are too apt to think that the conflict underlying a neurosis is brought to an end when the symptom has been formed. In reality the struggle can go on in many ways after this. Fresh instinctual components arise on both sides, and these prolong it. The symptom itself becomes an

---

[5]Cf. a similar instance in Lecture XVII of Freud's *Introductory Lectures* (1916-17).

object of this struggle; certain trends anxious to preserve it conflict with others which strive to remove it and to re-establish the *status quo ante*. Methods are often sought of rendering the symptom nugatory by trying to regain along other lines of approach what has been lost and is now withheld by the symptom. These facts throw much light on a statement made by C. G. Jung to the effect that a peculiar 'psychical inertia', which opposes change and progress, is the fundamental precondition of neurosis. This inertia is indeed most peculiar; it is not a general one, but is highly specialized; it is not even all-powerful within its own field, but fights against tendencies towards progress and recovery which remain active even after the formation of neurotic symptoms. If we search for the starting-point of this special inertia, we discover that it is the manifestation of very early linkages—linkages which it is hard to resolve—between instincts and impressions and the objects involved in those impressions. These linkages have the effect of bringing the development of the instincts concerned to a standstill. Or in other words, this specialized 'psychical inertia' is only a different term, though hardly a better one, for what in psycho-analysis we are accustomed to call a 'fixation'.[6]

---

[6]This tendency to fixation, or, as he called it elsewhere, 'adhesiveness of the libido', had been alluded to by Freud in the first edition of his *Three Essays* (1905*d*), *Standard Ed.*, **7**, 242-3. It was further discussed by him towards the end of his case history of the 'Wolf Man' (1918*b*), *Standard ed.*, **17**, 115-16, and in Lecture XXII of his *Introductory Lectures* (1916-17), both of which works were more or less contemporary with the present paper. He returned to it much later, in Section VI of his 'Analysis Terminable and Interminable' (1937*c*), where he himself made use of the term 'psychical inertia', and where he related the phenomenon to the 'resistance of the id' which is met with in psycho-analytic treatment, and which, in *Inhibitions, Symptoms and Anxiety* (1926*d*), Chapter XI, Section A(*a*), he had attributed to the power of the compulsion to repeat. A last allusion to 'psychical inertia' occurs near the end of Chapter VI of his posthumously published *Outline of Psycho-Analysis* (1940*a* [1938]).

5. Neuroses

Anxiety is the chief characteristic of the neuroses. It may be felt and expressed directly, or it may be controlled unconsciously and automatically by conversion, displacement, and various other psychological mechanisms. Generally, these mechanisms produce symptoms experienced as subjective distress from which the patient desires relief. The neuroses, as contrasted to the psychoses, manifest neither gross distortion or misinterpretation of external reality, nor gross personality disorganization.

Categories include the following: anxiety neurosis, characterized by anxious over-concern extending to panic and frequently associated with somatic symptoms; hysterical neurosis, characterized by an involuntary psychogenic loss or disorder of function with symptoms which characteristically begin and end suddenly in emotionally charged situations and which are symbolic of the underlying conflicts; phobic neurosis, characterized by intense fear of an object or situation which the patient consciously recognizes as no real danger to him, and manifested as faintness, fatigue, palpitations, perspiration, nausea, or tremor; obsessive compulsive neurosis, characterized by the persistent intrusion of unwanted thoughts, urges, or actions that the patient is unable to stop (such as repeated handwashing); depressive neurosis, manifested by an excessive reaction of depression due to an internal conflict or to an identifiable event such as the loss of a love object or cherished possession; neurasthenic neurosis, characterized by complaints of chronic weakness, easy fatigability, or exhaustion; depersonalization neurosis, dominated by a feeling of unreality and estrangement from the self, body, or surroundings; hypochondriacal neurosis, dominated by preoccupation with the body and with fear of presumed diseases of various organs; and other specific psychoneurotic disorders such as "writer's cramp" and certain occupational neuroses.

9. The Application of Learning Theory "As a Last Resort" in the Treatment of a Case of Anxiety Neurosis*

Joseph R. Cautela

Learning theory was employed in the treatment of an anxiety neurosis. The patient, a 33-year-old man who had developed anxiety reactions to a number of social situations, obtained relief from anxiety symptoms after two years of dynamically-oriented treatment in which he was said to have worked through some of his problems. He still retained, however, a fear of going to his work. Basing his decision on earlier studies of the treatment of behavior deviations, Cautela employed learning theory in the treatment of resistant anxiety. The therapist had a two-part plan for treatment: part 1 consisted of interfering with the unpleasant response to the work situation, and reinforcing a competing, more pleasant response to the work situation; part 2 employed a desensitizing technique to relieve the anxiety-producing work situation (i.e., instructing the patient to eat a candy bar whenever he felt fearful).

This case study is especially interesting because of the employment of the unusual combination of behavior therapy and insight therapy. Most behavior modification therapists neglect insight in the therapeutic procedure and concentrate on the behavior deviations through conditioning, extinguishing, and desensitization instead.

---

*Reprinted by permission of the author and publisher from the *Journal of Clinical Psychology*, 1965, **21**, 448-452.

INTRODUCTION

In recent years investigators such as Eysenck (3, 4, 5), Wolpe (12), Rachman (11), and Yates (13), have given conclusive evidence that the application of learning theory principles have been very effective in the treatment of abnormal behavior. Though the evidence is there for all to see, many psychologists engaged in some kind of therapeutic endeavor have not attempted to apply learning theory principles in the treatment of their patients. This writer has been a prime example of a sort of intellectual schizophrenia. The author has taught learning theory for a number of years and has been quite familiar with the recent literature on behavior therapy, but has never attempted to apply learning theory principles in the treatment of behavior problems. In retrospect, the main reason for this lack of transfer was that the learning theory approach seemed too simple for maladaptive behavior that appeared to develop in a very complex manner. Experience indicated that this undesirable behavior was due to faulty multiple causal relationships that existed for a relatively long time. It seemed logical that if the causal nature of the illness was complex and existed for some time, then the elimination of the illness has to be long and arduous. Actual work with behavior problems showed that this indeed seemed to be the case. This attitude on the part of the writer persisted until the remaining portion of a patient's maladaptive behavior seemed quite resistive to treatment. Then, learning theory was applied as "a last resort" and was successful. The details of the case are presented below.

CASE HISTORY

A 33-year-old male was referred by an industrial nurse. The patient had recently changed jobs within his plant, and soon after developed such a high degree of anxiety that he felt that he could no longer function in his work. An examination of the patient's history revealed that he suffered from chronic anxiety for the last five years. He became "dizzy and faint" in crowds, and in a store even if it was almost empty. If he had to stop at a traffic light and had to wait, he became extremely fearful and wanted to run out of the car. It seemed that any situation in which he had to relate to unfamiliar people made him tremble and he would feel like fainting. The patient revealed that he felt like a failure and was never able to complete anything he started out to accomplish. He resented his wife because she did not understand him and told him his fears were "all in his head." She thought his fears were a sign of weakness. The patient resented his wife's ability to relate well with other people. He changed jobs from a janitor to an inspector on an assembly line (he had seniority which allowed him to make the choice) to please his wife by making more money and having a more prestige position. Soon after he made the change to the new job his anxiety behavior became exacerbated and he reported his complaints to the plant nurse.

It became immediately evident that his parents, especially his mother, were a major factor in his illness. His mother was a neurotic woman who constantly screamed at the children, always criticized them severely for any failure, and never praised them. No matter what the patient did the mother never perceived it as good enough or successful. Regardless of the outcome of his problem-solving attempts they were almost always perceived as failures by the mother and now by the patient himself.

After the first interview with the patient, he arranged to have his old job back. He was treated for two years by arriving at the dynamics of his problems and working them through. At the end of this two-year period he was no longer fearful in crowds and no longer experienced panic while parked and waiting for the light to change. He enjoyed shopping and felt quite at ease in social relations. His relationship with his wife became very satisfactory. All his friends were amazed at the change in his behavior.

The one remaining problem area was his work. Though he was less anxious on his job than ever before and was able to appear well adjusted while working, he still complained about fear of going to work. He was still afraid that the foreman would criticize him or ask him to do something outside of his janitorial duties. The patient was still fearful that his fellow workers would discover that he was anxious and therefore take advantage of him. Leaving his job was no solution, for we both agreed he would be even more fearful in a new position. At least as janitor, when the anxiety became too great, he could go somewhere and be by himself. Even though all his non-work behavior was very satisfactory, it was reasoned that there must be some dynamic factor or factors that had been overlooked. These had to be discovered and worked through. Six months of trying to discover the proper dynamic factors that would eliminate this remaining maladaptive behavior proved fruitless. It was then decided "as a last resort" to try a learning theory approach.

TREATMENT

The first problem to consider was apparent lack of adequate generalization of extinction of the S(people)-R(anxiety) relationship from all other areas of the patient's life to the work situation. That there was some generalization there was no doubt. The patient did have less anxiety in the work situation than ever before, but apparently the generalization was not enough to overcome the reaction threshold.

From the beginning of the treatment the one apparent adaptive aspect of his behavior was his ability to enter into situations even though they were anxiety provoking. He continued his driving through the whole course of treatment. He used to go to dances with his wife. He never quit work (though he changed jobs within the plant). The repeated exposures to the anxiety-producing situations led to many reinforced trials and therefore to a strong development of habit strength. Though repeated exposures to one situation would generalize to other situations, each situation had its own habit strength. It can only be concluded that the thousands of reinforced trials over a five-year period in work led to the highest development of habit strength. The great habit strength resulted in very high reaction potential which was not sufficiently inhibited by extinction generalized from the other situations.

The problem then was to directly reduce the reaction potential (readiness to respond with anxiety)to work (S) situation. According to Guthrie (6), one way to weaken or eliminate a particular S-R relation is to present the S and prevent the R from occurring so that another R may be connected to the original S. In the Hullian model (7), the reaction potential to a stimulus may be forced below the reaction threshold by either building up total inhibitory potential or by reinforcing a competing response tendency to a greater degree than the original. A combination of the interference method of Guthrie and the reinforcement method of Hull has been adapted by Wolpe (12) in his reciprocal inhibition therapy. The first part of the treatment in this case encompassed both the interference and reinforcement model.

The patient was taught relaxation and autosuggestion. In the first session, while in a state of deep relaxation and autosuggestion in the therapist's office, the patient was asked to picture various scenes while at work in the plant. He was asked to suggest to himself that it was a pleasant feeling to be at the plant. He was instructed to smile when he felt pleasant while imagining his presence in the plant. When he smiled he was asked to visualize the foreman greeting him in a friendly way and joking with him. He was asked to smile when he felt at ease with this visualization. The same procedure was repeated for his relations with his fellow employees. In the second session, a week later, the above procedures were repeated for the first half hour. In the second half of the session it was suggested that even though his foreman and fellow employees were friendly toward him they sometimes would tease him and criticize him. He was asked to imagine that he would take the teasing good-naturedly and respond to the criticisms without fear. The procedure of the second session was followed in the next four sessions during the following four weeks. After the first session he was asked to repeat the procedures once a day at home.

The second part of the treatment consisted in asking the patient, after the first session, to eat a candy bar whenever he felt fearful at work. He had previously indicated he liked candy bars, and his janitorial work was flexible enough so that he could eat a candy bar almost any time. A vending machine was available on each floor for the purchase of the candy. It was reasoned that anxiety acted both in a response and drive producing capacity; thus starting a spiral of total drive (D) increasing reaction potentiality which caused a further increase in drive followed by an even further increase in reaction potential. Eating food would act to reduce the total drive state and to introduce a pleasant competing response to the fear stimulus. This is similar to the classic case described by Jones (8) and similar to the method of Lazarus (9). The hope was that this would stop the spiral effect and establish competing responses to allow autosuggestion techniques to exert their influence.

There was a problem involved in the candy bar procedure. Habit strength could generalize outside the work situation and cause obesity. To prevent the development of a strong anxiety-food habit, two procedures were adopted. The patient was told that the use of candy bars was specific to this situation while the autosuggestion procedure was being employed. He was also told that the candy bars would help him relax in this situation so that the autosuggestion could take over. The writer did not expect this technique to be very effective since the kind of conditioning involved in the anxiety-food situation was not on a verbal level. As a further check on the possible development of a habit that might lead to obesity, the patient was asked by some pretext not related to the treatment procedure to report his weight every week.

Results and Discussion

At the end of the first week the patient reported little or no change in his apprehension at work. By the middle of the second week, he began to notice that he wasn't as tense going to work as he had been previously. He also stated that he felt a little better at work. At the end of the third week, he reported a noticeable change in feelings at work. He seemed much less fearful than ever before. He didn't tremble so much when he talked to his foreman or fellow workers. By the end of the sixth week he reported that although he was not enthusiastic about his work, he had experienced whole days without an anxiety response. Once when he was criticized by his boss, his initial response was anxiety, but he recovered immediately and discussed the problem calmly with his foreman. At the end of the six-week period he was asked to continue the procedure on his own. At the end of the second week on his own, he reported that his job was no longer a problem as far as fear was concerned; but he would like to change jobs and felt confident that his fear responses would not generalize to another job. He left his job and began his new job with confidence. Six months after he started his new position he reported little or no anxiety in his working relationships. He reported that the work problem was all behind him now. He did not appear to have developed any other symptoms.

After the first session, the patient was asked to keep careful count of the number of candy bars he ate each day and to note it on a pad supplied to him. On the first day after the instructions concerning the candy bars the patient ate four bars. On the second day he consumed eight bars. The rise on the second day was probably due to the reinforcing effect of the candy during the first day. The rest of the week's intake varied from five to seven bars a day. There was a noticeable decrease the last week. One day he had two bars, the other days either one or no bars. It is difficult to ascertain whether the decrease in candy bar consumption was due to the decrease in anxiety-provoking stimuli or due to a satiation effect. No weight change was reported during the six-week period.

The lack of adequate control procedures in a case such as described in this paper calls for caution in interpreting the results. It is possible that the patient was in a state of latent learning before the learning theory principles were applied and the desired behavior might have emerged because of the previous therapeutic attempt using more conventional techniques. Also of course there is the possibility of spontaneous remission. The only reasons that allow for the interpretation of success due to the application of learning theory principles concern the reported successes by others (1, 2, 9, 10, 12) with the techniques used here with similar cases. Also, the coincidental gradual diminution of maladaptive behavior when the learning theory (behavior therapy) was used appears to be more than just a chance relationship.

REFERENCES

1. Ashem, B.: The treatment of a disaster phobia by systematic desensitization. *Behav. Res. Ther.,* 1963, **1**, 81-84.

2. Clark, D. F.: The treatment of monosymptomatic phobia by systematic desensitization. *Behav. Res. Ther.,* 1963, **1**, 63-68.

3. Eysenck, H. J.: Personality and behavior therapy. *Proc. Royal Soc. Med.,* 1960, **53**, 504-508.

4. Eysenck, H. J.: *Behavior Therapy and the Neuroses.* Oxford: Pergamon Press, 1960.

5. Eysenck, H. J.: *Handbook of Abnormal Psychology.* London: Pitmans, 1960.

6. Guthrie, E. R.: *The Psychology of Learning.* New York: Harper, pp. 70-73, 1935.

7. Hull, C. L.: *A Behaviour Theory Concerning the Individual Organism.* New Haven: Yale University Press, 1952.

8. Jones, M. C.: A laboratory study of fear: The case of Peter. *Pedagog. Sem.,* 1924, **31**, 308-315.

9. Lazarus, A.: The elimination of children's phobias by deconditioning. In Eysenck, H. J., (Ed.) *Behavior Therapy and the Neuroses.* Oxford: Pergamon Press, 1960, pp. 181-187.

10. Meyer, V.: The treatment of two phobic patients on the basis of learning theory. *J. abn. soc. Psychol.,* 1957, **55**, 261-265.

11. Rachman, S.: Treatment of anxiety and phobic reaction by desensitization. *J. abn. soc. Psychol.,* 1959, **102**, 421-427.

12. Wolpe, J.: *Psychotherapy by Reciprocal Inhibition.* Stanford: Stanford University Press, 1958.

13. Yates, A. J.: The application of learning theory to the treatment of tics. *J. abn. soc. Psychol.,* **56**, 175-182.

10. An Additional Study in Hysteria: The Case of Alice M.*

C. Scott Moss, Mary Margaret Thompson, and John Nolte

The case of Alice M. illustrates some of the psychoanalytic principles of hysteria and also provides an example of the use of hypnosis as an adjunct to treatment. Hypnoanalysis was used to explore a budding second personality and to uncover the history of certain of the symptom formations. The patient, a 31-year-old divorced woman, was voluntarily hospitalized for treatment following a six-month period during which she had strong feelings of depersonalization and convulsive seizures. The primary diagnosis was psychoneurotic reaction, conversion type (now classified as hysterical neurosis, conversion type).

The difficulties of differential diagnosis can be seen in this case. The development of a secondary personality (Alice developed a personality whom she called Joan Whitmier) is symptomatic of hysterical neurosis, dissociative type, while strong feelings of unreality are indicative of a more recent diagnostic classification, depersonalization neurosis. Also, Alice's infantile histrionic attention-seeking behavior which, in the past, was loosely called hysteria has, since the original publication of this case study, been classified as hysterical personality disorder. Unfortunately, the term "hysteria" has no specific diagnostic meaning and is often, as in the present case, used to describe symptomatology from any of the aforementioned disorders. The authors, using psychoanalytic theory, concluded that Alice had developed a generalized reliance on repressive defense mechanisms and that the convulsions were a motoric symbolization of

---

*Reprinted by permission of the authors and publisher from the *International Journal of Clinical and Experimental Hypnosis*, 1962, **10**, 59-74.

unconscious thought processes. They decided, at variance with Freud, that the treatment prognosis for "hysterics" like Alice is relatively poor because of the difficulty of changing the immature character structure.

It has been over 65 years since Breuer and Freud published their classic *Studies in Hysteria* (1895); a detailed account of Freud's first imaginative but fumbling psychotherapeutic efforts. Those authors discovered to their surprise that hysterical symptoms would disappear if they could effect a detailed recall of certain traumatic memories with sufficient vividness to cause the patient to react emotionally. They concluded that "the hysteric suffers mostly from reminiscences." The technique of choice was hypnosis, though Freud soon developed reservations regarding this approach, substituting first direct waking suggestion and then free association as techniques for facilitating recall of early memories.

It is not by chance, of course, that Freud's starting point in his study of psychopathology was the exploration of hysteria through the employment of hypnosis. The hysteric is generally naive and highly suggestible and as such has long been regarded as a "natural" somnambule, though recent studies suggest that he may not be the best possible subject (Eysenck, 1957; Gill & Brenman, 1959).[1] Hypnosis enables the hysteric to exhibit the power of unconscious motivation in the establishment of symptom formation with startling clarity.

Originally Freud used the discoveries derived from the study of hysteria as the paradigm for all mental illness; however, his expanding acquaintance with other disorders forced him to recognize that he had oversimplified the psychic structure involved. Nevertheless, there is no more convincing demonstration of the psychological genetics and dynamics of neurotic symptomatology. It is unfortunate from the viewpoint of students of psychopathology that hysteria occurs with decreased frequency and in diminished form, possibly as the consequence of a greater, widespread psychological sophistication today.[2, 3]

---

[1]Hypnosis is the use of suggestion to increase the suggestibility of people who are basically suggestible, hence its applicability with the hysteric.

[2]While the current incidence of hysteria is still debated, there is no question but that it is diagnosed less frequently. Chodoff and Lyons (1958) emphasize that through a process of *semantic encrustation* "hysteria" has acquired a variety of meanings. The term is currently used in at least five senses: (1) a pattern of behavior habitually exhibited by individuals said to be hysterical personalities or characters; (2) a particular kind of psychosomatic symptomatology called conversion reaction; (3) a psychoneurotic disorder characterized by phobias; (4) a particular psychopathological pattern; (5) a term of approbrium. The authors are primarily concerned

CASE STUDY OF ALICE

The patient, aged 31, Catholic, a divorcee and mother of three daughters (ages 11–17), was a voluntary hospital admission, diagnosed Psychoneurotic Reaction, Conversion Type. Her main complaints were of periodic feelings of unreality and "seizures," both of about six months' duration. These convulsive episodes were typically brief; she was said to scream and thrash about the floor and to claim amnesia for them. She had one previous hospitalization, five months earlier, staying only two weeks when her symptoms disappeared.

Individual psychotherapy was recommended and she was referred to a female staff psychologist. After 10 sessions the therapist asked for a consultation with the senior author. She related that Alice remained anxious, restless and complaining, and had recently manifested a major seizure during staff ward rounds. She also relayed the patient's request that hypnosis be employed in order to expedite treatment. The highlights of these first 10 sessions were summarized as follows:

1) Alice frequently complained of feelings of unreality, as expressed in the verbalization, "Nothing seems real around me. Even I don't feel real. It's like I'm running away from something and don't know what it is."

2) She often made reference of an autonomy-dependency conflict. While strongly resentful of treatment as an irresponsible child by people, she expressed frank fear of adult responsibilities. A seeming consequence was recurrent depressive episodes, in which she characterized herself as feeling "Like a small child, like a nothing."

3) Alice identified sex as a major problem. She stated, "I was a wife to my husband in every way except sexually—I couldn't stand to have him touch me." She recalled that while her mother reputedly despised men and rejected sex, she had frequent extramarital affairs. Alice re-

---

with the first two meanings. They present evidence that no single pattern of personality traits is to be found in individuals presenting conversion phenomena. On the other hand, a survey of psychiatric authorities resulted in identifying the following characteristics of the "hysterical personality." "The hysterical personality is a term applicable to persons who are vain and egocentric, who display labile and excitable but shallow affectivity, whose dramatic, attention seeking and histrionic behavior may go to the extremes of lying and even pseudologia phantastica, who are very conscious of sex, sexually provocative yet frigid, and who are dependently demanding in interpersonal situations." (p. 736).

[3]Ziegler et al. (1961) found in their study of 134 patients with conversion symptoms that the majority came from backward rural areas and simulated organic disease processes in a relatively crude manner commensurate with their lack of medical sophistication. However, a few better educated patients expertly simulated complicated disease entities. "We conclude that conversion reactions are molded by unconscious simulation of disease entities, and that symptom patterns change with changing medical knowledge of the patient and of his cultural milieu." (p. 903).

ported having always felt closer to her father and even having "double-dated" with him as a young teenager, though she also recounted a vague impression that as a little girl "he did something that frightened me." There was recall that at age six she had to repulse sexual advances by an older brother.

4) The patient also acknowledged that her relationship with her oldest daughter, Connie, constituted a considerable problem. She described Connie as resentful and rebellious. "I was always trying to win her love and never could. No matter what I'd do, it was never enough, she never showed any appreciation. I always tried so hard to give my girls what I never had."

While the preliminary sessions had been productive, it seemed likely that hypnosis could facilitate treatment. Alice proved to be a rather petite and attractive blond, quite feminine in a rather girlish manner. The initial impression was of an immature, unstable and passive-dependent personality. She was a moderately capable hypnotic subject. It was agreed to see her once a week and to employ hypnosis as a catalyst in the rapid uncovery of repressed content, while her primary therapist would continue a conventional therapy relationship on a three-times-per-week basis. The patient seemed quite accepting of this restructuring.

Intensive, long term psychotherapy designed to effect a personality reconstruction and directed at the goal of independent self-management seemed completely unrealistic and a more modest one was agreed upon by the two therapists. For a year Alice had been caught in a dilemma constituted of two men, her ex-husband, Frank, and a lover. Frank had been a competent provider but she had hated sexual relations with him; the second man made her feel "loved" and she enjoyed physical contact with him, but he was irresponsible and had been unable to make her feel materially secure. Material considerations were of especial importance because Alice wanted the three daughters with her. It was decided to focus on the psychological barriers which might prevent Alice from re-establishing a comfortable dependency in a marriage relationship.

An obvious item meriting scrutiny was Alice's Catholicism; however, this did not seem to occasion her much concern. She did state that her conversion to Catholicism five years earlier was attributable to a life-long fear of death, and volunteered a recurrent, extremely realistic and terrifying childhood dream, which was in some inexplicable fashion related to this fear. It was decided to use this dream as the initial entree into an exploration of the patient's problems.

> *Dream:* She walked into her bedroom and there in the dark stood a small furry white dog. Though it tried to be friendly and snuggle up to her, she was very frightened. She edged out of the bedroom

and when the dog tried to follow, she managed to close the door.
(The dream would invariably awaken her and she would sleep the
remainder of the night on the livingroom sofa.)

Hypnoanalysis of the dream yielded a seemingly clear example of the
disguise function of dream symbolism in a young child. The effort was
first made to help Alice decipher the symbol using a familiar movie
screen translation technique (Moss, 1960a, 1961); however, the mere
perception of the "puppy," even after 23 years, still occasioned her great
terror. A secondary method designed to increase emotional distance
and to also allow a more public representation of the symbol was instituted. In hypnosis Alice was handed a pencil and paper and told that
when she opened her eyes, she would "see" the dog-in-her-dream clearly
etched on the paper and that she was to carefully trace over this outline.
After successfully complying with these instructions, she was then told
that when she opened her eyes again she would see an outline of an image
representing the central meaning of the little dog, and she was to again
"trace these lines exactly as they appear there on the paper" (Figure 1).

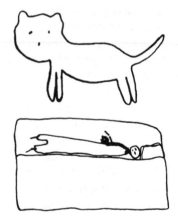

FIGURE 1.   Projected Desymbolization of a Dream Symbol

Upon completion, Alice suddenly recognized the full significance of
the drawings and abreacted strongly. She identified the second drawing
as her grandfather in his coffin, and the little white dog as a symbol of
death. She recalled that as a very small girl she and the grandfather had
close, affectionate ties, but that he died when she was six. However, she
did not fully comprehend the meaning of his death, and her parents had
told her he was "sleeping." When she was eight she observed the dead
body of a neighbor woman's baby, and suddenly, for the first time, she

experienced the full emotional impact of the loss of the beloved grand-father. That night she had the disturbing nightmare. To date she had been obsessed by the need to touch dead bodies, as if striving for some explanation of death in this manner (Moss, 1960b).

Asked the significance of the dog, she replied "Death is cold, black, ugly. It was a pretty, little white dog, but I was afraid of it. It wasn't large, black or cold; it was warm, cuddly and white. I think I must have rejected the idea of death and put something else in its place; something pretty and nice, something that wasn't horrible."[4]

An investigation of Alice's "feelings of unreality" led to the next major therapeutic development. These feelings antedated hospitalization by several months and were vaguely related to her seizures, which began about the same time. She began the session with a reference to the recent seizure experienced during ward rounds. "I got terribly upset," she recalled, "though I don't know why. I had told Dr. A. that I was ready to go home to my sister's and go to work, and he told me he had written to get her. I got awfully afraid and just went to pieces. And afterwards, for one whole day, I thought I was a Joan Whitmier. The thought scared me, 'cause I thought, supposing I wouldn't know my mother when she came, or the members of my family? It scared me so I pushed it out of my mind. I kept telling myself, 'No, I'm Alice M.' I was afraid if I didn't convince myself that I would become this Joan Whitmier and maybe stay her." Thus Alice revealed for the first time the presence of an embryonic second personality.

Through hypnosis direct contact with Joan was readily established, allowing a detailed characterization and comparison with the conscious, dominant personality. Joan described herself as the same age as Alice, but single, without children, and interested only in drinking, dancing, dating, nice clothes, and so forth. She was also fully conversant with Alice and her current difficulties. A most evident contrast was that Joan wanted absolutely no responsibilities. She explained that she came into existence as a consequence of Alice's extreme ambivalence about leaving the hospital and pursuing an independent existence. "Alice likes to be

---

[4]In attempting to depict death by its opposite, it is noteworthy that while her mind could alter the physiognomic qualities of the symbol, the emotional reaction remained appropriate to the covert meaning, again demonstrating the value of the associated affect as a clue to an understanding of the essential meaning of dream symbols. Several weeks later, the patient spontaneously recalled an event in which the dog-in-question actually had wandered into her bedroom, and the mother had interpreted this as a "sign" that a brother missing in service was alive. This experience assumedly accounted for the choice of the symbol and further clarified its meaning. Readers are referred to a recent investigation and discussion of the nature of dream symbolism (Moss, 1961).

a strong and good person and shoulder the responsibility of her children, and be a good mother to them, and take good care of them. She wants to set a good example in front of them, that they can live by, and grow up to be good girls. Yet, every now and then when she tries to do these things, I come along and keep her from it."

In an effort to achieve additional insight into the nature and existence of Joan, the technique of automatic writing was introduced with partial success. Joan first printed her name, drew her self-portrait, and then when asked for further clarification, repetitively reproduced two symbolic designs (Figure 2). Analysis through a series of suggested draw-

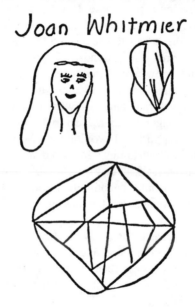

FIGURE 2. Automatic Drawings of a Secondary Personality

ings of increasing transparency of meaning led to the impression that the first design represented a preoccupation with sex (the outline depicted the head of a man Alice had intended to marry as a young girl but who had rejected her, and the internal lines represented sexual congress), while the second drawing symbolized Alice's feelings of confinement and frustration in an unmanageable marriage relationship. Later in the waking state, Alice immediately identified Joan's self-portrait (from the hair style) as herself when she was about 14. She recalled and was distressed by the conversation with Joan but seemed to accept an interpretation in terms of the conflict and dissociation of incompatible infantile and adult motives. Alice never again mentioned the existence of Joan, and the therapist felt it was strategic to avoid encouraging this dissociative tendency through further exploration.[5]

A third significant therapeutic advance was achieved three weeks later when the patient recalled her unhappy childhood and her intense jealousy of a younger sister whom she felt had deprived her of her mother's attention and love. She also affectionately recalled her grandfather as "The one I loved the most. He was just the loving kind. He always wanted me to sit on his lap and rock me. Mother never had time." When asked to examine her feelings towards her younger sister and to see if they had any application in the present, she immediately and for the first time confronted her hostile, jealous, competitive transference feelings toward her older daughter, Connie.

> *P:* She's been the sister that I hated, the sister I was jealous of, the sister that I didn't like. She even looked like her, talked like her, she was just like her in every way, that's why I didn't like her. . . . It seemed like everybody I ever loved has been taken away from me. . . . My grandfather, then my (older) sister left home—she ran off and got married, and then I didn't have her anymore, and then I was all alone again. So I ran off, just like she did, and got married, too. Then I had Frankie, and a home of my own, and someone to love me. Frankie loved me. Then I had Connie, and after that I had to share Frankie with her. And she took Frankie away, and I didn't have anyone.

---

[5]The question is almost invariably raised, are such multiple or dual personalities artifacts of psychotherapy? Certainly the essence of the psychological treatment is to differentially reinforce certain aspects of behavior while minimizing others, a process which could conceivably enhance the differences which reside within all personalities. Presumably hypnosis could encourage any dissociative tendencies, resulting in the gradual evocation of a fully developed secondary personality. Harriman (1943), for example, found that when he "erased" his subjects' primary personalities with hypnotic suggestion, that they spontaneously developed secondary personalities to fill the vacuum. On the other hand, it may be that dual personalities exist in much greater number than is generally supposed. Alexander (1929) wrote: "Therefore, when I describe the superego as a person, and neurotic conflict as a struggle between different persons, I mean it, and regard the descriptions as not just a figurative presentation . . . Furthermore, in the study of the neuroses there is no lack of such visible manifestations as a divided personality . . . In contrast to the emphasis laid on the varying roles of the analyst in the transference situation, little has been said about the varying role of the patient who may present to the analyst not one personality but many. The mechanism by which multiple personalities are established is as yet unknown. One may ask whether all acts of repression may not involve the creation of a larval form of a secondary personality" (p. 55).

T: So, when Connie told you, "Mother, I've never felt that you loved me," or when she said, "You were never really a mother to me, you were more of a sister," maybe she was closer to the truth than you were willing to admit?
P: I think she was. I didn't realize that I didn't love her, I thought I did.

The patient concluded the session with the recognition that a parallel existed between her relationship with Connie, and her relationship as a child with her own mother.

P: This is the same reason I didn't obey my mother, because I felt that she didn't want me, so I didn't care if I did what she wanted or not, and that's the way with Connie. Connie felt like I didn't love her and so she didn't care whether she did what I asked her or not. But with her daddy, it was a little different. She felt like her daddy loved her more than her mother, and she would do the things he asked her.

A critical insight into her relationships with her parents occurred several weeks later. She was again reminiscing about her childhood when she recalled her fear of an older man, a friend of her father's, "who always carried a little snake in his pocket." Age regression was employed and almost immediately she re-experienced in detail a very traumatic incident at age four when this man had taken her into a barn and used her as a stimulant for masturbation. The patient reacted to recall of this experience with a sizeable cathartic release. A synopsis of her verbalizations is quite revealing:

It seems strange now that I never remembered that. I guess it scared me so much that I didn't want to remember it. It was better *not* to remember it. . . . It looks like my mother should have taken better care of me when I was a little girl. Any mother that loves her daughter will protect her and take care of her, so that these things don't happen to her. I always protected my girls. If a mother doesn't care enough to protect you, then there just isn't anyone you can depend on. (She went on to express her resentment of her husband for the times he had forced sex relations on her.)

The day following the above session, Alice, in a state of considerable agitation, requested another meeting. She stated that she was vaguely aware of another, related episode but that it had proven elusive to recall. Hypnosis allowed her to immediately recapture in convincing detail an experience from age five. She vividly recalled being fondled and then ejaculated upon by her alcoholic father.

P: We were lying in bed, he reached over and pulled me up to him, and he put his hand on me, and I was so scared. And I cried, and I told my dad, "You're hurting me. Don't, don't do it!" Then he said, "Lay still and shut up!" I layed there and I didn't say anymore. And I cried, and I cried. And my mother came home, and I ran to the door. I hated my dad! And I was always afraid of him, for what he had done to me, because he made me lie there. And I was so afraid, because it had happened to me before, with this other man, and then my dad, and later my brother, all when I was four and five years old and I never wanted mother to leave me anymore with my dad.

T: It must have seemed that there wasn't any man you could trust.

P: There wasn't nobody except my grandfather. He was the only man I could trust.

Alice went on to again connect this episode with her hatred of her husband, her hostility towards her mother for not having protected her, and the attraction felt for her lover—like her grandfather, he had loved her for herself, not sex. The next few sessions brought increasing expression of homicidal feelings toward her husband and an exploration of the following event which had precipitated her hospitalization.

One night, when Alice and her husband were sleeping apart as usual, Connie came to her room crying and stated that she was afraid of her father. Instantly Alice *knew* that Frankie had molested the girl and went into the livingroom to accuse him. At this moment, without any awareness of its source, she had remarked, "I know just how she feels because my father tried that on me once." Her husband vehemently denied the accusation but she remained adamant, felt physically ill, and possessed of an intense hatred for him. "I told him I wanted to kill him. That a man who does that to his daughter isn't fit to live!" In the next couple of weeks the effort was made to work through this insight, and while recall of the childhood experience raised doubt in Alice's mind regarding the validity of her interpretation, she remained highly ambivalent.

The last major therapeutic progress was made in the exploration of the meaning of her seizure pattern, and came about as a result of a pending visit of her ex-husband which precipitated the first seizure since she began hypnotherapy. Hypnosis was used to regress her to the time of each of a half dozen seizures. The seizures were triggered off by direct suggestion and a detailed analysis was then made of the circumstances surrounding each event. The recurrent theme was a conflictual situation associated with overwhelming feelings of hopelessness and an appeal for help. The first seizure occurred two days after the situation in which Alice accused her husband of molesting their daughter. She had continued to press the issue and in a fit of rage he picked her up and threw her on the floor.

I remember thinking, "Oh, my God, I can't move, my back's broken!"
I couldn't move and I couldn't get up. *I couldn't get up!* And I
crawled across the floor, got to the phone and called the police.
And he just stood there and looked at me!

Additional questioning in a later session also elicited the fact that an
older sister had always been subject to "spells" and even as a young girl
Alice had the assignment of sitting on this sister's feet until the tremors
passed. Alice's seizures thus became her means of escaping from an im-
possibly desperate situation.

Unfortunately, this promising therapeutic beginning did not eventuate
in lasting improvement. Despite everything, the patient had never relinquished her wish for a reconciliation with her ex-husband; it was truly
a situation in which she couldn't live with or without him. She prevailed
upon the therapists to effect a meeting with him for the purpose of exploring this possibility. While expressing a desire to cooperate, Mr. M. gave
voice to his complete exasperation, and refused to even consider the
eventuality. Alice interpreted this action as one more in a long line of
rejections and reacted accordingly. She became dispirited and depressed,
lost her motivation for therapy, and her mood fluctuated widely and rapidly. She now openly expressed hatred of hospitalization and at the same
time was exceedingly fearful of the prospect of discharge. She associated
increasingly with another female patient, Maxine, whose behavior and
dynamics were somewhat similar, and with her discussed the possibility
of suicide. Alice also resumed the affair with her former lover. One
weekend she went home with Maxine and the two of them actually made
a half-hearted suicidal gesture.

The final episode occurred about one month later. Maxine signed
herself out of the hospital 'Against Medical Advice' and sought electroshock from a private psychiatrist. After a series of six EST she returned
to the hospital for a triumphal visit in a highly euphoric state, which
she represented to the other patients as miraculously reinstated, radiant
mental health. Alice thereupon demanded a similar treatment, and after
some hesitation it was decided to administer a course of hypnoshock
(Schafer, 1960; Guido & Jones, 1961). One actual full convulsive shock
was administered, and thereafter a series of seven simulated shocks were
instituted through hypnotic regression back to the original experience.
After the first three "shocks" Alice felt well enough to go on an extended
leave to her parent's home; the remainder were administered on an outpatient maintenance basis over a period of two months.

A comparison of the MMPI profiles of Maxine and Alice demonstrate that the effect of the two courses of treatment was similar. A six-

month followup revealed that both patients had maintained their improvement at least to the extent of remaining out of the hospital. Alice had married her lover, but unfortunately she contaminated a modern "miracle cure" when she and her new husband went to a private sanitarium and received several actual electro-shocks in an effort to resolve marital discord.

DISCUSSION

The dynamics of this case bear a remarkable similarity to those encountered by Freud early in his career as a psychotherapist, when he found that his hysterical patients gave frequent, detailed accounts of sexual seduction in childhood. Between 1900–1910, he concluded that these recitals were phantasied, though the reason for this re-evaluation was never clarified by him. It has been suggested that Freud could find no such incident in his self-analysis to account for his own neuroticism, and on this basis rejected the validity of these reports. The position could be assumed that it makes little difference clinically whether these sexual experiences actually transpired so long as they possess psychological reality for the patient. However, there are definite theoretical implications. Freud formulated a whole theory of personality development, predicated on the assumption that such recitals were a form of wish fulfillment and as such were evidence for the importance of infantile sexuality and the centrality of the oedipal conflict. It is unfortunate that such reports elude objective assessment.

Alice gives every evidence of developmental arrest at a very early age. As with the classical hysteric, she is characterizable as naive and suggestible, unreflective and impulsive, and in her relationships she is childishly clinging, affect-laden and unstable. There is a powerful capacity for dramatization, and aggressive impulses are repressed and displaced. A prominent feature of Alice's pathology is an intense and protracted autonomy-dependency conflict. She vascillates perpetually between a childlike dependency and a facade of responsible adulthood, wallowing in indecision and ambivalence, resulting in a perpetual indecision. While psychoanalytic theory assumes that the hysteric is fixated at the genital phase of infantile development with an incestuous attachment, there are many features of this case reminiscent of Marmor's contention that "fixations in the oedipal phase of development are themselves the outgrowth of pre-oedipal fixations, chiefly of an oral nature" (1953, p. 662). Alice's intense frustration of early dependency needs is reflected in her life's task of searching for another person who will assume responsibility for solving her problems. The dependency and passivity expressed in this solution contributes to the fact that the hysteric is typically female and the problem-solver a male. Her marriage at age 14 was an early manifestation of this form of problem solving.[6]

Alice seems attracted to men as a source of security rather than for sexual satisfaction, that is she searches for the "good father," a tender, impotent male who, like grandfather, will comfort, caress and provide for her without the burden of sexuality. Hers is a pseudosexuality in the sense that sex is viewed as a necessary evil, the price exacted from the female for need satisfaction from the male. In highly narcissistic fashion, Alice searches constantly for unqualified love but with an underlying conviction of eventual abandonment which contributes to her inability to reciprocate ('being loved is more important than loving').

Aggressive sexual advances, particularly from her husband, seem to have been unconsciously equated with the molestations experienced in childhood. It is a reflection of the strength of her dependency needs that Alice was willing to suffer 18 years of stressful married life and that only the direct reactivation of the oedipal conflict by her husband's assumed sexual advances to the daughter finally forced separation (and still Alice clung to the possibility of reconciliation). It is also noteworthy that despite the marked resentment felt towards her husband, the thought of sharing him precipitated an intense sibling rivalry with her own daughter.

Alice appears to have learned a generalized reliance on the repressive defense mechanism early in life as a way of grossly narrowing and constricting a threatening world into a more manageable form. The white dog dream graphically represents her effort as a young girl to distort and repress (shut the door on) unpleasant reality. Now, years later, Alice continues in her attempt to reject threatening reality, but succeeds largely in disrupting her ability to "feel like a real person." Both of the patient's major symptoms, her seizures and the associated feelings of unreality, are comprehensible in terms of her excessive reliance upon this mechanism.

It seems a reasonable assumption that people strive towards coordinated, integrated and consistent behavior. Experience can be handled in three ways: it is consciously symbolized and made meaningful, it is ignored and unrelated to the self-system, or it is disowned and distorted.

---

[6]Chodoff and Lyons (ibid) explain the predisposition of women to hysteria as attributable to the fact that the traits characteristic of this personality formation are typically feminine and thus more acceptable in women than men. They point out that the concept of "hysteria" is a picture of women in the words of male psychiatrists, and that the description amounts to a *caricature of femininity*. "A situation analagous to the one described might be imagined if women psychiatrists spent some generations coolly and rather inimically observing the less attractive foibles of males, and then put them together as the manifestations of a kind of personality characteristic of men!" (p. 739).

Maladjustment ensues as a consequence of a basic incongruence between experience and the self-structure. In Alice's case, an independent existence entails responsibility and responsibility stimulates anxiety; however, to avoid responsibility as a wife and mother, particularly in view of the extreme condemnation of her own mother, causes severe guilt. Because her answer is to engage in efforts at wholesale repression, there is no role in which she can be a genuine person. Current efforts at dissociation are flamboyantly represented in the depersonalized personality fragment of Joan.

Alice's seizures represent a prostration in the face of danger which annihilates the threatening perceptual image by temporarily rejecting consciousness itself, a mechanism not too dissimilar to the device of slamming an imaginary door in a dream. As with most symptoms, her seizures doubtlessly have multiple determinants: they certainly represent an expression of complete impotence and an appeal for help in a motoric manner; they are an expression of aggression in the form of an accusation ("Feel guilty, look what you have done to me!"); and finally, they seem to be a pantomimic repetition of traumatic physical and sexual assaults, possibly in an attempt at mastery.[7]

It might be re-emphasized in closing that the favorable prognosis of the hysteric is largely illusionary. Freud acknowledged in the *Studies in Hysteria* that psychotherapy can sometimes effect dramatic changes in the symptom picture, but the underlying character structure remains largely resistant to radical alteration. Psychotherapy, of course, is a highly reflective exercise requiring that a patient assume increasing responsibility for his own thoughts and actions, but experientially speaking, the hysteric has forsaken the world of reflection for impulsive action. Personal responsibility is discounted so that things "just happen" as-it-were, seemingly at the instigation of others or impersonal events. Resistance to psychotherapy was therefore to be anticipated, and in this case, the patient's preference for hypnotherapy by a male therapist is recognizable as an obvious expression of her ever-present desire for a magical cure by the fear-provoking, omnipotent male. It may be further conjectured that Alice's willingness to relinquish her repressive controls

---

[7] A major reason for the fluidity of hysterical symptoms may well be that they stem from what Sullivan calls a *happy thought* rather than a high grade id-superego conflict; that is, instigation is based on a sudden inspiration as how to get something for nothing. In this instance, through the device of becoming suddenly, dramatically ill, Alice undertook to retain her respectability while avoiding both adult responsibilities and the threatened emergence of highly ego-alien content. In order to keep her husband (i.e., security) she must show how helpless she is, without directly acknowledging this regressive dependency need, and at the same time she also punishes him for not loving and protecting her.

initially were not entirely a healthy effort at integration, but an expression of her willingness to again "pay the price" in terms of the coin demanded in order to attain satisfaction of her gross dependency needs.

Finally, there is the intriguing question of why we see fewer hysterics today than in the past. Has today's "psychological sophistication" really filtered down, to the lower middle classes? Or is it the psychotherapist who has become the more sophisticated, so that he now perceives the character deficiencies and the pregenital fixations behind what used to be called hysteria? A rereading of *Studies in Hysteria* gives rise to the impression that modern day psychotherapists might well debate the diagnosis of some of the cases reported therein.

References

1. Alexander, F.: *The psychoanalysis of the total personality.* Monogr. No. 52. New York: Nerv. & Mental Disease Publ. Co., 1929.

2. Breuer, J., and Freud, S.: *Studies in hysteria.* (A. A. Brill, Trans.) Boston: Beacon Press, 1950.

3. Chodoff, P., and Lyons, H.: Hysteria, the hysterical personality and "hysterical" conversion. *Amer. J. Psychiat.,* 1958, **114**, 734-740.

4. Eysenck, H.: *The dynamics of anxiety and hysteria.* New York: Frederick A. Praeger, 1957.

5. Gill, M., and Brenman, M.: *Hypnosis and related states.* New York: Int. Univer. Press, 1959.

6. Guido, J. A., and Jones, J.: "Placebo" (simulation) electroconvulsive therapy. *Amer. J. Psychiat.,* 1961, **117**, 838-839.

7. Harriman, P. L.: New approach to multiple personalities. *Amer. J. Orthopsychiat.,* 1949, **13**, 638-643.

8. Marmor, J.: Orality in the hysterical personality. *J. Amer. Psychoanal. Assoc.,* 1953, **1**, 657-671.

9. Moss, C. S.: Dream symbols as disguises: a further investigation. *Etc: J. Gen. Sem.,* 1960, **18**, 217-226.

10. Moss, C. S.: Brief successful psychotherapy of a chronic phobic reacaction. *J. abnorm. soc. Psychol.,* 1960, **60**, 266-270.

11. Moss, C. S.: Experimental paradigms for the hypnotic investigation of dream symbolism. *J. clin. exp. Hypnosis,* 1961, **9**, 105-117.

12. Schafer, D.: As-if electroshock therapy in hypnosis. *Amer. J. clin. Hypnosis,* 1960, **2**, 225-227.

13. Sullivan, H. S.: *Clinical studies in psychiatry.* New York: W. W. Norton, 1956.

14. Ziegler, F. J., Imboden, J. B., and Meyer, E.: Contemporary conversion reactions: a clinical study. *Amer. J. Psychiat.,* 1960, **116**, 901-910.

11. Isolation of a Conditioning Procedure as the Crucial Psychotherapeutic Factor: A Case Study*

Joseph Wolpe

The patient described by Wolpe is a 39-year-old woman who had developed a phobic reaction to automobile traffic, following an accident in which she was injured. The treatment of Mrs. C. is based on learning theory. Wolpe argues that the principles of behaviorism are well suited to the psychotherapy of neurotic disorders and that successes with this method are more readily demonstrated than successes in the psychoanalytic or psychodynamic schools. Psychoanalysis, for instance, sees the phobia as an outward projection of a feared sexual or aggressive impulse, which, when displaced to an external object, relieves the individual of the attendant anxiety. This explanation requires an acceptance of the psychosexual model of development and demands an analysis of the patient's early developmental period, his transference feelings toward the therapist, and the acquisition of insights concerning previously unconscious aspects of behavior.

Wolpe categorically rejects these psychodynamic hypotheses and suggests instead that the human neurosis is learned and, consequently, subject to the laws of learning which have been demonstrated in the experimental laboratory. Learning, to Wolpe, is based on conditioning theory that has its historical antecedents in the discoveries of Pavlov. Wolpe's treatment is based on the method of reciprocal inhibition. A phobic stimulus which produces extreme anxiety and is handled by the

*Reprinted by permission of the author and publisher from Wolpe, J., "Isolation of a Conditioning Procedure as the Crucial Psychotherapeutic Factor: A Case Study," *The Journal of Nervous and Mental Disease*, **134**:316-329. © 1962, The Williams and Wilkins Company, Baltimore, Maryland.

patient's avoidance of the stimulus is presented contiguously with a response incompatible with the anxiety, i.e., relaxation. Mrs. C., having been trained in deep muscular relaxation, was hypnotized and presented with a series of imaginary incidents related to the automobile accident. These scenes were presented with the least anxiety-producing stimulus first and with the desensitization proceeding gradually from the least through the most anxiety-eliciting of 36 levels of stimuli. Wolpe reported therapeutic success from this systematic desensitization method. Further, by isolating the conditioning procedure, he felt that steps had been taken to counter criticisms that the improvement might be due to incidentally gained insight, transference relationships, or suggestions, all features of the psychodynamic approach.

In a considerable number of publications (*e.g.,* 1–5, 7, 9, 11–13) it has been shown that methods based on principles of learning achieve striking in an elevator. Since these habits of emotional response have been acusually characterized by persistent habits of anxiety response to stimulus situations in which there is no objective danger—for example, the mere presence of superiors, being watched working, seeing people quarrel, riding in an elevator. Since these habits of emotional response have been acquired by learning (10, 11) it is only to be expected that they would be overcome by appropriate procedures designed to bring about unlearning. Most of the procedures that have been used have depended upon inhibition of anxiety through the evocation of other responses physiologically incompatible with it (reciprocal inhibition); for each occasion of such inhibition diminishes to some extent the strength of the anxiety response habit (11).

When "dynamic" psychiatrists are confronted with the therapeutic successes of behavioristic therapy they discount them on the ground that the results are "really" due to the operation of "mechanisms" postulated by *their* theory: transference, insight, suggestion, or de-repression. Despite the fact that it is now manifest (14, 15) that the basic "mechanisms" of psychoanalysis have no scientifically acceptable factual foundations, their proponents can still content themselves with saying that the *possibility* of their operation has not been excluded. Resort to this kind of comfortable refuge would be undermined if study of the therapeutic course of individual cases were to show *both* that there is a direct correlation between the use of conditioning procedures and recovery and that "dynamic mechanisms" are *not* so correlated, either because they cannot be inferred from the facts of the case or because even when they might be inferred they have no temporal relation to the emergence of change.

The case described below was made the subject of variation of several of the factors that are alleged from various standpoints to have therapeutic potency. A patient with a single severe phobia for automobiles was selected for the experiment because the presence of a single dimension of disturbance simplifies the estimation of change. It was found that a deconditioning technique—systematic desensitization (9, 11, 13)—alone was correlated with improvement, which was quantitatively related to the number of reinforcements given. At the same time, activities that might give any grounds for imputations of transference, insight, suggestion and de-repression were omitted or manipulated in such a way as to render the operation of these "mechanisms" exceedingly implausible. Furthermore, the conduct of therapy in several series of interviews separated by long intervals had results incompatible with "spontaneous recovery"—a possibility that might have been entertained if improvement during the intervals had been as great as during the treatment periods; but in fact virtually no change occurred during the intervals.

This case incidentally illustrates how difficult it can be to find stimulus situations that evoke sufficiently low anxiety to enable *commencement* of desensitization, and how the details of procedure must be tailored to the needs of the case.

THE CASE OF MRS. C.

The patient, a 39-year-old woman, complained of fear reactions to traffic situations. Dr. Richard W. Garnett, Jr., a senior staff psychiatrist, had referred her to me after interviewing her a few times. I first saw the patient at the University Hospital on April 6, 1960. Briefly her story was that on February 3, 1958, while her husband was taking her to work by car, they entered an intersection on the green light. On the left she noticed two girls standing at the curb waiting for the light to change, and then, suddenly, became aware of a large truck that had disregarded the red signal, bearing down upon the car. She remembered the moment of impact, being flung out of the car, flying through the air, and then losing consciousness. Her next recollection was of waking in the ambulance, seeing her husband, and telling him that everything was all right. She felt quite calm and remained so during the rest of the journey to the hospital. There she was found to have injuries to her knee and neck, for the treatment of which she spent a week in the hospital.

On the way home, by car, she felt unaccountably frightened. She stayed at home for two weeks, quite happily, and then, resuming normal activities, noticed that, while in a car, though relatively comfortable on the open road, she was always disturbed by seeing any car approach *from either side,* but not at all by vehicles straight ahead. Along city streets she had continuous anxiety, which, at the sight of a laterally approaching car less than half a block away, would rise to panic. She could, however, avoid such a reaction by closing her eyes before reaching an intersection. She was also distressed in other situations that in any sense involved lateral approaches of cars. Reactions were extraordinarily severe in relation to making a left turn in the face of approaching traffic on the highway. Execution of the turn, of course, momentarily placed the approaching vehicle to the right of her car, and there was a considerable rise in tension even when the vehicle was a mile or more ahead. Left turns in the city disturbed her less because of slower speeds. The entry of other cars from side streets even as far as two blocks ahead into the road in which she was traveling also constituted a "lateral threat." Besides her reactions while in a car, she was anxious while walking across streets, even at intersections with the traffic light in her favor, and even if the nearest approaching car were more than a block away.

During the first few months of Mrs. C.'s neurosis, her panic at the sight of a car approaching from the side would cause her to grasp the driver by the arm. Her awareness of the annoyance this occasioned subsequently led her to control this behavior, for the most part successfully, but the fear was not diminished.

Questioned about previous related traumatic experiences, she recalled that ten years previously a tractor had crashed into the side of a car in which she was a passenger. Nobody had been hurt, the car had continued its journey, and she had been aware of no emotional sequel. No one close to her had ever been involved in a serious accident. Though she had worked in the Workmen's Compensation Claims office, dealing with cases of injury had not been disturbing to her. She found it incomprehensible that she should have developed this phobia; in London during World War II, she had accepted the dangers of the blitz calmly, without ever needing to use soporifics or sedatives.

She had received no previous treatment for her phobia. During the previous few days, she had told her story to Dr. Garnett; and then a medical student had seen her daily and discussed various aspects of her life, such as her childhood and her life with her husband—all of which she had felt to be irrelevant.

The plan of therapy was to confine subsequent interviews as far as possible to the procedures of *systematic desensitization,* and to omit any further history-taking, probing, and analyzing. Systematic desensitization (1, 3–5, 9–13) is a method of therapy that has its roots in the experimental laboratory. It has been shown experimentally (6, 8, 11) that persistent unadaptive habits of anxiety response may be eliminated by counteracting (and thus inhibiting) individual evocations of the response by means of the simultaneous evocation of an incompatible response (reciprocal inhibition). Each such inhibition leads to some degree of weakening of the anxiety response habit.

In systematic desensitization, the emotional effects of deep muscle relaxation are employed to counteract the anxiety evoked by phobic and allied stimulus situations presented to the patient's *imagination*. Stimulus situations on the theme of the patient's neurotic anxiety are listed and then ranked according to the intensity of anxiety they evoke. The patient, having been relaxed, sometimes under hypnosis, is asked to imagine the weakest of the disturbing stimuli, repeatedly, until it ceases to evoke any anxiety. Then increasingly "strong" stimuli are introduced in turn, and similarly treated, until eventually even the "strongest" fails to evoke anxiety. This desensitizing to imaginary situations has been found to be correlated with disappearance of anxiety in the presence of the actual situation.

In the second interview, training in relaxation and the construction of hierarchies were both initiated. To begin with, Mrs. C. was schooled in relaxation of the arms and the muscles of the forehead. Two hierarchies were constructed. The first related to traffic situations in open country. There was allegedly a minimal reaction if she was in a car driven by her husband and they were 200 yards from a crossroads and if, 400 yards away, at right angles, another car was approaching. Anxiety increased with increasing proximity. The second hierarchy related to lateral approaches of other cars while that in which she was traveling had stopped at a city traffic light. The first signs of anxiety supposedly appeared when the other car was two blocks away. (This, as will be seen, was a gross understatement of the patient's reactions.) The interview concluded with an introductory desensitization session. Having hypnotized and relaxed Mrs. C., I presented to her imagination some presumably neutral stimuli. First she was asked to imagine herself walking across a baseball field and then that she was riding in a car in the country with no other cars in sight. Following this, she was presented with the allegedly weak phobic situation of being in a car 200 yards from an intersection and seeing another car 400 yards on the left. She afterwards reported no disturbances to any of the scenes.

The third interview was conducted in the presence of an audience of five physicians. The Willoughby Neuroticism Test gave a borderline score of 24. (Normal, for practical purposes, is under 20. About 80 per cent of patients have scores above 30 [11].) Instruction in relaxation of muscles of the shoulder was succeeded by a desensitization session in which the following scenes were presented:

1) The patient's car, driven by her husband, had stopped at an intersection, and another car was approaching at right angles two blocks away.

2) The highway scene of the previous session was suggested, except that now her car was 150 yards from the intersection and the other car 300 yards away. Because this produced a finger-raising (signaling felt anxiety), after a pause she was asked to imagine that she was 150 yards from the intersection and the other car 400 yards. Though she did not raise her finger at this, it was noticed that she moved her legs. (*It was subsequently found that these leg movements were a very sensitive indicator of emotional disturbance.*)

Consequently, at the fourth interview, I subjected Mrs. C. to further questioning about her reactions to automobiles, from which it emerged that she was continuously tense in cars but had not thought this worth reporting, so trifling was it beside the terror experienced at the lateral approach of a car. She now also stated that *all* the car scenes imagined during the sessions had aroused anxiety, but too little, she had felt, to deserve mention. While relaxed under hypnosis, Mrs. C. was asked to imagine that she was in a car about to be driven around an empty square. As there was no reaction to this, the next scene presented was being about to ride two blocks on a country road. This evoked considerable anxiety!

At the fifth interview, it was learned that even the thought of a journey raised Mrs. C's tension, so that if, for example, at 9 a.m. her husband were to say, "We are going out driving at 2 p.m.," she would be continuously apprehensive, and more so when actually in the car. During the desensitization session (fourth) at this interview, I asked her to imagine that she was at home expecting to go for a short drive in the country in four hours' time. This scene, presented five times, evoked anxiety that did not decrease on repetition. It was now obvious that scenes with the merest suspicion of exposure to traffic were producing more anxiety than could be mastered by Mrs. C.'s relaxation potential.

A new strategy therefore had to be devised. I introduced an artifice that lent itself to controlled manipulation. On a sheet of paper I drew an altogether imaginary completely enclosed square field, which was represented as being two blocks (200 yards) long (see Figure 3). At the southwest corner (lower left) I drew her car, facing north (upwards), in which she sat with her husband, and at the lower right corner another car, supposed to be Dr. Garnett's, which faced them at right angles. Dr. Garnett (hereafter "Dr. G.") was "used" because Mrs. C. regarded him as a trustworthy person.

This imaginary situation became the focus of the scenes presented in the sessions that followed. At the fifth desensitization session, Mrs. C. was asked to imagine Dr. G. announcing to her that he was going to drive

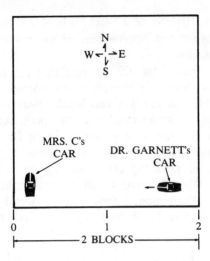

FIGURE 3. Imaginary enclosed square where Doctor Garnett makes progressively closer advances to Mrs. C.'s car.

his car a half-block towards her and then proceeding to do so while she sat in her parked car. As this elicited no reaction, she was next made to imagine him driving one block towards her, and then, as there was again no reaction, one and a quarter blocks. On perceiving a reaction to this scene, I repeated it three times, but without effecting any decrement in the reaction. I then "retreated," asking her to imagine Dr. G. stopping after traveling one block and two paces towards her. This produced a slighter reaction, and *this decreased on repeating the scene, disappearing at the fourth presentation.* This was the first evidence of change, and afforded grounds for a confident prediction of successful therapy.

At the sixth session, the imagined distance between Dr. G.'s stopping point and Mrs. C.'s car was decreased by two or three paces at a time, and at the end of the session he was able to stop seven-eighths of a block short of her (a total gain of about 10 paces). The following are the details of the progression. In parentheses is the number of presentations of each scene required to reduce the anxiety response to zero:

1) Dr. G. approaches four paces beyond one block (3).
2) Six paces beyond one block (3).
3) Nine paces beyond one block (2).
4) Twelve paces beyond one block, *i.e.,* one and one-eighth block (4).

At the seventh session, Mrs. C. was enabled to tolerate Dr. G.'s car reaching a point half a block short of her car without disturbance; at the eighth session, three-eighths of a block (about 37 yards); at the tenth, she was able to imagine him approaching within two yards of her without any reaction whatsoever.

The day after this, Mrs. C. reported that for the first time since her accident she had been able to walk across a street while an approaching car was in sight. The car was two blocks away but she was able to complete the crossing without quickening her pace. At this, the eleventh session, I began a new series of scenes in which Dr. G. drove in front of the car containing Mrs. C. instead of towards it, passing at first 30 yards ahead, and then gradually closer, cutting the distance eventually to about three yards. Desensitization to all this was rather rapidly achieved during this session. Thereupon, I drew two intersecting roads in the diagram of the field (Figure 4). A traffic light was indicated in the middle,

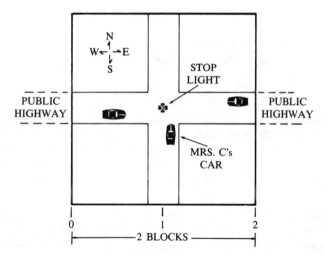

FIGURE 4.   Imaginary enclosed square with crossroads and traffic light added. Other cars pass while Mrs. C.'s car has stopped at the red light.

and the patient's car, as shown in the diagram, had "stopped" at the red signal. At first, Mrs. C. was asked to imagine Dr. G.'s car passing on the green light. As anticipated, she could at once accept this without anxiety; it was followed by Dr. G.'s car passing one way and a resident physician's car in the opposite direction. The slight anxiety this aroused was soon eliminated. In subsequent scenes, the resident's car was followed by an increasing number of students' cars, each scene being repeated until its emotional effect declined to zero.

At the twelfth session, the roadway at right angles to Mrs. C.'s car was made continuous with the public highway system (as indicated by the dotted lines) and now, starting off again with Dr. G., we added the cars of the resident and the students, and subsequently those of strangers. Imagining two unknown cars passing the intersection produced a fair degree of anxiety and she required five presentations at this session and five more at the next before she could accept it entirely calmly. However, once this was accomplished, it was relatively easy gradually to introduce several cars passing from both sides.

We now began a new series of scenes in which, with the traffic light in her favor, she was stepping off the curb to cross a city street while a car was slowly approaching. At first, the car was imagined a block away, but during succeeding sessions the distance gradually decreased to ten yards.

At this point, to check upon transfer from the imaginary to real life, I took Mrs. C. to the Charlottesville business center and observed her crossing streets at an intersection controlled by a traffic light. She went across repeatedly with apparent ease and reported no anxiety. But in the car, on the way there and back, she showed marked anxiety whenever a car from a side street threatened to enter the street in which we drove.

Soon afterwards, the opportunity arose for an experiment relevant to the question of "transference." A medical student had been present as an observer during four or five sessions. Early in May I had to leave town for a week to attend a conference. I decided to let the student continue therapy in my absence. Accordingly, I asked him to conduct the fifteenth desensitization session under my supervision. I corrected his errors by silently passing him written notes. Since he eventually performed quite well, he agreed to carry on treatment during my absence, and conducted the eighteenth to the twenty-third sessions entirely without supervision. His efforts were directed to a new series of scenes in which, while Mrs. C. was being driven by her husband along a city street, Dr. G.'s car made a right turn into that street from a cross street on their left. At first, Dr. G. was imagined making this entry two blocks ahead, but after several intervening stages it became possible for her to accept it calmly only half a block ahead. The student therapist then introduced a modification in which a student instead of Dr. G. drove the other car. The car was first visualized as entering two blocks ahead and the distance then gradually reduced to a half-block in the course of three sessions, requiring 63 scene presentations, most of which were needed in a very laborious advance from three-quarters of a block.

At this stage, the therapist experimentally inserted a scene in which Mrs. C.'s car was making a left turn in the city while Dr. G.'s car approached from the opposite direction four blocks ahead. This produced such a violent reaction that the therapist became apprehensive about continuing treatment. However, I returned the next day. Meanwhile, the point had been established that a substitute therapist could make satisfactory progress. (Under the writer's guidance, but not in his presence, the student therapist went on to conduct two entirely successful sessions the following week.)

I now made a detailed analysis of Mrs. C.'s reaction to left turns on the highway in the face of oncoming traffic. She reported anxiety at doing a left turn *if an oncoming car was in sight*. Even if it was two miles away she could not allow her husband to turn left in front of it.

To treat this most sensitive reaction, I again re-introduced Dr. G. into the picture. I started by making Mrs. C. imagine (while hypnotized and relaxed) that Dr. G.'s car was a mile ahead when her car began the turn. But this was too disturbing and several repetitions of the scene brought no diminution in the magnitude of anxiety evoked. It seemed possible that there would be less anxiety if the patient's husband were not the driver of the car, since his presence at the time of the accident might have made him a conditioned stimulus to anxiety. Thus I presented the scene with Mrs. C.'s *brother* as the driver of the car. With this altered feature, Dr. G.'s making a left turn a mile ahead evoked much less anxiety, and after four repetitions it declined to zero; we were gradually able to decrease the distance so that she could eventually imagine making the turn with Dr. G.'s car only about 150 yards away. Meanwhile, when she was able to "do" the turn with Dr. G. three-eighths of a mile away, I introduced two new left-turn series: a strange car approaching with her brother driving, and Dr. G. approaching with her husband driving—both a mile away initially. Work on all three series went on concurrently. When Mrs. C. could comfortably imagine her brother doing a left turn with the strange car five-eighths of a mile ahead, I resumed the original series in which her husband was the driver, starting with a left turn while the strange car was a mile ahead. This now evoked relatively little anxiety; progress could be predicted, and ensued. The interrelated decrements of reaction to this group of hierarchies are summarized in Figure 5.

Other series of related scenes were also subjected to desensitization. . . . One comprised left turns *in the city* in front of oncoming cars. Since cars in the city move relatively slowly, she felt less "danger" at a given distance. At first, we dealt with left turns while an approaching car was about two blocks away, and in the course of several sessions gradually decreased the distance until Mrs. C. could comfortably "do" a left turn with the other car slowly moving 15 yards ahead. The series where Mrs.

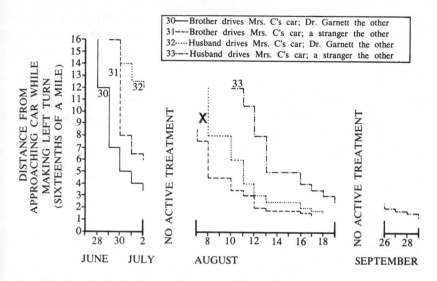

FIGURE 5. Temporal relations of "distances accomplished" in imagination in desensitization series 30, 31, 32 and 33. X: indicates some relapse in Hierarchy 31 following a taxi ride in which the driver insisted in exceeding the speed limit. The status of Hierarchy 32 was not tested before the relapse in 31 was overcome.

C. was crossing streets as a pedestrian was extended, and she was enabled in imagination to cross under all normal conditions. She reported complete transfer to the reality. A series that was started somewhat later involved driving down a through street with a car in a side street slowing to a stop. At first, the side street was "placed" two blocks ahead. The distance was gradually decreased as desensitization progressed, and eventually she could without anxiety drive past a car slowing to a stop. A series intercurrently employed to desensitize her in a general way to the feeling that a car was "bearing down upon her," was not part of any real situation. In our imaginary square field (Figure 3), I "placed" two parallel white lines, scaled to be about 20 feet long and 10 feet apart. During the session I said, "You are walking up and down along one white line and Dr. G. drives his car up to the other at one mile per hour. . . ." This was not disturbing; but at subsequent visualizings the speed was gradually increased and at an early stage the distance between the lines decreased to five feet. At four miles per hour there was some anxiety. This was soon eliminated, and several presentations of scenes from this series during each of 10 sessions made it possible for Mrs. C. calmly to imagine Dr. G. driving up to his white line at 18 miles per hour while she strolled along hers.

The total effect of desensitization to these interrelated series of stimulus situations was that Mrs. C. became completely at ease in all normal traffic situations—both in crossing streets as a pedestrian and riding in a car. Improvement in real situations took place in close relation with the improvements during sessions. A direct demonstration of the transfer of improvement with respect to crossing streets at traffic lights has been described above.

The patient's progress was slow but consistent. Because she lived about 100 miles away, her treatment took place episodically. At intervals of from four to six weeks she would come to Charlottesville for about two weeks and be seen almost every day. Noteworthy reduction in the range of real situations that could disturb her occurred in the course of each period of active treatment, and practically none during the intervals. She was instructed not to avoid exposing herself during these intervals to situations that might be expected to be only slightly disturbing: but if she anticipated being very disturbed to close her eyes, if feasible, for she could thus "ward off" the situation. Every now and then, particular incidents stood out as landmarks in her progress. One day in late August, driving with her brother in a through street in her home town, she saw a car slowing down before a stop sign as they passed it. Though the car did not quite stop, she had no reaction at all, though gazing at it continuously. This incident demonstrated the transfer to life of the desensitization to the relevant hierarchy which had been concluded shortly before. Since then, similar experiences had been consistently free from disturbance.

At the conclusion of Mrs. C.'s treatment, she was perfectly comfortable making a pedestrian crossing even though the traffic was creeping up to her. Left turns on a highway were quite comfortable with fast traffic up to about 150 yards ahead. When the closest approaching car was somewhat nearer, her reaction was slight anxiety, and not panic, as in the past. In all other traffic situations her feeling was entirely normal. Another effect of the treatment was that she no longer had headaches due to emotional tension.

In all, 57 desensitization sessions were conducted. The number of scene presentations at a session generally ranged from 25 to 40. . . . The last session took place on September 29, 1960. It was followed by the taking of Mrs. C.'s history [which] contains nothing to suggest that there were sexual problems underlying the automobile phobia.

When Mrs. C. was seen late in December, 1960, she was as well as she had been at the end of treatment. Her sexual relations with her husband were progressively improving. At a follow-up telephone call on June

6, 1961, she stated that she had fully maintained her recovery and had developed no new symptoms. Her relationship with her husband was excellent and sexually at least as satisfying as before the accident. A further call, on February 19, 1962, elicited the same report. . . .

DISCUSSION

Laboratory studies (6, 8, 11) have shown that experimental neuroses in animals are learned unadaptive habits characterized by anxiety that are remarkable for their persistence (resistance to the normal process of extinction). These neuroses can readily be eliminated through repeatedly inhibiting the neurotic responses by simultaneous evocations of incompatible responses (*i.e.,* by reciprocal inhibition of the neurotic responses) (6, 8, 11). The effectivenes of varied applications of this finding to human neuroses (*e.g.,* 1–5, 7–13) gives support to the view that human neuroses too are a particular category of habits acquired by learning.

In the systematic desensitization technique the effects of muscle relaxation are used to produce reciprocal inhibition of small evocations of anxiety and thereby build up conditioned inhibition of anxiety-responding to the particular stimulus combination. When (and only when) the evocations of anxiety are weakened by the counterposed relaxation does the anxiety response *habit* diminish. By systematic use of stimulus combinations whose anxiety-evoking potential is or has become weak, the habit strength of the whole neurotic theme is eliminated piecemeal.

The case of Mrs. C. illustrates with outstanding clarity how the course of change during systematic desensitization conforms to the expectations engendered by the reciprocal inhibition principle. Whenever a scene presented to the patient aroused a good deal of anxiety, that scene could be re-presented a dozen times without diminution of the anxiety. On the other hand, if the initial level of anxiety was lower, decrements in its intensity were achieved by successive presentations. It is a reasonable presumption that, as long as evoked anxiety was too great to be inhibited by the patient's relaxation, *no change* could occur; but when the anxiety was weak enough to be inhibited, repeated presentations of the scene led to progressive increments of *conditioned inhibition* of the anxiety-response habit, manifested by ever-weakening anxiety-responding. At every stage, each "quantum" of progress in relation to the subject matter of the desensitization sessions corresponded in specific detail to a small step towards recovery in an aspect of the real life difficulty. The fact that change occurred in this precise way in itself almost justifies the elimination of various "alternative explanations."

Mrs. C. had a total of 60 interviews, at each of which, except the first two and the last, a desensitization session was conducted. Including the initial three which proved to be unusable, 36 hierarchies entered into the sessions. All of these share the common theme of "car-approaching-from-the-side," but each has its own unique stimulus elements calling for separate desensitizing operations. The amount of attention a hierarchy needs is diminished by previous desensitization of other hierarchies that have elements in common with it. This is graphically illustrated in Figure 5. Hierarchies 30, 31, 32 and 33, each of which relates to turning left on the highway while another vehicle advances, differ, one from the next, in respect of a single stimulus condition and are in ascending order of anxiety arousal. Desensitization in overlapping sequences, starting with Hierarchy 30, shows parallel progressions. Now, desensitization of Hierarchy 33 was in fact first attempted before Hierarchy 30, from which it has three points of difference. At that time, presenting the approaching car at a distance of *one mile* evoked more anxiety than could be mastered by the patient's relaxation. But after Hierarchy 30 had been dealt with, and in Hierarchies 31 and 32, the "other car" could be tolerated at about one-half mile, it was possible to introduce Hierarchy 33 at three-quarters of a mile with very little anxiety. The increase in toleration was clearly attributable to desensitization to the stimulus elements that Hierarchy 33 *shared* with the three foregoing ones.

Figure 5 also illustrates the significant fact that *therapeutic change did not develop during the intervals when the patient was not receiving treatment,* and this was true even of reactions that were the main focus of treatment at the time. There is no drop, following the intervals, in the reactive level of any of the hierarchies represented. However, it is interesting to note that between July 2 and August 7 the reactive level of Hierarchy 31 has risen somewhat. This was not a "spontaneous" endogenously determined relapse, but due to the fact that, late in July, Mrs. C. had ridden in a taxi whose driver, despite her protests, had persisted in weaving among traffic at high speed. Immediately after this she was aware of increased reactivity. As can be seen, the lost ground was soon regained.

A question that may come to mind is this. What assurance did the therapist have of a correspondence between distances as imagined by Mrs. C. and objective measures of distance? The first and most important answer is that only rough correspondence was necessary, since what was always at issue was *distance as conceived by the patient.* The second answer is that a firm anchoring referent was the agreement between patient and therapist that a city block in Charlottesville would be considered 100 yards in length. Similar considerations apply to Mrs. C.'s conceptions of speed.

Among other explanations that may be brought forward to account for the recovery, the only one that, even at face value, would seem to deserve serious consideration in this case is *suggestion.* We shall take this usually ill-defined term to mean the instigation of changes in the patient's behavior by means of verbal or nonverbal cues from the therapist. In all psychotherapy there is at least an implied suggestion of, "This will make you well." Getting well under the impulse of such a general suggestion would not be related to particular therapeutic maneuvers, as was the case with Mrs. C. Another kind of suggestion has the form, "You will get well if. . . ." In commencing Mrs. C.'s desensitization, the therapist was careful to say no more than, "I am going to use a treatment that may help you." He did not say under what conditions it would help. During the first few sessions (and also several times later) when the scenes presented aroused considerable anxiety, repetition brought about no decrement of reaction. Decrement was noted consistently when anxiety was less. To sustain a hypothesis that suggestion was behind this would require evidence of the very specific instruction—"You will have decreasing anxiety only to situations that produce little anxiety in the first place." In fact, no such instruction was in any form conveyed. The patient could only have become aware *a posteriori* of the empirical relations of her changing reactions.

The relevance of the other "processes"—insight, de-repression, and transference—commonly invoked to explain away the effects of conditioning methods of therapy is negated by the absence of significant opportunity for such processes to have occurred. Any possible role of insight may be excluded by the fact that the only insight given to the patient was to tell her she was suffering from a conditioned fear reaction—and no change followed this disclosure. The possibility of de-repression may be ruled out by the non-emergence of forgotten material, and the de-emphasis of memory, even to the exclusion of the taking of a history during treatment—other than the history of the phobia's precipitation two years earlier and brief questioning about previous similar events, none of which had any effect on the neurosis.

The action of anything corresponding to "transference" is rendered implausible by the fact that interviews with the therapist led to improvement *only* when conditioning procedures were carried out in accordance with the requirements of reciprocal inhibition, and improvement was limited to the subject matter of the procedures of the time. Also, for a week, when the therapist was away, progress was effected by a medical student (20 years younger than the therapist) using the same conditioning techniques. In addition, the rather mechanical manner in which the sessions were conducted could hardly be said to favor the operation of transference effects; and certainly, the patient-therapist relationship was in no way ever analyzed. The third to the tenth interviews (and many others irregularly later) were conducted with the patient in full view of an unconcealed audience, without adverse effects on therapeutic progress.

The possibility of "spontaneous" recovery could be excluded with unusual confidence, since clinical improvement was a consequence of each of the periods of one to three weeks when the patient was being treated in Charlottesville, and was never noted during the four to six-week intervals the patient spent at home.

"Secondary gain," so often invoked in explanations of post-traumatic neurotic reactions, can have no credence as a factor in this case, either as a maintaining force or as determining recovery by its removal, for the patient did not receive any financial benefit, came for treatment eight months before litigation, became well two months before litigation, and did not relapse after a disappointing decision by the court.

REFERENCES

1. Bond, I. K. and Hutchinson, H. C.: Application of reciprocal inhibition therapy to exhibitionism. *Canad. Med. Assoc. J.*, 83:23-25, 1960.
2. Eysenck, H. J.: *Behavior Therapy and the Neuroses.* New York, Pergamon Press, 1960.
3. Lazarus, A. A.: New group techniques in the treatment of phobic conditions. *J. Abnorm. Soc. Psychol.* In press.
4. Lazarus, A. A. and Rachman, S.: The use of systematic desensitization in psychotherapy. *S. Afr. Med. J.*, 31:934-936, 1957.
5. Lazovik, A. D. and Lang, P. J.: A laboratory demonstration of systematic desensitization psychotherapy. *J. Psychol. Stud.*, 11:238-247, 1960.
6. Napalkov, A. V. and Karas, A. Y.: Elimination of pathological conditioned reflex connections in experimental hypertensive states. *Zh. Vyss. Nerv. Deiat. Pavlov.*, 7:402-409, 1957.
7. Rachman, S.: Sexual disorders and behavior therapy. *Amer. J. Psychiat.*, 118:235-240, 1961.
8. Wolpe, J.: Experimental neuroses as learned behavior. *Brit. J. Psychol.*, 43:243-268, 1952.
9. Wolpe, J.: Reciprocal inhibition as the main basis of psychotherapeutic effects. *A.M.A. Arch. Neurol. Psychiat.*, 72:205-226, 1954.
10. Wolpe, J.: Learning versus lesions as the basis of neurotic behavior. *Amer. J. Psychiat.*, 112:923-927, 1956.
11. Wolpe, J.: *Psychotherapy by Reciprocal Inhibition.* Stanford, California, Stanford Univ. Press, 1958.
12. Wolpe, J.: Psychotherapy based on the principle of reciprocal inhibition. In Burton, A., *Case Studies in Counseling and Psychotherapy.* Englewood Cliffs, New Jersey, Prentice-Hall, 1959.
13. Wolpe, J.: The systematic desensitization treatment of neuroses. *J. Nerv. Ment. Dis.*, 132:189-203, 1961.
14. Wolpe, J.: The prognosis in unpsychoanalyzed recovery from neurosis. *Amer. J. Psychiat.*, 118:35-39, 1961.
15. Wolpe, J. and Rachman, S.: Psychoanalytic evidence: A critique based on Freud's case of Little Hans. *J. Nerv. Ment. Dis.*, 131:135-148, 1960.

12. The Case of Clare*

Karen Horney

Karen Horney's psychoanalytic career began in the classical Freudian mold. Signs of her disparity with Freud soon became evident in her writings, when she took issue with his version of female psychology. Freud had postulated that in about the fourth year of childhood the boy's interest became focused on his penis, with concomitant attraction to the mother and resentment toward the father. During this stage of development, the boy feared retaliation and castration from the father (the Oedipal period). In the comparable age in the girl, however, there developed what Freud called "penis envy." He hypothesized that the girl's attachment to the father arose only after she was able to renounce her hopes of masculinity. Not only did Horney reject Freud's version of the Oedipal period, but she also objected to his belief that neurosis was a result of the damming up of the libido (principally a sexual drive energy) due to repression of sexual ideas during this stage. Horney believed that the etiology of the neurosis was primarily social rather than biological and that cultural conditions determined many neurotic conflicts. She felt that all neuroses were based upon disturbances in character which took their energy from the child's basic anxiety. Basic anxiety was seen as arising from the child's feeling of being small and helpless in a dangerous world. Such feelings were engendered in children by parents who did not provide the necessary warmth, protection, affection, and security. Such chil-

---

*dren, fearing desertion, repress their hostility, fail to assert themselves,
and lean on others but do not trust them.*

*Clare, Horney's female patient, had a background conducive to the
development of basic anxiety and neurotic trends. Horney felt that neurotic trends were coping mechanisms, developed to deal with life when
one felt helpless and isolated, central to psychic disturbance. In the
excerpts presented here, Horney, reviewing Clare's analysis, discusses
three neurotic trends and their implications in Clare's life. Because of
Horney's lack of specificity in diagnosis, the case study has been placed
under the broad category of neurosis. Horney has stated that neurotic
symptoms such as phobias, depression, and alcoholism result from conflicts exemplified by the analysis of neurotic trends. She also felt that
the essence of a neurosis lay in a neurotic character structure, the focal
points of which were neurotic trends.*

[Clare] was an unwanted child. The marriage was unhappy. After
having one child, a boy, the mother did not want any more children. Clare
was born after several unsuccessful attempts at an abortion. She was not
badly treated or neglected in any coarse sense: she was sent to schools
as good as those the brother attended, she received as many gifts as he
did, she had music lessons with the same teacher, and in all material
ways was treated as well. But in less tangible matters she received less
than the brother, less tenderness, less interest in school marks and in the
thousand little daily experiences of a child, less concern when she was ill,
less solicitude to have her around, less willingness to treat her as a con-
fidante, less admiration for looks and accomplishments. There was a
strong, though for a child intangible, community between the mother
and brother from which she was excluded. The father was no help. He
was absent most of the time, being a country doctor. Clare made some
pathetic attempts to get close to him but he was not interested in either
of the children. His affection was entirely focused on the mother in a kind
of helpless admiration. Finally, he was no help because he was openly
despised by the mother, who was sophisticated and attractive and beyond
doubt the dominating spirit in the family. The undisguised hatred and
contempt the mother felt for the father, including open death wishes
against him, contributed much to Clare's feeling that it was much safer
to be on the powerful side.

As a consequence of this situation Clare never had a good chance
to develop self-confidence. There was not enough of open injustice to provoke sustained rebellion, but she became discontented and cross and com-

plaining. As a result she was teased for always feeling herself a martyr. It never remotely occurred to either mother or brother that she might be right in feeling unfairly treated. They took it for granted that her attitude was a sign of an ugly disposition. And Clare, never having felt secure, easily yielded to the majority opinion about herself and began to feel that everything was her fault. Compared with the mother, whom everyone admired for her beauty and charm, and with the brother, who was cheerful and intelligent, she was an ugly duckling. She became deeply convinced that she was unlikable.

This shift from essentially true and warranted accusations of others to essentially untrue and unwarranted self-accusations had far-reaching consequences, as we shall see presently. And the shift entailed more than an acceptance of the majority estimate of herself. It meant also that she repressed all grievances against the mother. If everything was her own fault the grounds for bearing a grudge against the mother were pulled away from under her. From such repression of hostility it was merely a short step to join the group of those who admired the mother. In this further yielding to majority opinion she had a strong incentive in the mother's antagonism toward everything short of complete admiration: it was much safer to find shortcomings within herself than in the mother. If she, too, admired the mother she need no longer feel isolated and excluded but could hope to receive some affection, or at least be accepted. The hope for affection did not materialize, but she obtained instead a gift of doubtful value. The mother, like all those who thrive on the admiration of others, was generous in giving admiration in turn to those who adored her. Clare was no longer the disregarded ugly duckling, but became the wonderful daughter of a wonderful mother. Thus, in place of a badly shattered self-confidence, she built up the spurious pride that is founded on outside admiration.

Through this shift from true rebellion to untrue admiration Clare lost the feeble vestiges of self-confidence she had. To use a somewhat vague term, she lost herself. By admiring what in reality she resented, she became alienated from her own feelings. She no longer knew what she herself liked or wished or feared or resented. She lost all capacity to assert her wishes for love, or even any wishes. Despite a superficial pride her conviction of being unlovable was actually deepened. Hence, later on, when one or another person was fond of her, she could not take the affection at its face value but discarded it in various ways. Sometimes she would think that such a person misjudged her for something she was not; sometimes she would attribute the affection to gratitude for having been useful or to expectations of her future usefulness. This distrust deeply disturbed every human relationship she entered into. She lost, too, her capacity for critical judgment, acting on the unconscious maxim that it is safer to admire others than to be critical. This attitude shackled her intelligence, which was actually of a high order, and greatly contributed to her feeling stupid.

In consequence of all these factors three neurotic trends developed. One was a compulsive modesty as to her own wishes and demands. This entailed a compulsive tendency to put herself into second place, to think less of herself than of others, to think that others were right and she was wrong. But even in this restricted scope she could not feel safe unless there was someone on whom she could depend, someone who would protect and defend her, advise her, stimulate her, approve of her, be responsible for her, give her everything she needed. She needed all this because she had lost the capacity to take her life into her own hands. Thus she developed the need for a "partner"—friend, lover, husband—on whom she could depend. She would subordinate herself to him as she had toward the mother. But at the same time, by his undivided devotion to her, he would restore her crushed dignity. A third neurotic trend—a compulsive need to excel others and to triumph over them—likewise aimed at restoration of self-regard, but in addition absorbed all the vindictiveness accumulated through hurts and humiliations. . . .

Clare came for analytic treatment at the age of thirty, for various reasons. She was easily overcome by a paralyzing fatigue that interfered with her work and her social life. Also, she complained about having remarkably little self-confidence. She was the editor of a magazine, and though her professional career and her present position were satisfactory her ambition to write plays and stories was checked by insurmountable inhibitions. She could do her routine work but was unable to do productive work, though she was inclined to account for this latter inability by pointing out her probable lack of talent. She had been married at the age of twenty-three, but the husband had died after three years. After the marriage she had had a relationship with another man which continued during the analysis. According to her initial presentation both relationships were satisfactory sexually as well as otherwise.

The analysis stretched over a period of four and a half years. She was analyzed for one year and a half. This time was followed by an interruption of two years, in which she did a good deal of self-analysis, afterward returning to analysis for another year at irregular intervals.

Clare's analysis could be roughly divided into three phases: the discovery of her compulsive modesty; the discovery of her compulsive dependence on a partner; and finally, the discovery of her compulsive need to force others to recognize her superiority. None of these trends was apparent to herself or to others.

In the first period the data that suggested compulsive elements were as follows. She tended to minimize her own value and capacities: not only was she insecure about her assets but she tenaciously denied their existence, insisting that she was not intelligent, attractive, or gifted and tending to discard evidence to the contrary. Also, she tended to regard others as superior to herself. If there was a dissension of opinion she automatically believed that the others were right. She recalled that when her husband had started an affair with another woman she did nothing to remonstrate against it, though the experience was extremely painful to her; she managed to consider him justified in preferring the other on the grounds that the latter was more attractive and more loving. Moreover, it was almost impossible for her to spend money on herself: when she traveled with others she could enjoy living in expensive places, even though she contributed her share in the expenses, but as soon as she was on her own she could not bring herself to spend money on such things as trips, dresses, plays, books. Finally, though she was in an executive position, it was impossible for her to give orders: she would do so in an apologetic way if orders were unavoidable.

The conclusion reached from such data was that she had developed a compulsive modesty, that she felt compelled to constrict her life within narrow boundaries and to take always a second or third place. When this trend was once recognized, and its origin in childhood discussed, we began to search systematically for its manifestations and its consequences. What role did this trend actually play in her life?

She could not assert herself in any way. In discussions she was easily swayed by the opinions of others. Despite a good faculty for judging people she was incapable of taking any critical stand toward anyone or anything, except in editing, when a critical stand was expected of her. She had encountered serious difficulties, for instance, by failing to realize that a fellow worker was trying to undermine her position; when this situation was fully apparent to others she still regarded the other as her friend. Her compulsion to take second place appeared clearly in games: in tennis, for instance, she was usually too inhibited to play well, but occasionally she was able to play a good game and then, as soon as she became aware that she might win, she would begin to play badly. The wishes of others were more important than her own: she would be contented to take her holidays during the time that was least wanted by others, and she would do more work than she needed to if the others were dissatisfied with the amount of work to be done.

Most important was a general suppression of her feelings and wishes. Her inhibitions concerning expansive plans she regarded as particularly "realistic"—evidence that she never wanted things that were beyond reach. Actually she was as little "realistic" as someone with excessive expectations of life; she merely kept her wishes beneath the level of the attainable. She was unrealistic in living in every way beneath her means—

socially, economically, professionally, spiritually. It was attainable for her, as her later life showed, to be liked by many people, to look attractive, to write something that was valuable and original.

The most general consequences of this trend were a progressive lowering of self-confidence and a diffuse discontentment with life. Of the latter she had not been in the least aware, and could not be aware as long as everything was "good enough" for her and she was not clearly conscious of having wishes or of their not being fulfilled. The only way this general discontentment with life had shown itself was in trivial matters and in sudden spells of crying which had occurred from time to time and which had been quite beyond her understanding.

For quite a while she recognized only fragmentarily the truth of these findings; in important matters she made the silent reservation that I either overrated her or felt it to be good therapy to encourage her. Finally, however, she recognized in a rather dramatic fashion that real, intense anxiety lurked behind this façade of modesty. It was at a time when she was about to suggest an improvement in the magazine. She knew that her plan was good, that it would not meet with too much opposition, that everyone would be appreciative in the end. Before suggesting it, however, she had an intense panic which could not be rationalized in any way. At the beginning of the discussion she still felt panicky and had to leave the room because of a sudden diarrhea. But as the discussion turned increasingly in her favor the panic subsided. The plan was finally accepted and she received considerable recognition. She went home with a feeling of elation and was still in good spirits when she came to the next analytical hour.

I dropped a casual remark to the effect that this was quite a triumph for her, which she rejected with a slight annoyance. Naturally she had enjoyed the recognition, but her prevailing feeling was one of having escaped from a great danger. It was only after more than two years had elapsed that she could tackle the other elements involved in this experience, which were along the lines of ambition, dread of failure, triumph. At that time her feelings, as expressed in her associations, were all concentrated on the problem of modesty. She felt that she had been presumptuous to propound a new plan. Who was she to know better! But gradually she realized that this attitude was based on the fact that for her the suggesting of a different course of action meant a venturing out of the narrow artificial precincts that she had anxiously preserved. Only when she recognized the truth of this observation did she become fully convinced that her modesty was a façade to be maintained for the sake of safety. The result of this first phase of work was a beginning of faith in herself and a beginning of courage to feel and assert her wishes and opinions.

The second period was dedicated prevailingly to work on her dependency on a "partner." The majority of the problems involved she worked through by herself, as will be reported later on in greater detail. This dependency, despite its overwhelming strength, was still more deeply repressed than the previous trend. It had never occurred to her that anything was wrong in her relationships with men. On the contrary, she had believed them to be particularly good. The analysis gradually changed this picture.

There were three main factors that suggested compulsive dependence. The first was that she felt completely lost, like a small child in a strange wood, when a relationship ended or when she was temporarily separated from a person who was important to her. The first experience of this kind occurred after she left home at the age of twenty. She then felt like a feather blown around in the universe, and she wrote desperate letters to her mother, declaring that she could not live without her. This homesickness stopped when she developed a kind of crush on an older man, a successful writer who was interested in her work and furthered her in a patronizing way. Of course, this first experience of feeling lost when alone could be understood on the basis of her youth and the sheltered life she had lived. But later reactions were intrinsically the same, and formed a strange contrast to the rather successful professional career that she was achieving despite the difficulties mentioned before.

The second striking fact was that in any of these relationships the whole world around her became submerged and only the beloved had any importance. Thoughts and feelings centered around a call or a letter or a visit from him; hours that she spent without him were empty, filled only with waiting for him, with a pondering about his attitude to her, and above all with feeling utterly miserable about incidents which she felt as utter neglect or humiliating rejection. At these times other human relationships, her work, and other interests lost almost every value for her.

The third factor was a fantasy of a great and masterful man whose willing slave she was and who in turn gave her everything she wanted, from an abundance of material things to an abundance of mental stimulation, and made her a famous writer.

As the implications of these factors were gradually recognized the compulsive need to lean on a "partner" appeared and was worked through in its characteristics and its consequences. Its main feature was an entirely repressed parasitic attitude, an unconscious wish to feed on the partner, to expect him to supply the content of her life, to take responsibility for her, to solve all her difficulties and to make her a great person without her having to make efforts of her own. This trend had alienated her not only from other people but also from the partner himself, because the unavoidable disappointments she felt when her secret expectations of him remained unfulfilled gave rise to a deep inner irritation; most of this irritation was repressed for fear of losing the partner, but some of it emerged in occasional explosions. Another consequence was that she could not enjoy anything except when she shared it with the partner. The most general consequence of this trend was that her relationships served only to make her more insecure and more passive and to breed self-contempt.

The interrelations of this trend with the previous one were twofold. On the one hand, her compulsive modesty was one of the reasons that accounted for her need for a partner. Since she could not take care of her own wishes she had to have someone else who took care of them. Since she could not defend herself she needed someone else to defend her. Since she could not see her own values she needed someone else to affirm her worth. On the other hand, there was a sharp conflict between the compulsive modesty and the excessive expectations of the partner. Because of this unconscious conflict she had to distort the situation every time she was disappointed over unfulfilled expectations. In such situations she felt herself the victim of intolerably harsh and abusive treatment, and therefore felt miserable and hostile. Most of the hostility had to be repressed because of fear of desertion, but its existence undermined the relationship and turned her expectations into vindictive demands. The resulting upsets proved to have a great bearing on her fatigue and her inhibition toward productive work.

The result of this period of analytical work was that she overcame her parasitic helplessness and became capable of greater activity of her own. The fatigue was no longer continual but appeared only occasionally. She became capable of writing, though she still had to face strong resistances. Her relationships with people became more friendly, though they were still far from being spontaneous; she impressed others as being haughty while she herself still felt quite timid. An expression of the general change in her was contained in a dream in which she drove with her friend in a strange country and it occurred to her that she, too, might apply for a driver's license. Actually, she had a license and could drive as well as the friend. The dream symbolized a dawning insight that she had rights of her own and need not feel like a helpless appendage.

The third and last period of analytical work dealt with repressed ambitious strivings. There had been a period in her life when she had been obsessed by frantic ambition. This had lasted from her later years in grammar school up to her second year in college, and had then seemed to disappear. One could conclude only by inference that it still operated underground. This was suggested by the fact that she was elated and overjoyed at any recognition, by her dread of failure, and by the anxiety involved in any attempt at independent work.

This trend was more complicated in its structure than the two others. In contrast to the others, it constituted an attempt to master life actively, to take up a fight against adverse forces. This fact was one element in its continued existence: she felt herself that there had been a positive force in her ambition and wished repeatedly to be able to retrieve it. A second element feeding the ambition was the necessity to re-establish her lost self-esteem. The third element was vindictiveness; success meant a triumph over all those who had humiliated her, while failure meant disgraceful defeat. To understand the characteristics of this ambition we must go back in her history and discover the successive changes it underwent.

The fighting spirit involved in this trend appeared quite early in life. Indeed, it preceded the development of the other two trends. At this period of the analysis early memories occurred to her of opposition, rebellion, belligerent demands, all sorts of mischief. As we know, she lost this fight for her place in the sun because the odds against her were too great. Then, after a series of unhappy experiences, this spirit re-emerged when she was about eleven, in the form of a fierce ambition at school. Now, however, it was loaded with repressed hostility: it had absorbed the piled-up vindictiveness for the unfair deal she had received and for her downtrodden dignity. It had now acquired two of the elements mentioned above: through being on top she would re-establish her sunken self-confidence, and by defeating the others she would avenge her injuries. This grammar-school ambition, with all its compulsive and destructive elements, was nevertheless realistic in comparison with later developments, for it entailed efforts to surpass others through greater actual achievements. During high school she was still successful in being unquestionably the first. But in college, where she met greater competition, she rather suddenly dropped her ambition altogether, instead of making the greater efforts that the situation would have required if she still wanted to be first. There were three main reasons why she could not muster the courage to make these greater efforts. One was that because of her compulsive modesty she had to fight against constant doubts as to her intelligence. Another was the actual impairment in the free use of her intelligence through the repression of her critical faculties. Finally, she could not take the risk of failure because the need to excel the others was too compulsive.

The abandonment of her manifest ambition did not, however, diminish the impulse to triumph over others. She had to find a compromise solution, and this, in contrast to the frank ambition at school, was devious in character. In substance it was that she would triumph over the others without doing anything to bring about that triumph. She tried to achieve this impossible feat in three ways, all of which were deeply unconscious. One was to register whatever good luck she had in life as a triumph over others. This ranged from a conscious triumph at good weather on an excursion to an unconscious triumph over some "enemy" falling ill or dying. Conversely, she felt bad luck not simply as bad luck but as a disgraceful defeat. This attitude served to enhance her dread of life because it meant a reliance on factors that are beyond control. The second way was to shift the need for triumph to love relationships. To have a husband or lover was a triumph; to be alone was a shameful defeat. And the third way of achieving triumph without effort was the demand that husband or lover, like the masterful man in the fantasy, should make her great without her doing anything, possibly by merely giving her the chance to indulge vicariously in his success. These attitudes created insoluble conflicts in her personal relationships and considerably reinforced the need for a "partner," since he was to take over these all-important functions.

The consequences of this trend were worked through by recognizing the influence they had on her attitude toward life in general, toward work, toward others, and toward herself. The outstanding result of this examination was a diminution of her inhibitions toward work.

We then tackled the interrelations of this trend with the two others. There were, on the one hand, irreconcilable conflicts and, on the other hand, mutual reinforcements, evidence of how inextricably she was caught in her neurotic structure. Conflicts existed between the compulsion to assume a humble place and to triumph over others, between ambition to excel and parasitic dependency, the two drives necessarily clashing and either arousing anxiety or paralyzing each other. This paralyzing effect proved to be one of the deepest sources of the fatigue as well as of the inhibitions toward work. No less important, however, were the ways in which the trends reinforced one another. To be modest and to put herself into a humble place became all the more necessary as it served also as a cloak for the need for triumph. The partner, as already mentioned, became an all the more vital necessity as he had also to satisfy in a devious way the need for triumph. Moreover, the feelings of humiliation generated by the need to live beneath her emotional and mental capacities and by her dependency on the partner kept evoking new feelings of vindictiveness, and thus perpetuated and reinforced the need for triumph.

The analytical work consisted in disrupting step by step the vicious circles operating. The fact that her compulsive modesty had already given way to some measure of self-assertion was of great help because this progress automatically lessened also the need for triumph. Similarly, the partial solution of the dependency problem, having made her stronger and having removed many feelings of humiliation, made the need for triumph less stringent. Thus when she finally approached the issue of vindictiveness, which was deeply shocking to her, she could tackle with increased inner strength an already diminished problem. To have tackled it at the beginning would not have been feasible. In the first place we would not have understood it, and in the second place she could not have stood it.

The result of this last period was a general liberation of energies. Clare retrieved her lost ambition on a much sounder basis. It was now less compulsive and less destructive; its emphasis shifted from an interest in success to an interest in the subject matter. Her relationships with people, already improved after the second period, now lost the tenseness created by the former mixture of a false humility and a defensive haughtiness.

6. Personality and Other Nonpsychotic Mental Disorders

The personality disorders are characterized by deeply ingrained maladaptive patterns of behavior that are perceptibly different in quality from psychotic and neurotic symptoms. Generally, these are life-long patterns, often recognizable by the time of adolescence or earlier. Characteristic manifestations include such symptoms as hypersensitivity, shyness, excessive inhibition, aggressiveness, incapacity for enjoyment, and irresponsibility.

The category of sexual deviations is for individuals whose sexual interests are directed primarily toward objects other than people of the opposite sex, toward sexual acts not usually associated with coitus, or toward coitus performed under bizarre circumstances as in necrophilia, pedophilia, sexual sadism, and fetishism. Even though many find their practices distasteful, they remain unable to substitute normal sexual behavior for them.

The category of alcoholism is for patients whose alcohol intake is great enough to damage their physical health, or their personal or social functioning, or when it has become a prerequisite to normal functioning.

The category of drug dependence is for patients who are addicted to or dependent on drugs other than alcohol, tobacco, and ordinary caffeine-containing beverages.

13. Rebel without a Cause*

Robert M. Lindner

Hypnoanalysis, as the word suggests, is the combined use of psychoanalysis and hypnosis. Although some forms of hypnosis existed in antiquity,
the therapeutic use of hypnosis probably begins with Anton Mesmer
(1734–1815). Freud initially used hypnosis in his early investigation of
hysteria but abandoned it when he developed the technique of free association. It is debatable whether Freud relinquished hypnosis in treatment
because he found many patients incapable of being hypnotized, whether
he felt it antithetical to the change of mental state required for permanent relief from symptoms, or because, as some have suggested, he was a
poor hypnotist. Whatever the reason, his action seems to have influenced
the practice of psychotherapy, and until the 1950s, clinicians resisted the
use of the hypnotic method.

 Lindner's case study is a classic contribution to the reinstitution of
hypnosis in psychotherapy and foreshadows its current vitality as evidenced by the extensive research in experimental and clinical hypnosis.
Lindner had voiced objections, reflecting the feelings of substantial numbers of clinicians, that because of the length of therapy or the inadequacy
of free association in reaching the depths of the unconscious, orthodox
psychoanalysis did not meet the needs of countless patients. He therefore
attempted to demonstrate that permanent personality changes would accompany the use of hypnosis.

 The patient described, having a history of recidivism from the age
of twelve, was treated in prison. He was classified as a psychopath (a

---

*Reprinted by permission of Grune & Stratton, Inc., from *Rebel Without a Cause*.
(New York: Grune & Stratton, 1944). Pp. 25-31, 40-46, 141-148, 279-284.

diagnostic category now called antisocial personality). These sections from Lindner's book illustrate the concept of the antisocial character, the process by which the character is revealed, and the role analytic insight into the psychosexual etiology of the disorder played in the treatment.

The history of Harold, our subject, has been made available to the writer in many forms. Each of his delinquent acts when subject to court review was supplemented with detailed social service investigations according to the admirable latter-day judicial routine; and on the occasions of his incarcerations further study was made of the essential features of his home, family and personal life. Rarely has a clinician been provided with a more complete and documented anamnesis. This material proved eminently useful as a constant check and source during the hypnoanalysis, and provided a frame of reference, almost a topography, for the incidents and events elicited from the patient.

Harold's father, an unnaturalized Pole and a machinist by trade, came to the United States during the great exodus from Europe at the turn of the century. He was a big, bluff, hearty peasant of excellent work habits. Within a short time he met and married the native-born girl who became Harold's mother; and having settled in an industrial suburb of a large city in the East the couple soon became the parents of our subject and in time of two daughters. The father contracted an occupational disease early in his career, and the medical regimen imposed on him forced his abandonment of factory employment but permitted his occupation in a free-lance manner. His average earnings, computed over many years by social workers, were twenty-five dollars a week. Investigators described him as a hasty disciplinarian who is more ready with curses and unkind words than blows. He does not smoke or use intoxicants, is cut off from his family by reason of his unfamiliarity with English and his illiteracy (despite his long residence in this country); and the fact that his standards are, on the whole, old-world and markedly unprogressive. His reputation in the community is excellent and his affiliations with Polish-American organizations have resulted in firm if taciturn and blunt friendships with men of his own temper and kind. Now, at fifty-three, he is still pursuing his trade, more frequently, however, eyeing pastures he should have cultivated twenty years ago. He claims even at this date an interest in Harold, but investigators note his lack of patience toward his son's problems.

Harold's mother is today as she seems always to have been a symbol of patient and unrequited motherhood, a person who invites sentiment. A beautiful and buxom girl when she married at an early age, she is now a worn and tired woman, a product of housewifely routine and the monotonous drudgery of feeding, caring and worrying for a family in slightly above marginal economic circumstances. Her loyalty to her children and especially to Harold is famous among her acquaintances, and social workers note her over-solicitous, over-protective nature. This she has rationalized by pointing out the social limitations and barriers faced by Harold because of his peculiar physical defect. She is lavish in her statements of affection for the boy and admits to having saved him from pitfalls on many occasions. By all accounts, she is a sensible, intelligent and industrious woman in all affairs but those dealing with her son. She is a voracious reader of cheap romances and an ardent movie-goer, readily moved to tears and easily imposed upon. Her attention has for so long been fixed solely upon her family that she has but few friends; these she visits and entertains regularly with coffee and gossip. Her own family, including her mother, two married sisters and a brother, is bound by ties of mutual dependence in their unrelenting borderland of impoverishment.

Two younger sisters complete the family group. The elder of these is a pert, vivacious girl of nineteen who works steadily at a factory job and who contributes her entire wages to the parents; the youngest is a schoolgirl, bright and lively, the pet and joy of the old folks.

The whole family, with the exception of Harold, is well regarded by neighbors and friends. They practice the Roman-Catholic faith, own a car and are considered respectable additions to the neighborhood. The section in which they live is a crowded district of foreign-laborer families. They maintain a four-room apartment above a saloon in an old building with a few modern conveniences: rent is twelve dollars a month. The home is clean, modestly furnished in a comfortable if somewhat worn style. Beyond the youngest daughter's school-books, the mother's rental library romances, the eldest daughter's movie-fan pulps, and the Polish language newspaper, there are no books or periodicals in the apartment. A radio and some religious chromos complete the cultural scene.

Those relatives visited by investigators were cut from the same pattern and along the same lines as Harold's parents. The family history, so far as it can be traced, is negative for feeblemindedness or mental disorder of any variety, except for traces of alcoholism in the male members of the distaff branch.

The mother reports that Harold's birth, assisted by a midwife, was entirely normal following a labor of six hours duration. The child was healthy and there were no abnormal pre- or post-natal circumstances. At the age of one or two, Harold suffered measles, and between two and six other childhood exanthems were experienced. Tonsillectomy and adenoidectomy were performed when he was twelve. Except for these and his eye condition, his health was normal.

As to the optic disorder, it was the recorded opinion of two physicians whom his mother consulted that the diagnosis was *Nystagmus Amblyopia* resulting from the measles; another consultant diagnosed *congenital defective retinae* incorrectable, with ten per cent normal vision in the right eye and fifteen per cent in the left. The mother reports visits to numerous specialists in order to obtain some kind of favorable treatment. In all cases, however, results were unsatisfactory.

Harold attended public school from the first to the fourth grades in the city to which the family moved soon after his birth. Records from these years cannot be located, but his mother reports regular attendance and satisfactory performance. The fourth to the seventh grades were spent at a parochial school. The nuns who were his teachers have stated that he was a fair student and conducted himself passably well. He left parochial school to become a pupil in a special class for students with defective vision. At fifteen he graduated to High School, which he quit after one year. Officials and High School instructors considered his conduct fair but regretted that he did not produce to the level of his capabilities. At sixteen he renounced all scholastic pursuits and from that time forward worked fitfully on a relative's farm.

Harold's recorded criminal history began at the age of twelve when in the company of other small boys he broke into a grocery store and made off with almost seventy-five dollars worth of candy and tobacco. He was apprehended and sent to a juvenile institution for examination by specialists; but while awaiting his turn he escaped custody by leaping through a window. Again apprehended, he was placed on two years probation. At thirteen he was arrested for a trespassing offense and the Juvenile Court extended the probationary period.

After a two year respite Harold once more came into conflict with the law when he stole a sizable sum from a storekeeper. Probation was renewed. One month later, having made off with money from his mother's purse, he purchased a rifle and with it attempted to rob a couple in an automobile on a deserted city street. Tricked by his clever victim, he was held for the police who hailed him into Juvenile Court, where he was again probated for five years. Minor charges for trespassing, breaking and entering and vandalism were lodged during the following year. On one occasion he received a short sentence to a correctional institution; on another, a light jail term. Several similar charges and warrants were pending when he was arrested for the offense for which he is now serving. The details of this offense cannot, unfortunately, be revealed here, but it was a crime serious enough to carry a heavy penalty.

Many psychologists and psychiatrists have interviewed, examined and tested Harold. While they disagree on the causative factors in his case, all are in accord on the diagnosis of psychopathic personality complicated by social difficulties arising from the condition of the boy's eyes. One psychiatrist stressed the avoidance by other children which Harold probably experienced, stating that they undoubtedly considered him a freak and this, as a consequence, forced his mother's indulgence. Another specialist reported a need for productive occupation, and asociality and egocentricity as the leading factors in the clinical picture. Still another stated that Harold evinced pronounced feelings of inferiority in respect of his place in the family group, adding that he found the boy to be cowardly, unreliable and a schemer. This specialist also reported the presence of "subconscious jealousy of the father and a mother fixation." The last examiner's report closes with the statement: ". . . unless someone is able to psychoanalyze and reconstruct his personality from about three years of age on, the boy will continue on his career of crime and, because of his violent impulses, will become a more and more dangerous criminal." A final expert found Harold honest in his statements and fairly intelligent; and, questioning him closely on his sex habits, obtained an admission of masturbation and sexual relations with girls in the neighborhood.

On his arrival in the institution where the writer made his acquaintance, Harold showed a Mental Age of sixteen years and one month; an Intelligence Quotient of one-hundred and seven. He was found to be free of disease; serology was negative; weight 150 lb.; height 5 ft. 8 in.; ophthalmological diagnosis was *Nystagmus, Strabismus, Ptosis*; psychiatric diagnosis was *Psychopathic Personality*. The psychiatric initial summary revealed: ". . . a recidivist whose attitude toward officials and fellows is poor. . . . Since childhood he has had practically no respectable occupation or regular employment and it is evident he has matured without benefit of proper parental discipline. . . . During interview he presents the picture of a sullen, resentful, weak-willed, gullible, fidgety youth . . . lacks insight and judgment . . . enjoys using the language of the underworld and frequently lapses into gangland lingo when describing his escapades. . . . Prognosis for institutional adjustment and rehabilitation is guarded."

On a spring morning some time ago a prisoner sat apprehensively on a chair in the anteroom of the writer's office. He had been sent for at the urging of a clinical assistant who felt that at least some of the symptoms which the young man showed should be studied and treated. Since the inmate had no inkling of the reason for his call, he was filled with that nervous anticipation and foreboding of personal danger that only petitioners and clients of professional people can know. Several times he rose from his chair and paced the room with the curious litheness and agility common among psychopaths.

He was a moderately tall, sparingly built boy, wide-shouldered and narrow-hipped. The cast of his face would have evoked an impression of 'intelligent' from the layman; and there was a suggestion of competence in his large-knuckled hands. The one feature that attracted immediate attention was his heavy-lidded, continually fluttering eyes. These lent his appearance the almost mask-like quality of the totally blind, until the observer noted the restless, shifting play of the pupils and the quick winking of the lids.

During the interview and examination, Harold maintained a sneering sullenness modified by the abject disinterest such individuals often demonstrate in the presence of prison or hospital officials. He stated apathetically that he could foresee no benefits from any kind of treatment; that he had been dancing attendance on all varieties of medical specialists without reward; but that he would be willing to allow an examination and experiment with a new therapy. Accordingly, he was subjected to a complete physical check and another examination by a competent ophthalmologist. There was no change from his admission status.

A chance remark passed by Harold during the initial examination determined the writer first upon a therapeutic program based on posthypnotic suggestion. In response to the question, "Would you rather be blind than get so that you can keep your eyes open for longer periods?" Harold answered, "I'd rather be blind than to see some of the things I have seen." The presence and verbalization of so peculiar a remark, with its undertones suggestive of a pathological solution of conflict, settled the immediate initiation of a course of hypnotic therapy.

Harold entered the trance state rapidly and easily, obeying each instruction as it was issued. Various tests, ranging from hand-levitation to catelepsy to the production of anesthetic areas, were consummated successfully. Then, in response to the suggestion that his lids would open and remain fixed and steady while a strong light from an ophthalmoscope was directed into his eyes, Harold—who had never looked into daylight with open eyes and for whom an electric light was only a stimulus to rapid blinking—opened his eyes and stared directly before him as the sharp shaft played over his eyeballs. This convinced the writer that he had here to do with a condition which, although it was essentially physical, perhaps had been initiated by a traumatic assault on the organism at a crucial stage in its development. A course of treatment was begun and carried out faithfully for about two weeks. Each session concentrated on the lengthening of the post-hypnotic period during which Harold's eyes were to remain widely open and impervious to light. Results were not only highly satisfactory in respect of Harold's ability to control the mobility of his lids, but the writer noted the development of an increasingly favorable rapport.

All this time the author was keenly aware that he was attacking *symptoms* rather than *causes*. This, coupled with the temptation to capitalize on the rare, excellent rapport with a psychopath, (which was not understood at the time) prompted a resolve to attempt an analysis which, it was hoped, would for the first time ferret out the psychological factors responsible for the psychopathic pattern. The nature of the undertaking was described to Harold and he assented to being hypnoanalyzed.

It occurred to the writer that it would be invaluable to have a permanent and complete record of the entire transaction for the light it promised to throw on crime and psychopathy. A microphone was therefore concealed in the couch on which Harold was to lie during the sessions. Connection with a loudspeaker in another room was made, and there a competent stenographer of the writer's staff took down and subsequently transcribed the proceedings verbatim. This material, edited only to eliminate tiresome and meaningless repetitions and redundancies, is herewith made available to the reader.

But before we examine the transcript of the hypnoanalysis, a word needs to be said here concerning the peculiar ethical problems which beset the psychiatrist or psychologist practicing in a penal institution. Because of the fact that he is, to those of the inmates who consult him, someone who is unselfishly interested in their welfare, he is often made privy to information which his duty to the State or Government urges him to communicate to law-enforcement agencies, but which his sense of obligation to his patient and to his professional standards compels him to keep to himself. In the present instance, this insistent dilemma was happily resolved by the patient himself during the period of re-education which followed the hypnoanalysis. Not only did he grant permission to the writer to publish this material, he actually urged its publication: this because he had come to a genuine and sincere realization of the social importance and the dangerous significance of his condition . . .

The Third Hour

Yesterday I felt as if I was lying on a cloud somewhere with my head wrapped in cotton. I couldn't move it. I was as if I were up against a big stone cliff or something.

Why I said that I don't know. . . .

Yesterday I couldn't move my head. I don't know what it was. I still remember lying on this bed, or on a cloud. I felt as if my head was wrapped in cotton, so soft and yet so hard I couldn't move it. Sometimes it seemed as if my mind left my body and just went off by itself. . . .

Where the association is unimpeded by resistances, this is a common experience among patients.

I never had many friends on the outside. Usually I'd hang out by myself, go and sit on the guard-rail near the river and watch the river, the dark, dirty river go by. It rolls and rolls by. Then the river turns, it turns and you see it against the sky. The sky so clean and the water so dirty, just like someone took a paint brush and painted grease in a straight line.

I used to spend a lot of time on the river near my home where I had some small boats, just row boats. I never had no motor boat. And I used to play in the swamp, swampy, muddy grounds with bushes and weeds and some sandy spots. There were old logs and pipes laying around. I used to go there with a .22 and shoot bull frogs. One time I put a match on a tank and I tried to hit this match but the bullets always went over the tank or to the side. I always had a liking for guns. I don't know why. . . .

I used to get hitches on tug boats and barges and go up the river and back. I would just do nothing and waste a lot of time. Sometimes I would look for work but I would never find any. I never had a job, so I would just ignore it; wouldn't look for work at all; maybe spend a half day in a show and sleep a lot. It would get monotonous, and then I would read books. I used to read the wrong kind of books, I guess; detective magazines and crime stories just to pass the time. I used to listen to the radio a lot too. Most of the time to crime serials but once in a while to music. Not jazz music. Music. Music. Now I know it was classical music. I liked it. I don't know anything about it. I guess it is soothing to the emotions, makes a person free of everything.

I spent most of my nights on the outside with fellows. That was on account of my eyes. They don't blink at night.

When I was about twelve I used to hang around with fellows from my neighborhood and we used to shoot out street lights and lights on bill-boards with staples. There was a lunch wagon and we shot out its windows.

There was a fellow had a motor boat and we shot out all its windows and drilled two holes in the bottom of it. He used to go out fishing in it. One time he threw all the clothes of the fellows when they were swimming into the water, so that's why we got even with him. Me and another fellow one time stole a row boat, one that belonged to this fellow, and he threw a hammer and a saw at us but he didn't hit either one of us. We just ran.

There was a dock nearby where we went swimming and diving off poles. They were real high, forty feet or so. The water was deep there too. Maybe fifty feet. A lot of people used to go swimming there. There was a Park on the other side of the Boulevard from the river. I'd spend a lot of time there too. They had concerts in the summer on the baseball diamond and you would see the grandstand and the baseball diamond filled with people. Up across the street from the Park there was a stand where we used to get ice cream. We'd steal from two to five gallons every week, sometimes two or three big cans a week.

After I got a little older, all the older fellows used to come around to the gang. I must have been about sixteen then. There was a young kid that got his leg cut off, the right leg at the ankle. That stopped most of the fellows from going to the railroad yard. Right along side of the railroad was a coal company that had a big trestle where the freight cars full of coal used to be pushed. That trestle was on a grade, and they would tie the freight cars so they wouldn't roll down. One time we unhooked them. They started down the grade and rolled and rolled and rolled.

There was a church school I used to go to, and an order of sisters that ran it. It was an Irish Catholic school. I couldn't see the blackboard and I was sitting in the back of the classroom. So I kept the other children from doing their work and used to get beatings for not having my lessons prepared. I think that me and another fellow—he had a paralyzed arm—were the worst two fellows in the class. I used to pal around with the best student in the class too. He used to live about a block away from me. I remember one time we were coming home from school about 4 o'clock and I got hold of a newspaper and was reading it. He made a kind of sarcastic remark to me: "Don't take the print off." I never forgot that and we were not such good friends again. I recall how he used to tell me that I might get in trouble, that if I did anything they would give me time. I didn't pay any attention to him and one time told him to mind his own goddam business. This boy used to have a blackjack that he carried around with him and one time he hit me on the toe. It hurt bad. When we were about twelve his brother showed me the gun he carried. This brother was nineteen or twenty then. He was like a gorilla, hair all over and big muscles.

It seemed then that I had to have a gun too.

We had a clubhouse in an old barn near the railroad station. There was a big sword in the clubhouse, about three feet long, and a big shotgun, a muzzle-loader with a double barrel. We also had some fur skins that we stole from a nearby leather factory.

To me a lot of these fellows in the gang seemed awfully stupid and dumb. For instance, one time we had a checkbook and none of them knew how to fill out a check. I told them how to fill one out and they all wanted to have a check.

When I belonged to this gang, me and another fellow found two cans of paint in the cellar of an old house. We threw a match into one of the cans and when it blazed we turned the can upside down. It started smoking and black smoke came. The floor was just dirt and pebbles and stone, and the black smoke was all around, and we were gasping for air. Finally we found the stairs and ran. We heard the firemen coming and they rushed into the house. After a while they came out and said there was nothing there.

When I was still about twelve we used to build big fires on the river bank. Sometimes we'd catch crabs in the river, over on the other side, and cook them. One time at Christmas we got hold of a lot of trees, about fifty or more Christmas trees, and we piled them on the river bank and lighted them. It made a big fire, a great big flame, maybe a hundred feet high. The fire engines came down and even the fire boat and they put it out.

We used to steal keys every place we could get them, automobile keys, garage keys, all kinds of keys. We got them and tried to open a lot of locks. I never went inside a garage we opened. We used to steal a lot of batteries right off cars and trucks and sell them for one dollar apiece. That's how we got some money.

One time we broke into a paint shop. We pulled two or three boards out at the back of the building. Two of the fellows went inside. There was a police station right across the street from this place. A policeman came from the railroad station and went through the parking lot behind the paint shop. He had a flashlight and we knew it. So I told them to put the boards back in place and we lay down flat so when he would flash the light he wouldn't see us. He went by and didn't even flash his light. He went right through to the police station. We got nothing but paint, some ink, some pens, some old junk.

I remember one time we broke into a butcher stop.

Shop. A slip of the tongue. Orthodox analysts would regard this as a potent manifestation of resistance.

There were a lot of cigarettes. One of the fellows took about twenty packs. I told him to take them all; there were about three hundred. When the police found the place where we hid them in the barn the cigarettes were missing. Somebody must have stolen them from us.

Before I came here we had an apartment over a tavern. There was always a lot of noise and racket going on, but it was quiet when I came home at night. I would sleep, but the next day my mother would tell me about the noise and the racket. My mother now lives at grandmother's.

Directly across the street from my grandmother's house there is a lot. There are two garages on it. My father rents one of the garages and keeps one of his cars in the other. The other car he keeps out in the open. He said he bought this other car for my sister; my sister said to give it to me but he wouldn't do that, so my sister said she didn't want it.

My sister is about twenty now. She has a job: she likes to work and dress up and go out. She didn't go to High with me: she quit when she graduated from grammar school.

Me and Arty, the fellow who was on parole with me, used to hang out at a blacksmith's shop. We used to watch the blacksmith work and talk with him. About nothing, I guess. Then I stopped hanging around there. There was a trucking company right down the street from the smith's shop; they used to have crap games there. I never shot craps there: I couldn't see the dice.

I used to play pinochle with my cousin. He used to cheat me. My cousin John.

I'd stay out late a lot, go to a poolroom and play pool, listen to the radio, get drunk, do nothing at all. I'd stay out late and my mother would holler at me and hit me.

I got up early in the morning to get something to eat for my father before he went to work. I hardly ever spoke to my father. I don't know why. We never got along. He always jumped on me: he used to tell me how hard he had been working. Many times him and my mother would be arguing about me. I heard them but I made believe I never heard anything about it. When I write a letter home I hardly think of him and never even mention him. Sometimes my mother tells me how he feels; my sister does too. I never ask.

One time while he was busy fixing his car my mother told me to call him for supper. When I went to call him he didn't hear me, so I went nearer to call him again. He picked up a hammer and wanted to hit me with it. He said I had been cursing him. I guess I was about thirteen then.

I used to spend a lot of time at the park. There was a big bunch of fellows there on Saturday or Sunday night, all gambling and drinking, singing and making a lot of noise. Everybody would run in different directions when the radio car came around. I would go to the concerts there. All the girls from that neighborhood would go too. I tried to see how they would act when I talked to them. Most of them I discovered were just bums. I found that the girls who talked like ladies were the worst bums of all.

On Saturday and Sunday nights we had nothing to do and so three or four fellows would go to the show. We'd make a lot of noise and many times they threw us out. Whenever we would see several girls sitting together we'd sit near them and talk to them and make remarks until they got up and walked away.

Sometimes I used to just like to go and go and walk to the outskirts of the city. I liked to go away somewhere by myself. When I was at my aunt's home on the farm I'd go out in the woods sometimes and spend the whole day by myself. My uncle was the same way. He used to go and get away from everybody, way up in the mountains. It's cool up there, brooks run down the side of the mountain. In the winter I would go up into the mountains and chop wood. My aunt always liked to burn wood in her stove.

My uncle would eat a lot of meat. They always had chicken on the table and my aunt would find time to fry pancakes for him at every meal.

Sometimes I would go to my uncle's father's house. He had a big cherry orchard and on rainy or cloudy days when you couldn't do any work I would pick cherries. I'd eat more than I picked. I'd stay there all day long, just with my raincoat on. Lots of cherries in the trees. My uncle's father made cider and he'd get me drunk with it. My aunt didn't like it, didn't like it at all. There were a lot of arguments. He was an old man with grey hair and a grey mustache, an old thin man. He just said, "Well, it's nothing." My aunt used to yell and yell.

My uncle had a sister about two years and a half older than I was: I was sixteen and she was eighteen. She and some other girls would go out a lot. The fellows used to come around and take them out and lay them. One time, I remember, when she was in the kitchen, she called me in and she says she wants some love. I just turned around and I said, "No love today." And she said, "O yes, I forgot, you can't make love, you're blind." And I was so mad I held my penis and said, "This is blind too: it only has one eye." And my aunt heard it and came in and hit me. So when I came to go home from my aunt's house she came over to me and apologized. My uncle didn't say anything. That week I went home. I didn't want to be there anymore.

The last year I was there my father found some rubbers in my overalls pants. They were left from when I went around with Lila. He showed them to my uncle who burned them. My aunt told my mother and my mother hollered at me.

I can still hear my uncle's sister telling me that. I'll never forget it. She was not very fat: she had kind of brown hair with streaks of grey in it, or blond or something. She wasn't pretty: she was ugly. She had a friend who was big and fat. One time several fellows came to my uncle's house and brought a lot of whiskey with them. Everybody was drinking. Two of the fellows got drunk and they took the two girls outside but they came back very quickly. I don't think anything. . . .

THE TWENTY-FOURTH HOUR

As far back as I can remember I didn't like my father. I would never speak to him other than when it was necessary. For some reason I disliked him and I couldn't talk to him. I would tell my mother and sister to say things to him; I'd tell them and they'd tell him. My sister always got along with him. I got along best with my uncle. He and I were going to South America together when he received his bonus. He had a wife but he hadn't lived with her for eight years. He didn't get along very well with my father either. I guess it was because my father was quick-tempered and would argue with everybody. I know my father worked hard and didn't get much pay. He would always complain about something hurting him, his back or his head, and my mother babied him a lot.

When I was around twelve I got into trouble by breaking into a store with several other fellows and I went to the Juvenile Court and they sent me to the Home for three weeks. When I came back my father didn't say anything to me. He knew because my mother told him, and yet he didn't say anything about it. I figured he must be a pretty swell man if he didn't say anything to his son after he spent three weeks in a reform school. When I was older, around seventeen, he always wanted me to get a job. Whenever he'd see me he'd ask if I was looking for work. Usually I would lie to him and say yes, but he knew I was lying so he would turn around and call me a liar. That's why I would always try to be away from home when he came from work. I'd hear my father and mother arguing about me many times. When I was around seventeen I didn't have any job, no money, fed up with everything, so I figured I'd get money as easy and as quick as possible.

L: *'You were saying that your mother babied your father. Were you jealous of the attentions she showered on him?'*

When he had a sore back or something I didn't like the way she was so sorry for him.

L: *'Did you resent your mother's attentions to your father?'*

I always thought it was useless.

L: *'Did you ever have any distinct resentment against your father about that?'*

I think the only reason she was attentive to him was so he shouldn't be angry and start arguing with her. He always argued with her, that's the reason.

My father used to have two cars. He used one to go to work with; what the other car was bought for was because he wanted to get my sister interested in learning to drive and taking out a license. So one day she said to him in front of me, "What's the matter with him?" He said that he bought it for her, not for me. I guess I disliked him more after that. I guess he dislikes me too.

L: *'Why do you think he dislikes you?'*

I guess he couldn't hear very well so when he said something to me and I would answer him so he couldn't hear it he would think I'd given him a sarcastic answer.

L: *'Have you always disliked him or was there a time when you felt differently towards him?'*

I've always disliked him. He would always argue with somebody about something: he'd pick on me and my sister or my mother. Jesus! He'd even argue with my grandmother. I disliked him even more for that. Why should he argue with an old woman? But maybe there was a time when I liked him. I never talked to him because I felt he couldn't understand me. There are loads of reasons. One time I called him in to supper when he was fixing his car. He had a hammer in his hand and he said he would hit me in the head with it. I was about thirteen then. I didn't say anything, just let things go by. He told my mother about it and she argued with him. I could hear them.

When we lived on S——— Street we had four rooms; a kitchen, two bedrooms and a parlor. There was a door from one of the bedrooms to the parlor. I slept in the parlor sometimes and they slept in the next bedroom. My sister slept in the other bedroom. I—I— Sometimes I used to. I was sleeping in the bedroom next to their bedroom and I used to hear them moving over and—preparing for intercourse. Sometimes I heard my father tell my mother to—move—over and—and put her—legs up and . . . I hated to hear it. I would put the cover over my head and try not to listen. An action like that, it isn't nice for a son to hear. Many times I heard my father say to my mother, "What the hell do you think I married you for?" I'm not sure if I actually saw them doing anything like that.

> *There was marked overt resistance while the patient was speaking of physical relations between his parents. He twisted and squirmed on the couch, bit his lips and grimaced frequently.*

L: *'How do you suppose you would have felt if you had seen anything like that?'*

It's pretty hard to explain. I guess I hated to see him do anything like that in front of everybody. Sometimes when my sister used to get beatings from my father or mother—when she was younger she used to get hit sometimes for not listening to them—she would sit in the room crying, and I would go away by myself. I didn't like to see her get hit. My sister is a good girl. She works. She gives all her money to her mother. She doesn't play around with boys. My younger sister gets beaten a lot though. My mother beats her because she talks back. My mother is a timid woman; she cries right away. I guess I feel sorry for her, so I wanted to get away from everything and everybody and I'd leave home. I left home a lot of times; I can't remember how often but it was plenty.

L: *'If you had seen your parents during any intimacy, Harold, how do you suppose it would have appeared to you?'*

Well, it appeared that my father was hurting my mother. I guess it might have a lot of different meanings. Maybe I did see my father and mother do that. I can't recall. It must have been way back before I can remember. It might seem vulgar, brutal, filthy, dirty, or what not.

L: *'Is that the way a child would think?'*

Well, whenever we had to take a leak when we were little kids we would consider the penis dirty, nasty. My mother might have said that. She taught us that the genitals were dirty: she said that the penis was dirty.

I don't remember ever seeing my father naked. He strikes me as being the poor illiterate and ignorant European peasant type that come over to America to get something. They leave over there because there is nothing for them. He's a good mechanic but he doesn't know how to read or write. He has a big chest and a neck like a bull. He has a kind of pugilistic appearance. If I had ever seen anything like that it would make me feel as if he was hurting my mother, that he was choking her, killing her. But sometimes I know, when he was home and I was old enough to realize some things, I saw my father put his hands on my mother's buttocks. It didn't exactly appeal to me. I didn't think it was right. I guess I did feel a little resentment against my father for touching my mother.

L: *'You felt he shouldn't do it?'*

I disliked it when he did it in front of everybody. My mother would always tell him to look out for the children but he didn't care.

L: *'And you resented the fact that he handled your mother that way?'*

I certainly did.

L: *'You felt he had no right to?'*

Yes. But when I got older I saw it in a different light. I guess I know right from wrong.

L: *'You were jealous of him?'*

I must have thought that my father could at least be decent enough not to do anything like that in front of everybody.

L: *'You thought of your father's relationship with your mother as distasteful?'*

When I'd hear them in bed, hear them talk and him coaxing my mother I hated to listen to it. I'd put the covers over my head and try to shut out everything: sometimes I'd recite nursery rhymes to myself, just to forget, just to forget. I still sleep with the covers over my head. I hated to listen to it. I didn't want to. I didn't want to be around. I wanted to be away from there. I'd pull the covers over my head.

I don't remember much about my father and mother before that time. I got one severe beating from him for ruining his razor. He really beat me up: he lifted me from the ground and let me drop on the floor.

My mother told me that when they were first married he'd hit her. I hated him for that. I guess my mother was married to him about a week when she says she left him. They were living in B——— then and she came running back to my grandmother's; and my grandmother chased her back. My mother was about sixteen when they got married. Sometimes I wish my grandmother hadn't made her go back; she's had a very unhappy life with him.

Maybe he really is not as bad as I say he is. Maybe he treated my mother o.k. He always argued with my mother about me; why didn't I get a job, and this and that. When we lived on S——— Street, when I was about eleven, my mother would close the door between the parlor and the bedroom where I slept. She'd come in the room and just sit, read a book or look out the window. I didn't hear anything when she closed the door, but sometimes when it was warm the door would be opened and I'd have to sleep underneath the covers. Sometimes when my father came home from driving a truck he would have some kind of joke he would be aching to tell my mother, and I knew it must be a dirty joke of some kind. He would tell my mother to remind him to tell her and my mother would say, "If that's the kind of a joke I think it is I don't want to hear it." I knew it was a dirty joke when he would say anything like that and I disliked it; he shouldn't say anything like that to her. I guess I hated him. I remember when I was about eight or nine I was learning to ride a bicycle and there was a fellow that wanted to sell his for three dollars, so I asked my mother to buy it for me and she told me to ask my father. I didn't have guts enough to ask him; so finally I mentioned it at the table and he said, "What do you want to do, get killed?" So I never asked him for anything again. I have often wondered why I didn't want to ask him for anything. Now I think that's the reason.

I know my father used to chase a lot of women. My mother told me. My mother was born in this country and she could read and write and speak English good. I got along alright with her. My mother, my oldest sister and myself were always more like companions. O, we had a few arguments, but they were nothing. Sometimes my mother told me about the things my father used to do: how he used to hit her when they were first married. I was old enough then to think about such things. I didn't form any hasty opinions.

I think the reason my mother's godfather left us is that he had an argument with my father.

My father doesn't drink or smoke but my mother told me that he used to go around in his car picking up women. I don't know if she ever said anything to him. She said she knew he was doing it.

I'd tell myself when I saw how my mother and father fought that I'd never get married.

I always used to dress neatly, clean clothes; my mother always saw to it that we were clean. She'd try to help me with my ABC's, teach me how to add. My father never did anything like that.

Often I'd go to sleep on the davenport and when I woke up my mother'd be there. I guess she came in during the middle of the night to see if I was comfortable. She'd cry a lot too. She'd argue with my father; he would holler at her so she'd go somewheres by herself and cry and pay no attention to anybody or anything; and she would take my sister or me on her lap and cry. She'd never tell us why she was crying.

He used to say things about my eyes and curse me out.

My sister was a tomboy and he would say things about cutting off my penis and giving it to her.

L: 'Do you remember him actually saying that?'

When I was around eight or under he would say things like that. He was always telling dirty jokes. I feel there is something there. He said something like that. He used to say those kind of things then, lots of things.

L: 'Such as . . . ?'

A lot of dirty jokes. He would hint around at the table. When he was telling dirty jokes I didn't like to hear him tell them in front of my sister and myself. I didn't like to be around. My mother would holler at him to be quiet. He said something about cutting off my penis and giving it to my sister. She was a tomboy when she was a kid and he'd tease her about it. She'd fight with all the kids. One time there was a kid about my age she had a fight with because he said something about my eyes. She would always hold up like that for me when I was young. I know my father used to fix cars and he made a car once out of an old taxi. He changed the body and painted it up and sold it. I was afraid he'd change my body too. He always said he wished I was the girl instead of my sister. He likes her best. I remember when I was eight he said he wished she was the boy: that she was the best one; she would fight anybody and was afraid of nobody. He always said I ran to my mother in case anything happened. He would say I was the girl and she was the boy. I remember one time we had a dog, a little dog named Nellie. He would tell me that he would sic the dog on me and the dog would bite off my penis. The dog was a wild dog: she'd bite anybody; and she used to listen to my father and do what he told her. I don't know whether he actually did sic the dog on me but he said that once or twice. We had the dog for about two or three years when we lived on B——— Street. She got killed by a car: she always chased cars. I guess I was under eight when he said that. He used to threaten me about this dog. The dog bit me one time when I was running past the alley. He said it once or twice in Polish, never in English. In Polish he said he'd sic the dog on me so she'd bite off my penis. I remember one time at the table he said that. My mother came to my rescue and scolded him for saying it. Then she started telling me that Nellie wouldn't bite me and she called her over and told me to pat her head to see she wouldn't bite me. It might have been when I was seven. I remember I got along with the dog better after that: she was always with me. I was very small then. I guess my sister wasn't more than four.

I can see it all; like a picture. My sister, real small. I can see my hands. My sister has dirty-blond hair, straight, cut in front. It seems so real to me. I can see the knicker pants I've got on and I feel so small in the chair. My father looks like he always looked to me. I have a distaste for his appearance; he always needs a shave.

L: 'When your father made that threat, do you remember how you felt? Were you afraid he'd carry it out?'

Yes; I was afraid he would. I didn't know what to do. When he said that my mother was sitting on the other side of me. She told my father, "What do you want to say things like that for?" She touched my knee, put her hand on my knee and touched it and said, "Don't worry; Nellie wouldn't bite you." Then she called the dog over. The dog was dark-colored and white underneath the chin and neck and throat, and the dog's tail was wagging as my mother was patting him. She told me, "Pat him on the head, Harold." I was afraid of dogs for a while after that. His tail was wagging and she kept patting him and saying to me, "He won't bite you." The dog looked at me with such pitiful eyes and he put his head under my leg when I kept on patting him.

L: 'Was Nellie a he or a she?'

She was a female dog . . .

THE FORTY-SIXTH HOUR

L: 'Harold; have you been thinking about the things we've been discussing?'

Yes. I've been thinking about it, and I was also thinking how it really does connect. I know they do connect because sometimes I can't think of anything right in this room and when I am four or five hours by myself sometimes it will just come to me and I can refer to it, associate it with something we said here. Everything we said is true. I know something has happened to my eyes. I don't know what it is but they never looked before like they look now. The lenses are contracted and I can read small print now and they wink about half as much as they did before. But the most important thing is what's happened to me. Now that I know all these things I feel like a different person. I get along better with people now and I understand why I do things and I don't anymore act without thinking. There's lots of chance to get messed up in here, and now that I know why I want to do something I can keep myself from doing it. Before I would just do it and not think of why or what was going to happen. But about my eyes . . . A lot of specialists, doctors who treat nothing except diseases of the eye, they all said that the nerves are all good, that there is no reason my eyes were like that. My mother always thought it was due to the measles. Will measles have that effect on people's eyes?

L: *'Yes; measles can have an effect on the eyes; it may make them more sensitive to light. But it is very doubtful that such was the complete situation in your case. As a matter of fact, we know that your eyes were winking before you had the measles: therefore your winking certainly could not have been due to it. The measles, though, might well have reenforced the original condition. You had this traumatic, that is, shocklike, incident in your early life, and that appears to be the original cause of your winking. Now when you got the measles, this condition was undoubtedly aggravated. You see, physicians tell us that many diseases follow this process: the disease affects what is called the 'area of least resistance' in your body. Suppose, for instance, that a germ enters your body, and there already is a weakness (let us say) in your kidneys. It's quite likely, then, that this germ will settle in your kidney because its natural powers of resistance are already weakened. Now in your case it's perfectly possible that the measles may have affected your eyes, because your eyes were already weakened.'*

But now, within the last few months and especially the last few weeks, they wink much less. Before I could never keep them open at all for more than a second or so. They wink much less and I can see a lot better . . .

Doc, I wonder if you would please go through the whole thing, like a summary of the whole business?

L: *'If you wish.*

'It all goes back to that morning. Now the night before; I think we can say with assurance that the night before was a Saturday night, and that evening you went to the moving pictures with your mother and your father. You were between six and eight months old. You were in your mother's arm, half-sitting, half-lying, and your father was sitting on the other side. You were looking across your mother and saw your father. The theatre was dark except for the lights coming from the projecting booth. Now on the screen you saw the face and figure of a dog or a wolf (probably a dog, probably Rin-tin-tin who was popular around that time), so that the face of the dog became closely associated with the light from the projecting room. You could see the light shining, as it were, directly

on the dog. You were frightened by the dog, by what you saw, and you may or may not have been crying—whether you were or were not is unimportant: you were afraid.

'Now the following morning you awaken early. Your mother is lying on the right side of her bed; your cradle is near her. You look across— the same way as you looked across from your mother's arms the evening before—and you see your father. You see him, and it looks as if he is hurting your mother. As a matter of fact he is lying on her. His face is hard; his eyes are hard; but your mother's eyes are tender and she looks as if she is being hurt. As your father withdraws, you see his penis. It looks to you like a strange, vicious animal. It looks like an instrument that can hurt, for you immediately apprehend that it is this which is hurting your mother. And you were afraid of it because you dimly knew that seeing your father and mother in that position was something you weren't supposed to see: and the reason you knew you weren't supposed to see it was because your mother pushed your father off and pointed to you, and he stopped what he was doing and removed himself. And then you were afraid of it because you thought it was going to hurt you.*

'Now your mother gets out of bed. She comes over to your cradle and takes you out and into the other room, to the breakfast table. Your father comes in. At the breakfast table you look at your father; and immediately the shock of what just happened and the shock of the events of the night before, become associated directly with him. You look at him and you are afraid of him, of him and of his penis. Everything he does reminds you of these things that have happened. There is an awful amount of fear there. As a child, you feel it, and you start to cry. And as you start to cry it seems to you as if the whole room is getting black. All these events have served to remind you (since with a child so young all time is condensed and there are no sharp lines to divide time) of the night before, at the moving picture, where the blackness was pierced by the light from the projecting room. Now you seem to see it coming from your father's eyes. His face seems all 'cut-up' just like the face of the dog you saw in the movie.*

'Your mother placates you and calms you. But immediately you are completely alienated from your father, afraid of him. He reminds you of the things that caused you discomfort, fear, terror. And the fear of his penis, which seemed to be a threatening, dangerous and brutal weapon, thrusts you even more upon your mother, whom you believed it had hurt.*

'So you closed your eyes. You ran away from it. The winking has come from the association of all this fear with the event you had witnessed. As we have seen, one way of running away from something is to* *close your eyes to it. Because for you the whole thing centered in your eyes. The eyes were the guilty organs. They were guilty of having seen that which they were forbidden to see. Now the fear of your father's penis—and all it meant—followed you through all your life. You have always felt afraid and inadequate and aggressive toward your father because your weapon was not as big or as powerful as your father's. So you later played with knives and guns: you stole money to buy guns. You were trying to convince yourself that you had a penis; trying to prove yourself as good as your father. And all the while the original dependence upon your mother became re-enforced as it became increasingly evident that you could never accept your father's relations with your mother, or reconcile yourself to him in view of your fear of him.*

"*Now every male child—or at any rate most male children—go through a period of such 'castration fears,' fears of losing the penis. You were afraid your father would steal this thing from you, would take it away. Your father actually threatened to have his dog bite it off.*'

Yes; it was my father's dog. It would only listen to him . . .

L: '*And remember: when you saw your father that morning, he reminded you of the dog in the show the night before.*

'*All your life you have been haunted by these castration fears and anxieties. That's one reason why you masturbated frequently. It was a very good way of convincing yourself from time to time that you were still manly, you still had a penis. And always it was closely associated with your eyes. It always has been. You even thought later on that when people looked at your eyes they could tell that you had been masturbating. So that's really why you closed your eyes: to shut out that first sight, that first knowledge. You had a deep feeling of guilt and you were afraid . . . so you hid your eyes. All through your life this relationship—your father's eyes and his penis to your eyes and your fear of his penis—has been following you.*'

Yes—yes. I can see it all. I can see it all now. That's why I took those knives and that pen knife from him.

I always thought I couldn't get along with my father, talk to him in a sensible way. When I'd say anything to him he'd always be right and I'd always be wrong. I always thought that was one way to keep apart, one reason we didn't talk together much; but I see now I had reasons to show him that I was as good as he was. He was stronger than me, so I was afraid of him. He'd tell me I was wrong so I wouldn't say anything to him.

L: '*And you were always afraid he'd have you castrated.*'

O, yes. Maybe two years ago they were going to sterilize all convicts, people said. I laughed it off in front of everybody but I thought about it and thought about it. I never told anyone but I was afraid, so afraid. As a matter of fact, that idea has been in the back of my head for as long as I can remember . . .

My mother was always good to me. I always could talk to my mother. When my father threatened to sic the dog on me to bite my penis off my mother comforted me and said the dog wouldn't do it. She called the dog over, and when the dog had its paws on my lap I was afraid of him. Later on I started petting him myself . . .

L: *'To a child, things of that sort are very serious, crucial. It had, in your case, plenty of background as well. The soil was well prepared. First there was that very traumatic incident accompanied by the fear of your father's organ; then the deep fixation on your mother; then the castration fears. As a result, all your life you've felt inadequate, castrated. You could never do anything, never get anywhere.'*

Even when I was growing up, from the time I was fourteen, I remember I always used to think in the back of my mind that the other fellows were better than me at driving a car, or swimming, or making some pretty girls, or in school. I was really a bright kid in school though, the best of all the boys in most of my classes. And swimming—I could swim and drive a car pretty well but . . . As a matter of fact, when I had intercourse with a girl I never liked to look at or touch her genitals, because they made me think of a castrated man, or made me think about not having genitals myself . . .

And then that—accident . . . I see I did it to get rid of my father somehow without really having to get rid of *him*. The whole thing fits. I'm sorry about that. I wish . . .

L: *'And the stealing?'*

The stealing? It—I—it was because I—wanted my mother and that was . . . I wasn't allowed to have her. So I stole things. I went into houses alone because I—didn't—want anybody else to—have her . . .

Yes. It's all right now. I even *feel* it now.

L: *'Now that you understand these things, Harold, we shall have to have a period of re-education before we are finished. We want to accomplish a complete change in your attitude toward yourself and the rest of the world. The eyes will take care of themselves. They are unimportant compared with the complete overhauling of your personality and life. There is nothing more to fear now.'*

I can see everything as it went by . . . All the years. All the things changed, the symbols changed and that's all; but what they stood for was still there. I used to be so afraid of his big arms and hands, afraid he'd beat me with them, so I went through many things. I can see now how it—all—made steps, all along, all the ways up . . .

Here Harold was placed in a deep hypnotic sleep. Under hypnosis, he was requested to review the entire case and demonstrate his understanding of it. He was also asked to review the writer's summary and his own remarks as they occurred in the final hour. Finally, his comprehension was re-enforced by suggestion . . .

14. The Existential Therapeutic Approach to Homosexuality*

George Serban

Psychologists and psychiatrists supporting various nonanalytic treatments of homosexuality frequently cite the failure of psychoanalysis to bring about or contribute to the changing of homosexual behavior. Those who criticize Freudian psychology do so for a variety of reasons. Behaviorists, for example, who do not generally concern themselves with unconscious and emotional fixation, would therefore treat homosexuality as a learned response vulnerable to experimental extinction. Existential psychotherapists also disagree with the Freudian concept of preheterosexual fixation in development, but they are more concerned with the authenticity of the individual and the choices he has made which may have led to an inauthentic existence. Believing that man has the freedom to choose an authentic existence, this type of therapy must deal with these choices.

Serban has applied the principles of existentialism in the treatment of a homosexual man. Homosexuality represented, in this patient, inauthenticity. Homosexuality was a mode of life chosen to avoid feeling nonmasculine and it tended to perpetuate the feelings it was constructed to avoid. The patient felt ineffective as a man and sought homosexual relations with physically strong men. Although this gave him a brief feeling of possessing a strong masculine body, his satisfaction was, at the same time, negated by his thoughts of himself as a homosexual. The despair and anguish in which he had been trapped by his choices and

*Presented at a meeting of the New York Ontoanalytic Association, May, 1967. Reprinted by permission of The Association for the Advancement of Psychotherapy from the *American Journal of Psychotherapy*, 1968, **22**, 491-501.

magical thinking reached a peak when he considered the value of his existence and the choice of self-extinction and non-being. At that point he sought help. The value of phenomenology, which emphasizes the meaning of personal experience in the understanding of behavior, is demonstrated as a tool of the existential psychotherapist in the successful treatment reported here.

Freud's concept of homosexuality, which was acclaimed by its protagonists as a breakthrough in the understanding of human sexuality by opening new avenues for the treatment of patients, has proved to be of little clinical value. In fact, the ambiguous and pessimistic position taken by Freud in later years in his famous letter addressed to an American mother made any attempt to treat homosexuality a disheartening, if not impossible, effort (1). Moreover, his theories about homosexuality—keynotes in the psychoanalytic conceptualization of human sexual development—have increasingly been attacked by his own followers. The less the theories fitted the clinical realities, the more they required re-examination and modification, to the point of total revision. However, all those who attacked Freud, like Sullivan, Karen Horney, Rado, and Bergler, have only changed the emphasis of approach from the oedipal level to the interpersonal sphere of love, without any ability to liberate themselves from the basic framework of their hypothetical assumptions of the main body of Freudian theories.

To the extent to which the theories failed to provide a clear formulation, the therapy was left confused, with speculative interpretations of a haphazard nature. The best hope was to reconcile the patient to his condition by alleviating his guilt. A mutual sense of hopelessness made the treatment merely palliative. For example, the most recent statistics of I. Bieber show a 10 per cent success with exclusively homosexual patients and 27 per cent for the whole group (2). These discouraging results leave open to question not only the theoretical psychoanalytic framework of interpretation of sexual conflict, but psychoanalysis per se as a method of treatment of homosexuality.

For this reason, I will try to present a new therapeutic concept based on the phenomenological interpretation of the homosexual condition. It has evolved during the process of treating 25 homosexuals. I will describe the essential aspects of therapeutic interest of one case, in an attempt to answer the following questions:

What interplay of forces made the individual choose, among other choices, this particular mode of existence? Is it only a sexual mode of existence or a whole world of being?

What is the meaning for the being of this particular mode of existence?

CASE HISTORY

The patient, in his mid-twenties, was the only son of a low middle income family. The father, a house painter, was somewhat detached, disinterested in family affairs, and apparently argued continuously with his wife; he separated from her a few times until he finally divorced her when the patient was nine. The patient had only a vague recollection of his father, since the father was always away and never showed any real interest in him. His mother, cold, aggressive, neglected him emotionally because she was more concerned with her own love affairs until she remarried when he was about ten. The stepfather was described as pleasant; he took care of him but was uncommunicative, brusque, rude, and sometimes violent.

The patient spent most of his early childhood outdoors, playing all year round under the California sun. His life in the family was monotonous and uneventful, sometimes punctuated by outbursts of arguments between his parents, or between him and his two older sisters who were supposed to look after him. The only meaningful memories to him are related to the short periods he spent with his grandmother who gave him a sense of being wanted and loved.

The patient claims that his first memories are related to his behavior in kindergarten. At that time some of the other boys frightened or abused him. He felt too weak to fight back and preferred "to keep his distance." During elementary school his relationships with other children improved to some degree, but mainly because he did not get involved with them and was subservient. In junior high school he had the feeling that his body, against his expectations, did not grow "quite well." He felt small, unattractive, and weak. His problem was compounded by the fact that he had to wear glasses, which gave him a sense of fragility. He remembers being ashamed to undress in front of the other boys and refusing to expose his naked body at gym. He could never forget when his two sisters made fun of him by calling him "funny ribs." Apparently, he was skinny and his lower ribs protruded ungraciously. Uncomfortable and self-conscious about his body, he tried to hide it under smart clothing. Ungainly, wearing glasses, he retreated from the other boys' games, an outside observer, resented and at the same time admiring them. "I could not play basketball or baseball. I felt clumsy. They laughed at me, at the way I threw the ball. They used to ignore me. I admired and envied those good at games. The girls talked to them and the same girls ignored me. I wanted the friendship of one of the players very much; I wanted one of those strong guys to be my pal."

Above average in intelligence, but withdrawn, shy, without real friends, he became more and more involved with himself. He daydreamed about "wonderful things happening" to him. He identified with public heroes, wondered about their exploits, and dreamed of becoming one of them. Books took him out of this world and gave him a maximum of gratification because he relived the lives of his heroes in his own imagination. Generally, his heroes were artists or actors. Particularly actors held a fascination for him; he enjoyed going to the movies and could integrate them easily in his daydreams, especially Westerners.

Unable to express his being, to belong to this world, unable to hold ground on it, he tried to escape beyond the world into a different one which he could master and enjoy because it fitted his needs. Addicted to daydreaming, the real world melted into an unreal one, that of fantasy and wish fulfillment.

He went through high school detached, disinterested, without friends, and with a deep complex about lacking that unidentifiable quality of maleness. With the upsurge of sexuality his sexual gratification was restricted to masturbatory fantasies of being involved in amorous situations of a chivalrous nature, but without any notion of lovemaking. Even later on he could not conceive the idea that somebody might want him. With girls he was very conscious of his alleged ungainly body, ashamed of his looks, and toward boys he had mixed feelings of admiration and inferiority. He felt unable to offer anything to anybody, to compete with boys, or to try to conquer a girl, because either way "I was not a man. I could not talk tough like other boys. I lacked conviction and authority. I listened to their exploits without having anything to say. Sometimes I walked away. They didn't care either way. I wanted to be one of them. With girls I didn't even know what I was supposed to do on a date. I felt a stranger, an outsider. As a mark of distinction, I cultivated my strangeness which became a kind of eccentricity for them."

Therefore, when he was drafted into the Army, he was excited and at the same time afraid that everyone would laugh at him, especially when seeing his body in various Army situations. Obsessively, throughout the years he tried to conceive a type of male behavior which would compensate for his alleged physical deficiencies. In fact, he succeeded in improving his diction and in acquiring an aristocratic, condescending manner which, combined with an air of aloofness, would have given him, he thought, a relative sense of security. In the Army he was afraid that the mock screen would fall and that his true self, "the mouse," as he called himself, would be revealed. His first pleasant surprise was to see that everybody treated him properly and somehow he managed to make a few friends. But he felt that this situation was due to the close association in Army life in which they had "to put up with each other."

However, the most unusual thing happened to him when one of his casual friends, after a week end drinking spree, showed an emotional interest in his body. That man wanted and was excited by his body. Naturally, this led to mutual masturbatory activity. It was the first time that someone had expressed a genuine interest in him and his body. It became the first revelation of his body existence for others, though outside of any social, conventional, formal relationships. But, as he said: "I was an outsider anyway. I shared secretly in a kind of intimate conspiracy something with somebody and that something was always rejected before." The highly prized quality of experience gave a sense and direction to his life. Finally, one year later, after being suspected of homosexual activities, he was released from the Army with an honorable discharge. But the meaningfulness of the relationship gave him a feeling of a deep participation with others who previously had rejected him in games, or despised and ridiculed him throughout the years. In a sense he became a man, at least like these men.

Discharged from the Army, with a new sense of value of his body and himself, he saw a new world opening to him where he could find emotional support. With any new boy friend he reinforced his old need for body recognition and sexual want. He felt that the long search for the sense of belonging and fulfillment had ended now. "Surprisingly enough, men better off than me, with nice bodies, handsome, intelligent, became friendly with me. They wanted me, they appreciated me, and I sensed why. I had something for them, a large penis, something which they wanted very much."

After a change of various menial or clerical jobs, he decided under the influence of one of his lovers, an actor, to become what he had dreamed about during the lonely years—an actor. Now, since he was not only accepted by men in bed, but was found cute, if not attractive, he felt no compunction in trying to expose his body on the stage—it was like a symbolic need for a mass acceptance. He started to play with various small companies in small theaters. On the stage, he felt that all the applause was directed at him as a sign that he and his body were accepted. In the theater he became what he was not but should have been: the hero. Love and hate, grandeur and failure, old frustrations and repressed feelings were consummated on the stage. The other self came to life in the floodlights of the theater and with the encouragement of a supporting audience. Theatrical successes made him feel wanted, important, and loved, although, from a "distance," without others seeing his real self. But everything was a mock dream because "outside of the glittering lights of the stage I felt lost." Alone, he again saw his real body-look, otherwise carefully concealed under the external appearance of would-be maleness.

To him the most desirable thing was to look masculine to others, and to this pursuit he dedicated his free time. He cultivated his voice, calculated his posture and gait, and pondered his behavior for the utmost, allegedly masculine effect. Fascinated by classical sculptures, he used to spend hours either looking through art books or visiting museums. The hope of building up his body at gym was a constant preoccupation of his. At other times at home he would browse through male model magazines for hours, stirring up powerful sexual fantasies which led to sexual self-stimulation. The world became focused on an obsessive want to catch the illusive mysterious fragrance, the essence of maleness. Thought and action, fantasy and reality, were interpreted through the prism of its virile meaning and its sexual connotation.

However, the doubts were there, always questioning his intentions, always berating his efforts. At the end of each day's effort at capturing that masculine image, he looked at his body despisingly. He hated it. The old body gestalt of his childhood and adolescence was revived, painfully and dramatically. Then a feeling of hopelessness would overcome him. The need for reaffirmation of his body's qualities would sometimes take on obsessive proportions. It drove him on to compare it with another male body in the contest of love. In a state of frenzy, he had to find a man. If nobody was available among his friends, the long, subtle, devious, and dangerous search—though abhorrent to him—of finding a partner through "cruising" would start. "I would work myself up to a state of trance. I wanted somebody to possess my body, to tell me nice things about my body, my penis. I wanted to hold a strong body, to touch and feel it, to have it given to me. It was like being under a spell." Only handsome strong males interested him, because only they could offer him the best proof of acceptance. The sexual moment was a climactic gratification of possessing and being possessed as a body. Afterwards, the meaning of the relationship was lost; it reminded him only of being a homosexual. "I hated myself and the other. I wanted to run away. A gap, a void, stood between us." Any communication was superfluous. When the fascination was gone, a deep feeling of emptiness would surround him. He felt that the majority of his lovers were either conceited or "faggots," and he hated their mask and mannerisms, their imperceptible homosexual airs. He fully realized that he was wanted sexually, in terms of his well developed penis. He could hardly overlook the other's interest, fascination, and craving for his large penis. It was like a mutual trade of deep-seated longing. "They wanted my impressive penis and I wanted their body. A mutual envy was present in the deal; a mutual resentment concluded it."

The world design of sex was confused. Women were seen blurred, far away, untouchable and unattainable. He started to wonder what kind of experience men might have with them. He rejected being a homosexual and resented the women who he felt did not accept him. He wondered whether his inability to relate to women, at least socially, was not due to his homosexual outlook or his airs, as conveyed by his body. Within his own theatrical group, in order to discourage any personal intimacy with women who might find out "terrible things about him," he behaved arrogantly, caustically, wittily, and distantly. In general, he put a wall between himself and others and hid himself behind it under an air of abstract intellectualism or transcendental preoccupations.

Alone, with the mask off, he felt lonely and depressed. Even when his theatrical career moved somewhat toward success, his loneliness became unbearable. The longing for love in a meaningful emotional communication became a dream unattainable to reach. At one time he thought he was in love with another man. However, he felt that the situation was unrewarding, implying a sense of sham in which each lover tries to find or impose his maleness at the expense of his partner. He felt that the deep resentment for their existing situation would make the love totally unstable and unpredictable. The search for the ideal partner from whom he could finally extract that elusive masculinity, vanishing as soon as the orgasm was over, became an endless project of his life. And with it the sense of isolation and inability to reach for himself estranged him from the world. A paralyzing feeling of emptiness and disintegration would overtake him from time to time. He felt himself sinking into non-existence in which he would lose the sense of his being and of his life expression. The flow of time became more frightening to face as present, or projected into the future. Any future anticipation was anxiety creating by his inability to surpass the established pattern. In reality, his denial of the possibilities of his being, as a man, brought him closer to nothingness. His inability to transcend his falling into non-being undermined his freedom, the very foundation of his being. Unable to break the chains which limited his existence to a self-defeating goal, unable to free his being from his mirage-pursuit, he concealed it in the duplicity[1] of his consciousness. He was a man, with his maleness proven only in a homosexual situation which in itself destroyed the very idea of being a man.

When his emotional anguish reached the high point of questioning the value of his existence and its purpose, the fantasy of self-extinction

---

[1] The coexistential consciousness of being the deceived and the deceiver of his own being.

overcame him. It became obsessively present, frightening, and at the same time relieved his mind. It was a future possibility, a final solution, the ultimate act of freedom in the service of non-being for total annihilation of his being. But the dread of death at the same time made the patient realize the possible loss of all other possibilities which could have preceded the final one. By questioning his position toward his mode of existence, the patient asked for help. He wanted to find out what went wrong with him, since he felt condemned by this inability to express his freedom of decision in making his own choice of life.

In this short fragment of phenomenological analysis, I have tried to show the central drama of his conflict progressively evolving—despair versus duplicity of consciousness as related to his concept of maleness.

DISCUSSION

The therapeutic approach was directed toward the solution of this very conflict. But in order to do so, the patient's problem had to be reduced to its essence, that is, his inability to convince himself without a shadow of doubt of the maleness of his body, sexually or otherwise. To the extent to which he was unable to do so, his life became a long series of events related or directed, in the totality of a life project, toward relieving his ontological anxiety of non-being itself. His mode of existence became dedicated to this cause: the pursuit of would-be masculinity. His world became restricted to his goal, and his reality distorted by his own created needs: a continuous struggle and competition for sexual identification through sexual expression with others.

Theoretically, two possibilities were open to him, either to prove this sexual identification in relationship to the opposite sex, or in context with his own sex. In order to comprehend the full meaning of his actions, one first has to clarify the concept of sexuality which the patient developed with the advent of puberty and thereafter. Important to note in this case is that the maturated sex organ, instead of becoming contingent on the psychic body in order to express harmoniously the upsurge of his new emotional need of relating to the opposite sex, became separated due to the patient's inability to accept his body as sexually desirous to the other sex. Unable to do so, the sexual organ, instead of expressing any definite image of sexuality, was used purely for physiologic self-relief. The sexual desire toward the opposite sex could not have been carried because of the psychic body image which denied its value for the opposite sex. Under this condition the sexual organ as an instrument for sex could have carried only the type of sexual desire directed toward the confirmation of the body's search for identification (3). And he wanted the boys because in them he could find a meaning to his unaccepted masculinity; with them, the line of communication was open. He was solicited by them in one way or another in the close relationships of the Army. The gratification of the body gave to his sexual drive a specific direction of expression of his dormant sexuality for others. Logically, his solution was perfect, for his age at that time at least, but socially and ontologically it led him to bankruptcy. It could give him only instant satisfaction, but otherwise everlasting denial of maleness as a biologic force, which in reality has the need to be reinforced by the opposite sex.

Thus the patient found himself caught in a strange psychic mechanism, that of a duality of consciousness. He tried to maintain simultaneously a balance between two opposite ideas, between a thesis—that of maleness, and its antithesis—that of homosexuality, between a concept and its negation (3). Obsessively, he tried to reach for a synthesis of the two. But he never succeeded in doing so. To conceptualize his thinking, one might say that the patient developed and used a pattern of logic in which, while differentiating between the facticity[2] of an idea and its transcendence, he changed their logical position, replacing one with the other, in the process of doing. In other words, he strove to prove the maleness of his body in the sexual contest with another man, but by doing so he negated the very thesis under exploration.

How was it possible for him to do this? Under close scrutiny, one finds that he introduced surreptitiously into his mechanism of thinking an element foreign to our commonly acceptable logic, an element of magical, supernatural belief which became an accepted premise for him, directing the outcome of his actions. He gave his body to others as if through a supernatural power he could have rubbed off the other one's masculinity; at the end of the game he came out less of a man due to the facticity of his own action, the transcendence of which he negated. In essence, we might say that the patient used an operational concept of ambiguity toward himself. The distortion of the logic made him be what he was, a homosexual, a product of his past experiences, and at the same time, to want to be what he had not been, a man, by dissociating himself from the past and recreating it over and over again in the future.

But how and why did the patient use this particular logic—let us call it metalogic. This was not a decision taken as such, not an elaborated, sophisticated system of lying; it was a pattern of thinking, evolved from a system of seeing and being seen in the world. It can be safely said at this point that if the thinking of the schizophrenic is paralogical, the thinking of the neurotic—the homosexual—is metalogical. The structure of the thinking is obviously based on this imponderable element of super-

---

[2]"The characteristic of Dasin's being which has been taken up into existence . . . ." (4).

natural want, hope, and belief. It defies the Aristotelian laws of logic. The metalogical thinking operates with either ambiguous or contradictory premises, where the conclusions are reached by the patient's introduction of an extra element of personal belief, unrelated to the judgment in itself, but used as a categorical proposition in the totality of his thinking. This type of thinking has been loosely identified in the past by psychiatrists as emotional thinking, a formulation which is vague and psychologically meaningless. The metalogic has gradually developed to serve a purpose, to enable the patient to escape from a crushing reality of not being what he pretends to be and is not. This type of thinking has evolved over the years, surreptitiously taking over his being, and making the patient surround himself with a frail reality and veil of evidence to support his ambivalent position.

But the duplicity of thinking created this duplicity of the world. His world was ambiguous and gay, a self-made world of inauthenticity which led him to despair and nothingness, because it was based on the negation of the world design of sex. The negation of his being made him untrue to himself and brought out the feelings of despair and depression.

Accepting his destiny in the Freudian tradition of unconscious determinism would mean to consider himself arrested, fixated at one period of life. To become reconciled with it, to try to make the best of it, would mean to lose his freedom of choice, would mean to restrict himself to non-being. Paradoxically, from the point of view of therapy, it would mean to reinforce his metalogical thinking by offering more rationalizations based at this time on alleged unconscious motivation which supposedly commands and controls his drives. But, can the patient truly deny that all his impulses are set free without his conscious consent? (3). Can the patient sincerely accept that any new commitment to action is outside of his responsibility, without any meaningful value attached to it? Obviously not. Otherwise, the patient would not be in therapy. The only thing which he can do is not to deny the responsibility for the act, but by splitting his consciousness in the moment of duplicity, to place the meaning of the act in the past, away from the present. The future is clear, until it becomes anguishing past in the process of redoing.

What then should the therapeutic method be for his despair of nonbeing? Certainly, to break the vicious cycle which suffocated the true emotional expression of the patient. The therapeutic sessions tried to uncover methodically and progressively the factors involved in his early formulation of his body concept with its sexual connotation for others as they had emerged from his metalogical thinking. Since for the patient the body had become the unique point of reference toward the world, with the resulting mode of sexuality as an expression of it, a detailed analysis of his projected quality of the body was required. The way the patient wanted his body to be seen by others in various situations of his life history became the object of inquiry and evaluation. The others' reactions to his body were carefully studied—to the extent to which the interaction between the reflection of his body in the others' eyes, as conveyed to them by him and his after-response to it, has defined the patient's whole concept of masculinity and sexuality. At this point, interesting to note was the patient's initial inability to relate and compare the maleness of his body with a woman's body, instead of with his own sex. He had always seen the qualities of his body only in inter-male competition, but not as they might have been evaluated under feminine scrutiny. The critical re-evaluation of his understanding of his own body led him to a new concept of sexual relationships with others which were reformulated in adult terms of masculine versus feminine body acceptance.

Since the distorted consciousness of his body was his consciousness of the world, the metalogical *Weltanschauung*—with the rationalization of his attitude, the absurdity of his beliefs, the supernatural tinge of his judgment—were questioned, analyzed, and re-evaluated to the point of total disintegration. The thinking of the patient was reoriented toward a rationally integrated logic. For him, in the past, the psychology of feelings, needs, and emotional reactions of women were vague, if not unknown entities. Any relationships based on an intimate communication were puzzling and uninspiring due to a prevailing sensation of being rejected by them. Once he felt free of any sense of inadequacy toward women, he was able to give a new meaning to the relationship with them. His ability to encounter them on an equal basis of sharing experiences and emotions lifted the veil of mystery and fear, in communication. There was not any more a need for duplicity toward himself in order to avoid any direct feminine relationships, since he could see them with an adult eye, that of a man relating to a woman in an emotional and biologic need for each other. But the redefining of his being in the terms of the new meaningful approach to things, free from its ambiguity of the past, led the patient inevitably toward the final question.

To what extent could his body's inadequacy of his adolescence influence his present inability to relate sexually to the opposite sex? True, the potentiality of the drive toward the opposite sex was present; but in actuality, its physiologic mechanism was dormant because of non-use. The change of the concept of thinking, the change of his mode of existence, the envisioning of a new world of being for himself and for others, the realization of his true masculinity did not enable the patient, who never had relationships with the opposite sex, to relate instantly in a new sexual situation, alien to himself. In this case, as in many others with the same type of personality and inexperience, a mental reorientation is required to the sexual stimuli necessary for arousal in the process of lovemaking with the opposite sex.

Therapists, using various methods of persuasion and reassured by the patient's cooperation, are convinced that the simple attempt of the patient to sleep with a woman will immediately and naturally result in intercourse. Unfortunately, when it does not occur and the patient feels rejected, the therapist attributes the failure to the patient's unconscious resistance. In reality, the most important element, the psychic response evoked by the sensorial stimulation of the sexual body, was therapeutically forgotten, and this factor happens to be the most important and basic element for any unfolding of a sexual situation. In this respect, the homosexual is in a strange situation, that of having to readjust his sexual life to a new, somewhat different, set of corporeal stimuli. He has to reorient himself toward a new sexual physiognomy which has to take on new sexual meaning for him. To start with, different tactile and olfactory sensory reactions have to take on a different sexual significance and to be assimilated in the process of his "warming up." A unique world of sensations faces the patient; for instance, the silkiness of the hair, the softness of the skin, the configuration of the body, with its female genitalia. Even the sexual situation requires a different approach, behavior, and motions.

In general, the patient has to integrate new types of erotic perceptions into the total sexual representation of the act (5). While in any heterosexual situation the peripheral sexual automatism follows the intentional representation of the sexual act in the conscious mind, here one is faced with a reverse process. First the patient, in relating to women, operates with a purely peripheral genital automatism of gratification which afterwards creates the necessary stimulation for a new cerebral representation of it, based on a repeated evocation of the new erotic perceptions. In other words, psychically the patient has to replace the former stimulating male erogenous zones with which he dealt in the past with the new feminine ones, in the process of his genital sexual stimulation. It means that, at the beginning, the patient has to approximate the same type of technical approaches to which he was used, in order to be successfully aroused physiologically for a sexual response. In these terms, vaginal intercourse will become a variant form of his former anal intercourse. The sphere of sexual activity is enlarged progressively on a subtly differentiated scale until it reaches a total heterosexual response.

Finally, the patient has reached for his freedom, to be what he wants to be, a man using emotionally and sexually his body and masculinity according to his free choice, and ability of commitment. From this vantage point he can see that his present depends on him and his decisions, without ambiguity or dramatization of his destiny.

The therapy gave him a flexibility in carrying out his project of life, in relating to himself and to the world without the ever-present shadow of his sexual non-being. The affirmation of his newly integrated sexuality gave him a sense of power, of real equality with others, and, more than anything else, a sense of fulfillment of his most secret desire—to be free, to decide on his own whether or not to be a homosexual.

REFERENCES

1. Freud, S.: Letter to an American mother. *Am. J. Psychiat.,* 107:786, 1951.
2. Bieber, I.: *Homosexuality.* New York, Vintage Books, 1965, pp. 275-319.
3. Sartre, J. P.: *Being and Nothingness.* New York, Philosophical Library, 1956, pp. 384-386; 55-59; 47-49.
4. Heidegger, M.: *Being and Time.* New York, Harper & Row, 1962, p. 174.
5. Merleau-Ponty, M.: *Phenomenologie de la Perception.* Paris, Gallimard, 1966, pp. 181-189.

15. The Application of Faradic Aversion Conditioning in a Case of Transvestism[*]

C. B. Blakemore, J. G. Thorpe,
J. C. Barker, C. G. Conway, and N. I. Lavin

Transvestites wear the clothing of the opposite sex, a behavior that may be considered a combination of homosexuality and fetishism. The authors report the treatment of a well-educated, 33-year-old male transvestite. The patient had previously received six years of psychotherapy plus medication for his anxiety, but the basic symptom remained unmodified. The study describes treatment by aversive faradic (electric current) conditioning and reviews past studies which have used aversive chemical agents. This literature indicated that because the essential timing of the conditioned stimuli and the unconditioned response in classical conditioning is extremely difficult with the use of a chemical agent, electric shock was preferable. Further, electric shock permitted the use of operant learning as well as Pavlovian conditioning in the treatment. The therapists employed the classical conditioning procedure, pairing the stages of dressing in female attire with an electric shock and buzzer. Thus, an activity once related to sexual pleasure became associated with discomfort. Operant behavior was used in the following way: the patient was given intermittent electric shocks while removing female garments, with the removal of all female clothing bringing about cessation of the shock. The patient was reported symptom-free six months after the completion of treatment.

---

[*]Reprinted by permission of the authors and publisher from *Behaviour Research and Therapy*, 1963, **1**, 29-34. Copyright 1963, Pergamon Press, Inc.

INTRODUCTION

Attempts to treat transvestism by means of symptomatic behaviour therapy have been described by Davies and Morgenstern (1960), Barker *et al.* (1961), Lavin *et al.* (1961) and Glynn and Harper (1961). In each of these studies the treatment has been based on some form of Pavlovian classical conditioning procedure, in which the aim has been to establish an aversive response to certain behavioural aspects of the symptom. This has been achieved by associating stimuli related to the symptom with the unpleasant effects following upon the administration of a chemical agent, customarily apomorphine or emetine hydrochloride.

In their discussion of this method Lavin *et al.* (1961) point out some of the many difficulties accompanying this technique. At a practical level it is difficult to time correctly the important relationship between the presentation of the symptom-related stimuli (the conditioned stimulus) and the onset of the vomiting response (the unconditioned response), from which the conditioned aversion response is to be developed. Such practical difficulties are important also at the theoretical level, for they complicate any explanation of the exact nature of the learning process involved, and upon which the treatment is supposed to be rationally based. Despite the apparent success of Lavin *et al.* in the treatment of their patient,[1] this critical evaluation of their procedure remains appropriate. Similar criticisms of this technique have been made by Eysenck (1960) and Rachman (1961), both of whom suggest that the substitution of electric shock for the use of a chemical agent may overcome most of the difficulties involved in timing the onset of the noxious stimulus. In addition to overcoming these practical difficulties, adoption of this suggestion should also make it possible to introduce greater flexibility into the treatment procedure; for example, it becomes possible to utilize the actual symptomatic behaviour of the patient in a more realistic way, rather than depending upon the use of stimuli related to the symptom in the kind of artificial situation which the employment of emetic drugs necessitates.

In the study to be reported we have attempted to incorporate these considerations into the treatment of a further case of transvestism by behaviour therapy, in which aversive conditioning was aimed at by coupling the actual act of cross-dressing with the unpleasant experience associated with faradic stimulation. This treatment was structured in such a way that an explanation of the efficacy of the technique could be based on learning models other than the straightforward classical conditioning paradigm.

---

[1]Lavin *et al.* (1961) report no relapse after a six months follow-up. After an eighteen months follow-up their patient remains, to the best of their knowledge, symptom free (Personal communication).

CASE HISTORY

The patient, aged 33, was the son of a coalminer. Although the other members of his family were physically healthy, he alleged that his father was neurotic and his older sister "highly strung," and he blamed them for a discontented childhood. At school he preferred female to male company, but a nervous disposition prevented him from forming lasting friendships. He obtained School Certificate, subsequently trained as an engineer, and has had a successful career in the Civil Service. He married four years ago and has one son aged two years.

His earliest recollection of transvestism was of an incident at the age of four, when he remembered deriving pleasure from wearing his grandmother's shoes. Thereafter he dressed frequently in his mother's and sister's clothing in secret, which was always a pleasurable experience. Whilst wearing a corset at the age of twelve he experienced emission and afterwards found cross-dressing more satisfactory when accompanied by masturbation. Transvestism occurred approximately fortnightly between the ages of twelve and eighteen years and was usually, but not invariably, accompanied by masturbation. He obtained sexual gratification from observing his mirror image when dressed in female attire, and also from feeling the clothes next to his skin. He did not derive pleasure from handling clothing, but observed that wearing black court shoes and black stockings produced greater erotic stimulation than any other garment.

National Service with the R.A.F. between the ages of eighteen and twenty prevented indulgence in transvestism, although he masturbated frequently with transvestite phantasies. During this period he developed a duodenal ulcer, which perforated at the end of his service. Subsequently he indulged frequently in transvestism, and developed the compulsion to appear in public in female attire, complete with make-up and wig. This compulsion invariably occurred at night, and although unaccompanied by sexual satisfaction it reduced tension and conferred a sense of relief.

Because of a deep sense of guilt leading occasionally to suicidal preoccupation, he destroyed all his female clothing on several occasions, but was forced to buy more to relieve the resulting tension. He deliberately delayed marriage until the age of twenty-nine because of his transvestism. Although intercourse was possible he preferred to cross-dress, and initially he had to resort to dressing up in his wife's clothing during intercourse to obtain an erection. His wife's revulsion forced him to abandon this practice, and of late normal coitus seemed to give him greater sexual satisfaction than dressing up. However, his transvestite behaviour has persisted, and he freely returned to it as his only form of sexual outlet when intercourse was precluded during his wife's pregnancy.

His motives for seeking treatment included a fear that his young son would discover his abnormality, consideration for his wife, possible legal consequences of his being discovered in public dressed in female clothes, and a wish to be rid of his perversion in the hope that this would reduce associated chronic anxiety. He seemed genuinely anxious to be cured and had read widely on the subject and was well acquainted with different methods of treatment.

Prior to entering Banstead Hospital for behaviour therapy, he had received six years of supportive psychotherapy at two other hospitals. Initially stilboestrol had been prescribed, which he had not taken. He had been sedated mainly by sodium amytal grns. 1½ t.d.s., which had helped to overcome tension, although he had become addicted to this drug. His basic symptom was however entirely unmodified by all the treatment that he had received during this time.

On examination he was a tall, asthenic man (height 6 ft, weight 10 st. 5 lb), with normal genitalia and secondary sexual characteristics. He was physically fit and looked younger than his years. His intelligence was well above average (Full scale I.Q. = 127). On the Maudsley Personality Inventory he was found to have a high neuroticism score.

TREATMENT

Apparatus. The treatment was carried out in one of the side-rooms of an admission ward. This room, which measured 12 ft × 7½ ft, was situated at one end of a quiet corridor and remained shuttered throughout the treatment. A standard, movable bed-screen divided the room. One half of the room was furnished with a chair, a full-length tailor's mirror and an electric floor grid. The other half of the room contained the generator for the grid and a buzzer sounding device.

The electric grid was made from a 4 ft × 3 ft rubber mat, the upper side of which had a corrugated surface. Tinned copper wire, one-tenth inch in diameter, was laid and stapled lengthwise in the grooves of this mat at approximately half-inch intervals. Alternate wires were connected to the two terminals of the electric current generator. This was a hand-operated G.P.O.-type generator which produced a current of approximately 100 V a.c. when resistances of 10,000 Ω and upwards were introduced onto the grid surface. It was found that two quick turns of the generator handle were sufficient to give a sharp and unpleasant electric shock to the feet and ankles of anyone standing on the grid.

Procedure. The procedure adopted in the treatment of this patient resembles in certain respects the paradigm involved in instrumental conditioning, in addition to the classical conditioning model employed in earlier studies (Kimble, 1961). Although the cross-dressing behaviour was followed by the onset of the noxious stimulus, as in the classical conditioning situation, the procedure to be described has much in common with escape learning in the absence of a warning signal, and in which the patient's subsequent behaviour was 'shaped' by verbal instructions.

The treatment was organized in such a way that the patient was seen on a daily basis, with his attending hospital from 9.00 a.m. until late afternoon each day, while spending the evening and sleeping at home. Throughout each day treatment sessions were administered at thirty minute intervals, each session consisting of five trials. The number of trials per day varied between 65 and 75, until 400 trials had been given over a total period of six days. The duration of this treatment was not continuous, however, for a weekend break of two days, which the patient spent at home, intervened between the fourth and fifth treatment days.

At the beginning of each session the patient, dressed only in a dressing-gown, was brought into the specially prepared room and was told to stand on the grid behind the screen. On the chair beside him was his 'favourite outfit' of female clothing, which he had been told to bring with him at his first attendance. These clothes had not been tampered with for the most part, with the exception that slits had been cut in the feet of nylon stockings, and a metal plate fitted into the soles of the black court shoes to act as a conductor. Each trial commenced with the instruction to start dressing, at which he removed the dressing-gown and began to put on the female clothing. At some point during the course of dressing, he received a signal to start undressing irrespective of the number of garments he was wearing at that time. This signal was either a shock from the electric grid or the sound of a buzzer, and these were randomly ordered on a fifty per cent basis over the 400 trials. The shock or buzzer recurred at intervals until he had completed his undressing. He was allowed a one minute rest period between each of the five trials which made up a treatment session.

In order that the number of garments put on should not be constant from trial to trial, the time allowed from the start of dressing to the onset of the recurrent shock or buzzer was randomly varied between one and three minutes among the trials. It was possible, also, that the patient's undressing behaviour would become stereotyped if the interval between the successive shocks or soundings of the buzzer remained constant from trial to trial; therefore, while these intervals were kept constant within a trial, they were randomly varied between 5, 10 and 15 seconds among trials. The explanation of the procedure given to the patient before treatment commenced did not contain any reference to the randomization of these variables, and did not include any instructions pertaining to the speed of undressing. At the start of each new trial the patient did not know, therefore, how long it would be before he received the signal to undress, whether this would be a shock or the buzzer, or the frequency with which these would recur during his undressing.

Prior to the commencement of the treatment it was predicted, for reasons to be discussed below, that towards the end of the treatment the patient's undressing behaviour might be characterized by a differential response to the shock and the buzzer. To check this prediction his time taken to undress was recorded for each trial during the last day of treatment. During these 75 trials the patient behaved in no way differently to the shock and buzzer, and there was no significant difference between the times taken to undress during repeated presentation of these two stimuli.

PROGRESS

During the first four days of treatment it was obvious that the patient found the procedure unpleasant, arduous and stressful. As a result his motivation declined, and when he left hospital at the end of the fourth day, to spend the weekend at home, it was felt that there was every possibility that he would not return to complete the remaining sessions. He did come back, however, and stated that as a result of his experiences during the weekend he now believed that the treatment was likely to be successful. He explained that he had found himself in a number of situations which previously would have stimulated him to cross-dress, but that when these occurred during the weekend he had felt no desire to do so. He had experienced, however, a dull pain in his testicles while in these situations.

He has been seen on two occasions since his discharge from hospital, the second of which was six months after the completion of treatment. He reports that he has not indulged in any kind of transvestite behaviour since he left hospital, and that he has had no desire to experience what was at one time his most satisfying form of sexual outlet. He claims that his relationship with his wife has improved during these six months, that he is generally less anxious, and that he is taking less sodium amytal than at any time for a number of years. In certain situations, in which formerly he would have cross-dressed, he sometimes experiences a dull testicular pain and sexual tension, which is relieved only by intercourse with his wife or by masturbation.

DISCUSSION

Our aim in this study was to condition the patient in such a way that he would develop an aversion for transvestite behaviour. The criterion by which to measure our success must be, therefore, his behaviour after treatment in relation to putting on and wearing female clothing. In this respect our efforts would appear to have been successful for a period of at least six months. Although it can be argued that this may be only a temporary improvement, and that he might relapse into his previous transvestite behaviour pattern at some later date, he has, nevertheless, remained symptom-free for a longer period following this treatment than at any time during the past ten years.

It is difficult to establish exactly how this conditioned aversion was brought about. Of the two possible explanations which most readily present themselves, either separately or in combination, one would utilize a learning process associated with the act of dressing, while the other would involve aversion developed during undressing and escape from female clothing. In the first of these the patient received an unpleasant electric shock during the actual act of putting on female garments; this provides us with the basic essentials for the development of a conditioned aversion response along classical Pavlovian lines. The variation of the time allowed for dressing would ensure that the patient was not handling or wearing the same garments on each trial, and thus the aversion would be generalized. In the second of the possible processes responsible, the patient was repeatedly shocked during the act of undressing, and therefore was positively reinforced by the cessation of these shocks, for behaviour which involved the escape from and avoidance of female clothing. Here we have the basic requirements for the development of an instrumental conditioned avoidance response.

When we designed the programme for the treatment we thought it probable that the patient would discriminate in his behaviour between the shock and the buzzer, and would take longer to undress when the buzzer was being sounded than when he was receiving electric shock. Under these circumstances he would have experienced a reduction of tension and anxiety when hearing the buzzer, for he would then know that this was a non-shock trial, and this would have been associated with the avoidance of female clothing. This prediction was not borne out by the facts, for during the last 75 of the 400 trials there was no significant difference in his undressing behaviour to the shock or the buzzer.

The role of the buzzer incorporated into the design may provide some indication, however, as to which of the possible explanations outlined above was making the greater contribution to the treatment procedure. It might be argued that one effect resulting from the inclusion of the buzzer trials in the design was that the total number of trials were only partially reinforced with actual aversion (shock) trials. It is known, moreover, that while instrumental learning can take place under a schedule of partial reinforcement, and resistance to extinction of the learned response is thereby facilitated, the establishment of a classical Pavlovian conditioned response becomes much more difficult, if not impossible, by the use of partial reinforcement (Kimble, 1961). These considerations would appear to offer some little support for a contention that the learning factors contributing to the success of our treatment, were more closely related to instrumental than to Pavlovian classical conditioning.

One final explanation of the learning process underlying this treatment, which should not be overlooked, involves the possible role of massed practice. It is known that repeated practice of certain learned responses will lead to their temporary inhibition. In our case the patient dressed and undressed in female clothing 400 times in six days, and the habit may have become temporarily inhibited as a result of this alone. It is impossible to say to what extent this contributed to our findings, or if it is a relevant factor in this type of situation, and further research is called for to elucidate any such relationship.

REFERENCES

1. Barker, J. C., Thorpe, J. G., Blakemore, C. B., Lavin, N. I. and Conway, C. G.: (1961) Behaviour therapy in a case of transvestism. *Lancet* **1**, 510.

2. Davies, B. M. and Morgenstern, F. S.: (1960) Temporal lobe epilepsy and transvestism. *J. Neurol. Neurosurg. Psychiat.* **23**, 247-249.

3. Eysenck, H. J.: (1960) Summary and conclusions, in *Behaviour Therapy and the Neuroses*. London, Pergamon Press.

4. Glynn, J. D. and Harper, P.: (1961) Behaviour therapy in a case of transvestism. *Lancet* **1**, 619-620.

5. Kimble, G. A.: (1961) *Hilgard and Marquis' Conditioning and Learning*. New York, Appleton-Century-Crofts.

6. Lavin, N. I., Thorpe, J. G., Barker, J. C., Blakemore, C. B. and Conway, C. G.: (1961) Behaviour therapy in a case of transvestism. *J. Nerv. Ment. Dis.* **133**, 346-353.

7. Rachman, S.: (1961) Sexual disorders and behaviour therapy. *Amer. J. Psychiat.* **118**, 235-240.

16. Psychodynamics of Alcoholism in a Woman*

Douglas Noble

Although the use of alcoholic beverages dates to the earliest recorded history of man, and alcoholism as a problem has been noted for centuries, the scientific study of drinking as a personal problem is a twentieth century phenomenon. Considerable research has been done to delineate physiological, cultural, and personality factors which may contribute to the excessive use of alcohol. Investigators have noted significantly different ratios of alcoholism among Swedes, Irish, and Jews, as well as other sociocultural groups. Genetic-biochemical factors have been posited, but success in identifying them has been limited. Research in personality factors gives some indication that a variety of emotional disorders are related to alcoholism, and that the majority of alcoholics are dependent, passive, aggressive individuals. Alcoholism may be symptomatic in neurotic and psychotic reactions. In psychoanalytic theory, alcoholics are viewed as oral and narcissistic personalities with marked oral frustration as a result of unmet dependency needs of childhood. Alcoholism is far less common in women than men but thought to be more pernicious for women.

Noble's case study of a 32-year-old female reviews the family history and relationships in a psychoanalytic approach to symptomatic alcoholism. The clinical history indicates that parental as well as parent-child conflict created a matrix for the patient's disturbing tensions. The patient developed strong guilt feelings about her own sexual feelings in juxtaposi-

---

tion to what she felt was her mother's condemnation of them. Further, she seemed to feel unloved by the mother and subsequently identified with the father. Her intense drinking began when she felt betrayed by both her father and her lover. During analysis, the intensive drinking recurred periodically, when recovery of unconscious material created peaks of tension and anxiety. Noble provides a psychoanalytic interpretation of the transference process and the patient's dreams, and demonstrates how she became aware of the nature of her dependency on her parents (with its concomitant frustration and hostility) and of her identification with, and ambivalence toward, her father. The author believed the outpatient psychotherapy was successful.

Symptomatic alcoholism in the male has been carefully studied by various writers in its etiological relationship to family background. Prominent among these investigations are those of Knight,[1] whose studies of essential alcoholism in men indicate that this syndrome is genetically related to a combination of a possessive, over-indulgent mother and a harsh inconsistent father. Chassell,[2] in a detailed study of a young man whose alcoholism was accompanied by manifestations of anxiety hysteria, stressed the role of a highly seductive and covertly hostile mother.

The fact that there is limited material in the literature on alcoholism in the female occasioned this review of the history and treatment of a woman patient in whom alcoholism appeared as a symptom of her third emotional illness.

CLINICAL HISTORY

The patient's first illness was characterized by depression and hysterical manifestations; the second, by frank conversion symptoms; and the third, by depression, phobic manifestations, and alcoholism.

The patient was a 32-year-old, six-foot-tall career woman who came to the hospital and asked to see a psychiatrist. She complained of suicidal impulses, of fears that some accident would befall her parents, and said that she had been drinking excessively for several years. Her parents had at first opposed her consulting the psychiatrist, but she finally persuaded her father to accompany her.

---

[1] Robert P. Knight, "The Dynamics and Treatment of Chronic Alcohol Addiction." *Bull. Menninger Clinic* (1937) 1:233-250.

[2] Joseph O. Chassell, "Family Constellation in the Etiology of Essential Alcoholism," *Psychiatry* (1938) 1:473-503.

In the initial interview she said, "I believe my trouble goes back to high school days when, because of my height, I was forced to take men's parts in the school plays." The patient appeared depressed and said that this was related to the failure of her plans to marry a man of psychopathic tendencies who had told her that he intended to secure a divorce and marry her. Whenever the time came to do so, however, he had repeatedly met the patient's pressures with excuses. Incidentally, the patient had lent him a large sum of money to finance the divorce proceedings. Her drinking had begun soon after she had left home, at her father's suggestion, to work in this man's office. She began to see him socially and attracted considerable criticism in the small community where they lived. The patient met this criticism with the attitude that she must stick closer to her man in fighting the intolerance of the world. Sexual intercourse took place only when the patient had been drinking and was followed by extreme guilt and depression. She made repeated attempts to break the relationship but did so only after moving to another town and arranging for her younger brother to live with her. Her drinking diminished while her brother was with her; but after he moved to another city to join his fiancée, the patient resumed correspondence with her former lover and began to drink heavily. This led to serious difficulties in her work so that when treatment began her employer was about to ask for her resignation and did so, in fact, later. This employer, for whom the patient professed great admiration, was a middle-aged woman who had told the patient that she herself had been disappointed in men and had given up hopes of happiness in life: she had advised the patient to seek satisfaction in working 20 hours a day.

In recounting her history further, the patient stated that she had experienced two previous emotional illnesses. The first of these occurred when she was 17 and followed a disappointment in a relationship with a boy of her own age. She was depressed, would go away by herself for long periods, hold her breath, and hope that she would die. She had wishes that a tidal wave would engulf the town.

Her second illness occurred four years later at the age of 21. In describing it, the patient recalled that she had been disturbed over three problems. First, her father had sustained such serious financial losses that she was doubtful of being able to finish college. Second, her father had been showing marked irritability towards her mother and younger brother. Third, she felt rejected in a minor love affair with a fellow-student. Her most prominent symptoms were those of a lump in the throat and pulsations in her neck. She consulted an internist who was acquainted with her family and who suggested that her symptoms were of emotional origin. He further remarked that they might be connected with her resentment of her parents' dominating attitudes. The patient angrily left the physician's office. Her fears that she would not finish college did not materialize, and after she had graduated and obtained regular employment, her symptoms subsided.

Subsequently, her employment record had been unusually good, and when treatment commenced, she held an important executive post. Most of her jobs had, however, been obtained with some help from her father; and although she was actually earning a higher salary than he, she doubted her ability to succeed without his influence. She felt that her father resented the fact that her earnings exceeded his and added that her mother was very critical of women who "took men's jobs."

She also stated that her anxiety over her father's increasing irritability with her mother had persisted. Her mother was five years older than the father but looked considerably more than that and for years had been letting herself go. She was quiet-spoken and had dominated the patient with an appearance of sweetness which had favorably impressed the patient's friends but had left the patient baffled and filled with fear of her mother's disapproval. In recent years, the patient and her father had been ashamed of the mother's appearance.

The father was a tall, upright man who had spent his life in various public activities and had at one time been a member of the vice commission in the city where he lived. He was strict, self-educated, and he boasted that his family worked together as a team. He took pride in his youthful appearance and was flattered when his friends told him that the patient looked more like his sister than his daughter.

The patient felt guilty because she had not lived up to the precepts taught her by her parents. Her mother had been extremely critical of her relationship with a married man but her father had shown more tolerance saying, "You and I are people of the world. We understand." The mother's attitude towards the patient's drinking was expressed in such comments as: "I would rather see you dead than alcoholic like your uncle or your brother," and "when people drink it hurts their parents terribly."

The brother to whom the mother had loosely applied the term "alcoholic" was the patient's only sibling, three years younger than she. He had not been intemperate in drinking but had shown marked irregularity in his working record; because of his persistent unwillingness to study or attend classes while at the university the father had refused to allow him to continue. The patient recalled many violent scenes between her brother and the father. Some years earlier, the patient had made a strong effort to induce her brother to cooperate with the father's plans, had had many talks with him, and had assisted him financially at college. She had been shocked to discover that he was consistently wasting his own time and her money. After he had been forced to leave college, and the patient had started to drink, the brother came to live with her.

Returning to discussion of her parents, the patient said that she had always been aware of their suppressed feelings of resentment toward each other. These feelings, she believed, had been greatly increased by the advent of the grandmother into the home when she, the patient, was 12. She recalled feeling very strongly her mother's and her grandmother's disapproval at that time and said that she would often awaken in the mornings with fears of her mother's admonitions and the constant question in her mind, "What have I done?"

It developed that the guilt and anxiety associated with experiences such as these were basic to the patient's symptom formation and specifically to her alcoholism. When the patient was first interviewed, sanitarium treatment was recommended; but since she declined to enter the hospital, the physician agreed to attempt extra-mural psychotherapy. Subsequently it developed that as critical situations arose in treatment, the patient would manifest anxiety conversion symptoms, depression, or more frequently episodes of drinking. These episodes were sometimes very severe. The patient was arrested twice and was discharged from two positions. During her drinking episodes the patient usually entered the sanitarium; but only once, after her second attempt to work had failed, did she remain for an extended period of four months. In the latter part of treatment she would come to the sanitarium when she felt her anxiety mounting in order to protect herself from drinking.

The circumstances which precipitated her alcoholic episodes were studied in detail during the analysis with the result that considerable insight was gained. The therapist made no recommendation at any time during the treatment regarding the patient's drinking; but soon after treatment commenced, the patient of her own volition reduced her drinking greatly. Subsequently, her alcoholic episodes were related to critical phases in the therapeutic situation. These episodes were usually preceded by experiences in which the patient felt rejected by one or more people who were significant to her. The study of the patient's relationship with these people revealed the basis of her symptomatic alcoholism, and the data which emerged from the analysis of these conflicting relationships is summarized for clarity under several headings which follow.

Attitudes Toward Mother

The patient had experienced immense guilt over her feelings toward her mother. "There is a feeling like a monitor hanging over me—I feel it after I have been drinking." In a quiet sort of a way, she said, her mother had kept her constantly busy with menial household tasks while criticizing her self-chosen activities, particularly her reading, which was characterized as "dirty-filthy sex." There were many quarrels over the patient's choice of clothing, the patient feeling that she should make the most of her height, the mother that she should conceal it. The patient had developed a defense of docility in relation with her mother and mother substitutes, the hostile basis of which was, however, clearly revealed in her dreams and during episodes of drinking.

The mother had always been insecure in her relationship with the patient's father. She had told the patient that during their long engagement she had not expected the patient's father to marry her, believing that he would be attracted to a younger woman; she had added that her own father was a total abstainer but had had a weakness for women.

The mother had marked fears of cancer and of blindness and at times of stress, would clutch her breast or complain that she was going blind. These symptoms greatly accentuated the patient's guilt over her death wishes toward her mother which revealed themselves as fears that her mother would develop cancer, go blind, or die. Feelings of resentment were augmented by the fact that the mother supported the brother in his quarrels with the father. This contrasted with the mother's wish to keep the patient constantly at work.

The maximum anxiety was, however, provoked in the patient by the mother's expressed attitudes toward sexual problems, "the terrible role of woman, the agonies of menstruation and the horrors of childbirth." In treatment the patient said that thoughts of menstruation made her feel guilty and that she experienced the same feeling after drinking.

Shortly after treatment began, she mentioned that it was difficult for her to talk to the therapist about menstruation and she criticized him for discussing the subject freely. She then recalled that she had wanted to keep the onset of menstruation a secret from her father and had been very angry with her mother for telling him of it.

Her attitude of extreme anxiety and inhibition over sexual matters had been reinforced by certain significant experiences. The patient recalled that at the age of 11 she had spent the summer at the home of an aunt, her father's sister, who had praised the patient for her modesty in concealing her body remarking to her mother, "I hope she will always be like this."

During that summer, a feeble-minded cousin who lived on the farm had shown the patient some suppositories; this had horrified her. About this time, she became embarrassed in mixed company and developed an especial fear of kissing games. She felt that this withdrawal from relationships with boys was approved by her mother. "I began to feel different from other girls." At this time, she developed a compulsion—which persisted for several years—to steal compacts and cosmetics: When she was

17, she had accumulated 200 stolen compacts, but when her mother gave her one at that time, she threw it away.

Thus, the patient's difficulties in relation with her mother contributed in a major way to the development of her anxieties over sexuality, her fears of intercourse and of pregnancy. As she grew up, she noted that she chose for her companions men of shy withdrawn personalities. She withdrew from men who showed an active interest in her and on two occasions when marriage was in the offing, broke off the relationships.

Later she found herself developing an intimate relationship with a thoroughly unsuitable married man—a psychopath. She became pregnant by him, and he deserted her when, under sordid circumstances, she had an abortion the horrors of which realized all of the fears of woman's suffering which the mother had described. It was following the abortion that the patient's excessive drinking began.

In the latter part of the patient's analysis it was revealed that beneath the patient's expressed hostility toward the mother there lay a deep wish for maternal affection. After this longing had been exposed and worked through, the patient—who had been taking a post-graduate course at the University—decided that it was time for her to be self-supporting and obtain full-time employment. She did so and at that time was able to recognize good qualities both in her mother and in her former employer. Interestingly enough, she also had a dream in which her former employer, a mother figure, became a heroine.

ATTITUDES TOWARD FATHER

There were many areas of the patient's life experience in which she felt rejected by her father. She felt that he was dissatisfied with her appearance, with the trend of her interests, and probably with her sex. Several months after treatment began the patient surprised the therapist by suddenly remarking, "I think you believe that I have no ear for music."

This manifestation of transference led to several significant associations. The patient recalled that while her father was away from home during the First World War she, as a little girl, had learned to play a piece on the piano which she had practiced assiduously for his return. When he finally did return, he showed no interest in her playing: he did, however, tell her that he had become very much interested in a little French girl while he was overseas and gave the patient a doll which, he said, he had named after the French girl.

The patient kept this doll for several years and then broke it in a fit of anger. Further, the patient stated that her father was a good singer but that she had never been able to hold a tune. She had, on the other hand, bought books of folksongs such as her father liked and had studied these in her room. It is interesting to note that after discussing these problems, the patient began to take part in group singing at the sanitarium.

The patient added that her father continued to complain, while she was growing up, that she was unappreciative of the opportunities afforded her, but that he was indifferent to the interests that she did develop.

In this respect she felt that he gave more encouragement to her brother. She said that he was greatly concerned about her height and she felt that he regarded this as a deformity which she also came to do. His practice of urging her as a child into boyish feats of daring increased her dissatisfaction with herself as a girl.

Later in life, the father pushed her into taking various jobs in which she was only partially interested. She became dependent upon her father's help in securing work but was never satisfied with what she did.

When the patient first returned to work during treatment, she encountered many difficulties as a result of her drinking and her resignation was requested. In discussing this matter, the patient said that she felt that the therapist was urging her to work and that she felt "she had to prove her intelligence." She added that she had always felt a need to show her parents that she was intelligent and responsible, but that she also wished to be irresponsible. Soon after this there was another episode of drinking in which the patient made a suicidal gesture. She said that she had developed intense inward resentment which she had not been able to express to the therapist over the fact that he had not, in appreciation of her creative abilities, offered her a job in the handicraft department of the sanitarium.

Parenthetically, it was not until the latter part of treatment that the patient, acting upon a wish to find a job for herself, obtained a job without her father's help and proved successful in it. In this position she found expression for both her creative and administrative talents.

The patient's problems with her father had seriously interfered with her relationship with other men. She stated that she often found herself drinking with men with whom her father had quarreled, men whom he had characterized as "stuffed shirts." She said, "Now I know who was the stuffed shirt." Her father had a tendency to kid her about imaginary boy friends. On one occasion when she was at high school and sensitive about her height, he pinned a number of love letters on the Christmas tree purportedly sent by her admirers.

During her high school years the patient had evolved what she described as a compensatory idealization of her father. This, she said, kept her away from contacts with boys: she felt that she would find "one man" like her father whom she would love always.

Discussions of her relationship with her father were often accompanied by exacerbations of drinking. Following one of these occasions, the patient had a dream, "I was talking to a Congressman; I was afraid he was going to blackmail me: I was afraid he would find out about my suicidal thoughts, perhaps from my former employer."

In association, the patient recalled the period of depression she had experienced at the age of 17. She said that she had had suicidal thoughts and that her father "felt hurt" when she told him about them: "I wanted to hurt my father." She then remembered that shortly before this period of depression she had overheard her parents having intercourse. She said that she became extremely anxious and for several weeks put cotton wool in her ears so that she would not hear them again. The feelings aroused by this were associated with earlier and later feelings of rejection from the father. The patient reported that sometime after she left home she began to receive frequent letters from her father asking that she come home for the week end because "her mother needed her," and that he, the father, had to be away on business. The patient discovered that her father was carrying on a love affair with a woman in another city and was using her, the patient, to facilitate his plans.

She herself then began to carry on a sexual affair with the psychopathic married man; and shortly after this, when she had become pregnant and had an abortion, her drinking began. Repeatedly feelings of rejection and depression were associated in the analysis with drinking, noticeably so when the therapist was away or when her father was out of town leaving her at home with her mother. On those occasions she would develop murderous thoughts towards her mother, her former fiancé and would feel "unreasoned rages" at the baby next door. Following these rages, she would experience hang-overs or try to obtain nembutal as she was accustomed to do after she had been drinking. The relation between the patient's feelings of rejection from the father and her symptomatic drinking was gradually worked through in the transference. It was then discovered that much of the patient's disappointment in her father was a secondary development of her feelings of rejection by the mother. Her resentment of her father's penuriousness was, for example, revealed both as a wish for his love and for the love which her mother gave to him and to her brother.

Attitudes Toward Brother

The patient felt that both parents, especially her mother, favored the brother. As a reaction against her jealous feelings the patient developed a "sisterly protective" attitude toward the brother. During his high-school and college days when he was involved in difficulties with his father, the patient tried to induce her brother to cooperate with the father's plans. She went for long walks with her brother and left her favorite books in his rooms with passages marked which she regarded as appropriate to his needs.

Beneath the patient's protective attitude toward her brother, there was a wish for dependence upon him such as existed in relation with her father. During the period that her brother was living with her, the patient stopped drinking, but when he left, she resumed correspondence with her former fiancé and again began to drink.

In the transference relationship the patient recognized through her feelings about other patients the antagonism that she felt toward her brother. She saw that the "sisterly" attitude carried over to her relations with other men but that "underneath, she was chronically angry with them." She related her shyness with men to this unrecognized anger.

The patient's jealousy of the brother was associated with a wish to be treated as he was by the parents. Some of the evidences of real favoritism on the part of the parents had strengthened the patient's jealousy. The mother, for instance, had protected the brother against his father's anger, helped to keep him dependent and had refused to believe that the brother was ever at fault. The patient herself felt that there was a rejection of her by both parents and discovered a strong wish to be protected by her mother as her brother had been.

PARENTS' PROBLEMS

Consideration of the parental background is of importance in the understanding of the patient's alcoholism. The paternal grandfather had died, supposedly from alcoholism, when the father was eight years old. In consequence, the father had been conditioned strongly against alcohol by his mother who frequently pointed to the grandfather as an example. In telling her of this, her father had said to the patient, "At times I hated my father."

It has been mentioned previously that this grandmother who was so strongly opposed to drinking moved into her son's home when the patient was 12, and that at that time, the patient became aware of increased guilt and anxiety. The tension between the parents was undoubtedly heightened at this time and, additionally so, because of the father's ambivalent attitude towards his mother. This increase in tension was noted by the patient and exploited for her own ends.

Late in treatment, the patient recognized that her chronic anxiety over her parents' dissatisfaction with each other was associated with her own wish to provoke and to participate in quarrels between them.

The father's relationship with his two sisters is of importance. His older sister, after whom the patient was named, had been her father's teacher and mentor and had maintained a close relationship with him. On one occasion she had, as did the patient many years later, secured a position in the same government agency as the father, doing similar work. The patient realized that her tendency to identify with this aunt pleased the father and annoyed her mother. The father's younger sister, on the other hand, had temper tantrums and was called "crazy": When the patient became angry her mother would say, "Now you are acting like your aunt."

There is little doubt but that the father's attachment for his mother had conditioned his choice of an older woman for his wife. The mother felt insecure as a woman and as a wife and mother. She had told the patient that she was jealous of her younger and more beautiful sister. She had not expected the patient's father to marry her after their prolonged engagement thinking he would have availed himself of an opportunity he had to marry a younger, more attractive woman. This attitude must have strengthened her resentment of her husband's attachment to his own sister and of his frequent boast that his friends told him that the patient looked more like his sister than his daughter.

After their marriage, the mother was unwilling to participate in the semiprofessional social events that were a part of her husband's work. This seems to have been due to her fear that she could not compete with the other wives. She had told the patient that during the period of courtship, not expecting to marry, she had attempted to consolidate her position in the business world. (She complained of women who took "men's jobs.") The mother's need for financial security was an important motive in her marriage and a probable source of guilt. In talking with the patient, she exaggerated the financial problems that arose in the family. If she were refusing a request of the patient's for money she would play the martyr and gesture dramatically as though she were going to die. The mother's tendency to "let herself go," which was accentuated when the paternal grandmother came to live in the home, revealed her lack of self-regard and was, at the same time, a manifestation of her resentment of her husband and of his mother.

Both parents had acquired from their own families strong prejudices against drinking. The mother's attitude was especially complicated. Frequently, the mother had warned the patient that she was in danger of becoming an alcoholic like the mother's brother. She had applied the same term "alcoholic" to the irresponsible behavior of the patient's brother. It happened that a few months after the analysis began, the "alcoholic" uncle, of whom the mother had spoken, came to visit the family. He turned out to be a man whose business career had been consistently successful and who drank temperately. The mother, following his arrival, boasted to all the neighbors of his great business success. It can only be concluded that the mother was involved in an ambivalent relationship with him and that she rationalized her resentment as an objection to his "alcoholism."

Throughout the treatment, both parents emphasized the hurt to them in the patient's drinking which had the effect of increasing its symptomatic value as an effective expression of revenge.

TRANSFERENCE PROBLEMS AND DREAMS

When vital problems were exposed through the transference situation, the patient sometimes reacted with conversion symptoms or depression but most frequently with resort to sedatives or alcohol. In association with her drinking there was much acting out of her problems; but following the alcoholic episodes much important analytic work was done. The patient experienced considerable guilt and anxiety at those times and was especially willing to analyze the circumstances which had precipitated her drinking. It was repeatedly observed that crises in treatment developed around situations in which the patient felt rejected by the therapist, and that her sensitivity to rejection was an expression of her great unconscious demands. By getting drunk, she expressed her helplessness, her demand, and her resentment. Transference attitudes were clearly revealed in much of her acting-out as well as in her dreams some of which, for this reason, are reported in this section.

Some months after the beginning of treatment, the patient, who was living at home, reported that her real wish was to live in the sanitarium and have her parents pay for her analysis. Soon after, a drinking episode resulted in her admission to the sanitarium; but, feeling guilty about her dependence upon and interest in the therapist, she left impulsively saying it was necessary that she go to work. She obtained an administrative post but continued to complain that the therapist was pushing her into work. She resumed drinking and returned for a brief stay in the sanitarium. Discussion of the episode revealed that at the time she returned to work thoughts of love and sex in relation to the analyst were coming into her mind. She felt rejected and said, "That is the business of my high-school days all over again." Because of her drinking and her inability to get along with her woman superior, her resignation from the new post was soon requested. Further analysis of this experience brought out that her feeling of being pushed into work by the therapist related to many similar experiences with her father with whose aid she had obtained various administrative positions. She herself had always felt, however, that her major talent lay in creative activities and that in these pursuits, her father had not encouraged her. Nevertheless, her interest in her father, with its unconscious erotic elements, her desire to gain his approval, and her resentment against her mother had led her to take "men's jobs" in which she had never found satisfaction. The dependency and magical thinking which existed beneath her identification with her father was revealed later in the analysis. Following a period of drinking which was accompanied by a suicidal gesture, the patient said that she deeply resented the fact that the therapist had not recommended her for a job at the sanitarium in the art department and that his failure to do so was because he regarded her mind as a "garbage heap." As a matter of fact there had been no prior discussion of her wish to obtain work at the sanitarium and there was no vacancy.

As this problem was being analyzed, the patient made more demands upon the therapist, especially that she be given sedatives. One of the administrative physicians had occasionally prescribed therapeutic doses of sodium amytal.

The patient intentionally took a small overdose following which, in a dramatic gesture, she threw away photographs of her father and of the French girl to whom he had become attached when overseas.

She then had a dream.

> *Dream:* The analyst was giving her sodium amytal. She already had some in her hand but was asking for more. She was requesting more because she knew that she or the analyst was going to be absent for some time and she would not have a chance to obtain sedatives. Another physician [the one who had previously given her amytal] appeared and her therapist disappeared. The second physician had a forceful, sarcastic attitude and said, "What are the tablets you have in your hand?" He seemed to believe that she was attempting to deceive the therapist. The patient tried to explain that she had told the therapist about the tablets but the second physician was not convinced. She then got mad and struck him on the head. Furious, she threw things around including a golden chair. There was nothing in the room except a large bottle of sodium amytal from which the doctor was going to dispense the drug.

Associations: The patient said that she was angry with the therapist because she had not been able to establish a sisterly protective relationship with him "in which she could conceal a part of herself."

She accepted the interpretation that this related to her feelings for her brother and said with feeling, "I hate my brother." (She added that her shyness with men was associated with her mixed feelings about her brother.) She felt that the therapist had a contemptuous attitude toward her because she had given up her work and become a post-graduate student. The patient felt guilty because of her own and her father's attitude towards her brother's indolent behavior. Those attitudes, she felt, must be shared by the therapist.

As the patient became more aware of her dependency and of the resentment underlying it there were stormy sessions both with her parents and with the therapist, and some drinking episodes. There were delays in payment of the therapist's fees and much resentment of her father who, while she was not employed, was advancing money to her to pay for part of her treatment but at the same time was complaining considerably about it.

It was felt that the patient's own resentment at paying the physician provoked many of these difficulties; but this problem was not clearly exposed until the patient returned to regular work. The therapist then strongly recommended that she pay her current bills from her salary while gradually reducing the accumulated indebtedness; this action helped considerably in the resolution of her dependent attitudes.

Another dream, which related to the working through of the problem with her father, is reported.

> *Dream:* I was summoned to a conference for doing too much talking. I met a Flight Commander in the Air Corps. He was mentally sick. I recognized him as a man I had known when I was 21 years of age. I found myself in the War Department going from place to place and I was being followed by a time bomb which seemed as if it would go off at any moment.

Associations: "I had a good conversation with my father: he said, 'All girls get married eventually; what you need to do is get married and have your own home.' I felt angry and embarrassed at what he said. One of the men patients said to me last night that his doctor had said to him, 'You must never talk about your analyst.' " In the preceding interview the patient had reported that, for many years, she had had fantasies of her father as a ladies' man. In the same hour, she had expressed anger with the therapist at his failure to comment upon her greatly improved figure and had quoted her mother as saying, "With your figure you cannot wear a blouse." She had also said that she had been doing some drinking and had returned to the sanitarium because she was angry with the therapist over the fact that he had cancelled the appointment on the day before, a public holiday. She felt rejected by the physician and had developed symptoms of a lump in her throat and pulsations in her neck, similar to the symptoms of her illness at 21. It developed that the conflict which had existed in her mind during that illness centered in her attachment to a 21-year-old man and her concurrent unconscious attachment to her father. At the same time she greatly resented her father's interest in other women and his inaccessibility to her. These problems were complicated by the mother's criticism of her as unattractive. The father's suggestion that she get married had embarrassed her because of her deep guilt about sexuality, which was associated with her mixed attraction and resentment toward her father. These feelings had reappeared in association with the therapist so that she had been disturbed by the remark of the other patient, "You must never talk about your therapist." In further association, the patient said, "I become disturbed as soon as I recognize sexual feelings. That relates to my drinking."

The analysis of the patient's compulsive need to re-enact her problems with her father in her relationship with other men was followed by a marked improvement in the patient's professional and social relations with men. Incidentally, she obtained a position without the help of her father. In her work, she utilized the postgraduate training she had received as well as her creative talents.

Concurrently with the analysis of her relationship with her father, references to her mother appeared with increasing frequency in the patient's dreams and associations.

Dream: She was at a department store. Her former employer came in and said, "I have not seen you for a long time." Patient got up raving mad and said, "I'll have you know I'm insane." She left the store. She found herself in a tenement house. She had to get by a doctor who was standing with his back to her. This doctor was a composite of two of the doctors at the sanitarium, one of whom was her therapist.

Associations: She said that she had been bothered the night before by a sexual emotion which she could not tolerate. Her parents had insisted that she invite her former woman employer to dinner. She was disturbed over the fact that she had had a severe quarrel with her parents, particularly with her father who had complained about her drinking and her neglect of her mother. The mother had called them into the house; the patient went into a tantrum in which she screamed at her father. She said that her father left the room but later in the evening came down and said his attitudes had been conditioned by his mother's violent antagonism to drinking. Following this the patient said that she had always gotten into one quarrel after another with people who were important to her, "I didn't realize what I was doing, I might have ruined my own career." As treatment proceeded it developed that her resentment of and dependence on her father, her brother, and the analyst were related basically to her feelings regarding her mother. In this connection a dream is of interest.

Dream: The patient was in a church. At first the church looked like an impressive cathedral. Later it took on the appearance of an ordinary Catholic Church with wax figures around it. Finally, she found herself by a small shrine. A Polish woman was kneeling in front of this shrine praying about a dead man. The prayers sounded like whinings and mutterings, a recital of the man's faults and misdeeds. She listened. The analyst was kneeling beside the Polish woman.

The patient's father approached and in a loud voice which caused her mingled surprise and fear said, "I want to talk with you a few minutes, doctor." The analyst seemed angry but got up and went away.

In the same hour, the patient reported another dream:

She was having an interview with the analyst in which he was asking for an increase in her fee. He did not state what the amount of the increase was to be but that mystery seemed to irritate her.

Associations: The patient recalled an incident that happened several years earlier when she had been required to investigate conditions in the home of a Polish woman, who was said to be misusing funds provided by the welfare department. This woman was also said to have had an illegitimate son by a priest. As a result of the patient's inquiry, letters were written to the newspaper complaining about the officious conduct of social workers. One of the letters stated that the patient, following her professional visit, had been seen in the park necking with her boy friend. The patient said that this referred to her father who had accompanied her and had parked his car a block away from the house. She said that in talking of this episode she had had feelings similar to those which were awakened when her mother had talked to her about menstruation and which were similar to those aroused when drinking was discussed. Further associations revealed the nature of the patient's identification with her father.

This identification in which there was much unrecognized resentment had manifested itself in her idealization of her father and in her choice of professional work: It had led, however, to serious interferences in her relations with men in that she felt guilty because of her erotic interest in and resentment of the father. Her drinking made it possible for her to admit sex feelings into awareness and to have intercourse. At the same time, however, her resentment toward men also came into awareness increasing her guilt and "hang-over." Parenthetically, this hang-over feeling was later associated with the feelings she had had when her mother had talked with her about sex. The patient's basic wish was for maternal protection and care and it was the maternal rejection to which she reacted so strongly in her life situations and in the transference relationship.

A dream which the patient reported early in her analysis is relevant to this problem.

Dream: I had a wild dream, like a surrealist picture. I had returned to my own city from the sanitarium. I was watching a fire engine going over the water. I saw a woman in a rowboat and recognized a former associate—a social worker—this woman split into two people—one of these people remained in one part of the boat—that person disappeared—I was in another part of the boat floating down the water. I knew I was to disappear—then I saw J—my former fiancé—he was waving to me from behind a fence—I knew that he couldn't reach me. Then I woke up. I suppose I disappeared.

Associations: "I had a frightened feeling on awakening and a sinking feeling in the stomach." This reaction was similar to feelings experienced by the patient when sexual matters had been discussed.

It was felt that this dream revealed the split with the mother and the unsuccessful attempt to deal with the hostility toward the mother by identification with the father. Definite improvement occurred when, following the analysis of her ambivalence toward her father, the patient was able to face and to resolve the deeper resentments toward her mother and mother substitutes.

PROGRESS IN TREATMENT

Treatment lasted for approximately three years. The patient's ups and downs became less marked as treatment progressed; and as she worked through the basis of her feelings of rejection, she became less sensitive and more adaptable. The therapist did not advise the patient against drinking at any time, but on her own initiative she reduced her drinking considerably soon after treatment began. Thereafter, periods of drinking occurred when marked anxieties were aroused, but as insight was gained these episodes became less frequent and less severe.

About one year after treatment began the patient, having lost a job because of her drinking, decided not to work for awhile but to study for an advanced degree. She had always intended to complete her technical training but had never done so because of her involvement in administrative work. She had envied other women who were technically trained. The completion of her post-graduate work qualified her for a professional appointment in which she was able to progress without her father's help and in which she utilized her creative talents. She discharged her financial indebtedness to the sanitarium and to the analyst.

The marriage of her therapist during the analysis aroused sharp feelings of rejection which were analyzed without return of drinking. Shortly before the termination of treatment, she learned that the therapist's wife had had a child. This led to the expression of feelings of resentment and jealousy and to the activation of some unresolved sibling rivalry. After these problems had been studied in a series of interviews, the patient expressed the feeling that she had gone as far as she could with her analyst. It was agreed that treatment could be interrupted and that she could return later if she wished. She promised to write the therapist after a period of a few months to inform him of her progress. There was no return of drinking following the separation from the physician.

Her professional work progressed very satisfactorily during the next year despite the fact that plans she had made were interrupted by her father's being forced into premature retirement through illness. The patient felt obligated to help in the support of her family and she moved with them to another state where her brother resided, obtaining a small house for herself and her parents.

Two years after treatment was terminated, she wrote the therapist at his request. The letter indicated that she was working steadily and had developed an active professional and social life. She said that she was moderately happy and in excellent physical health. There had been no return of alcoholism or other disabling symptoms.

DISCUSSION

Why did the patient add to her existing difficulties the disorganizing symptom of alcoholism?

In attempting to understand this problem it is helpful to reconsider the circumstances under which the patient's excessive drinking began. She had left home for the first time, at her father's suggestion, to work in another town. Here, with her father's acquiescence, she became involved with a man who despite a plausible exterior, manifested all of the least pleasing characteristics of her father. In her new situation, away from her family, and in a community whose antagonism she had aroused by her unconventional behavior, she became more and more insecure. Added to her problem was her discovery that her father was carrying on an extramarital affair, and was using her to facilitate his plans. The patient was therefore disappointed in both men to whom she was attached and her identification with them, which had hitherto proven an effective aid to her security, was seriously shaken. Further, the circumstances of her abortion realized the worst fears of sexuality that her mother had predicted. The patient needed help from her mother but was indeed caught in her own rebellion. Guilt, intense resentment, and an equally intense oral demand upon the parents eventuated.

Alcoholism was an attempt to express and to resolve these problems. It relieved, temporarily, her guilt over sexuality and did bring the patient considerable solicitude from her parents.

Moreover, her attempt to solve her problem by separation from the man with whom she was involved was not successful since she found herself, by unconscious choice, working for a woman who closely resembled her mother. Her conflict, and her attempt to resolve it by drinking, were thus perpetuated.

Alcoholism was a very effective means of taking revenge upon the parents, particularly upon the mother who had frequently said to the patient, "I would rather see you dead than alcoholic." Depression was less adequate than alcoholism in the patient's attempt to deal with her unrecognized resentment and guilt, and her accumulated anxiety was too great to be masked by conversion symptoms. As more disorganization of her personality occurred, more desperate methods were resorted to in the effort to maintain equilibrium.

These factors may contribute to the understanding of the various types of alcoholism, the symptomatic types, and the "essential alcoholism." The distinction between these types is, perhaps, a matter of degree. Therapy becomes progressively more difficult according to the extent to which the patient has been able to dissociate feeling from personal relationships, to remain unaware of anxiety, and to mask dependency beneath a plausible attitude of independence.

Most alcoholic patients show to a greater or lesser degree this mask of plausibility; it is most prominent in the so-called "essential alcoholic" who, because of the family constellation, has been able to remain dependent. In all instances, however, the symptom formation is related to oral demand, usually, upon the mother. The history of the woman patient which has been reported does not seem to indicate a different basic problem from that which exists in men patients. In both instances there is an intense early and cumulative disappointment in the mother, "oral frustration."

It seems likely that the subsequent life-course of any such patient is dependent upon the degree to which constructive interpersonal experience is accessible within or possibly without the family.

In the history reported, the patient, although severely frustrated by her mother, had available to her a relationship with the father which, though far from satisfactory and characterized by identification and overvaluation, possessed some real constructive elements.

In the course of treatment, the patient was able to work through her disappointment in the father and to see him as a human being with virtues and failings. Moreover, as it later developed, there were favorable elements in the relationship with the mother. Her mother had some qualities which the patient admired and because of which the mother could respect herself. Both parents were able to mobilize sufficient adaptive capacity to modify their attitudes towards the patient during her treatment.

It is probable then in the history of the "essential alcoholic" that these favorable influences are lacking. In this connection, a general observation regarding alcoholism as a symptom might be made. The destructive behavior of the alcoholic arouses such resentment in the members of his family that it becomes extremely difficult for them to give consideration to it as a symptom of anxiety. Because of this resentment and because of the attitude of our culture towards drinking, it is readily possible for them to rationalize their own unrecognized and possibly etiological resentments toward the patient.

The opportunity for resolution of mutual difficulties is much less than in those instances where the patient is more obviously "sick." With the alcoholic, irrational condemnatory attitudes are considered justified and are perpetuated. This seems to have occurred in the families of both parents in the history reported. One wonders whether the idea that alcoholism is hereditary might not be related to this fact.

Lastly, the experience of the patient described was of interest in view of the commonly expressed opinion that the alcoholic requires prolonged hospitalization.

In the treatment of the patient reported, extra-mural treatment was the goal and the hospital was utilized as a help in tiding the patient over critical periods of anxiety. There was only one occasion in which the patient remained in the hospital for an extended period. At the end of this time there was evidence that the patient was becoming dependent upon the hospital and she progressed more rapidly after she had been discharged.

The extent to which the alcoholic patient is capable of assuming responsibility is always a difficult problem. It appears that extra-mural psychotherapy is the goal with hospital treatment as an adjunct. It is important, however, that, during periods in the hospital, the patient continue regular therapeutic interviews with her own analyst. Otherwise valuable opportunities for analyzing the precipitating circumstances of the alcoholic episodes will be lost.

7. Psychophysiologic Disorders

This group of disorders is characterized by physical symptoms that are caused by emotional factors and involve a single organ system, usually under autonomic nervous system innervation. The physiological changes involved are those that normally accompany certain emotional states, but in these disorders the changes are more intense and sustained and the individual may not be consciously aware of his emotional state.

Subcategories include psychophysiologic skin disorders, including such skin reactions as neurodermatosis and hyperhydrosis, in which emotional factors play a causative role; psychophysiologic musculoskeletal disorders such as backache, muscle cramps, and tension headaches; psychophysiologic respiratory disorders such as bronchial asthma, hyperventilation syndromes, and hiccoughs; psychophysiologic cardiovascular disorders like hypertension, vascular spasms, or paroxysmal tachycardia; psychophysiologic hemic and lymphatic disorders; psychophysiologic gastro-intestinal disorders including peptic ulcer, constipation, or "heartburn"; psychophysiologic genito-urinary disorders such as disturbances in menstruation; and psychophysiologic endocrine disorders.

17. Adlerian Approach to Headache*

Alfred Adler

As early as 1910, Alfred Adler described psychosomatic disorders such as migraine, a cardiovascular disturbance, as being related to emotional stress. Since his early description, a number of clinical observers have suggested a personality description of migraine sufferers that is very similar to Adler's, as discussed in this case study. In general terms, patients with migraine are said to be competitive, hostile, aggressive, ambitious, perfectionistic, and intelligent. In these patients there is usually a buildup of frustration tension and headaches are triggered by some external event which has increased the resentfulness. Adler, who broke with Freud mainly because they disagreed on the importance of infantile sexuality, also discounted the importance of the unconscious. Therefore, as seen here, no mention is made of unconscious factors such as repression of hostility. Rather, Adler, who believed that man's basic drive is for superiority, demonstrated how his patient strove for superiority in a neurotic rather than in a normal way. The patient, in trying to dominate her fiance, did so by utilizing the headaches to force him to obtain a divorce so that he could marry her. Adler felt that the urgency in her demand was in response to a competitive feeling toward her younger sister, who was engaged to be married. Adler demonstrated how the life style the patient had molded during her first few years inclined her toward a domineering attitude and conquest by temper. He felt that the striving for superiority as a means of overcoming the early inferiority felt by

---

*Reprinted from Alfred Adler, *The Problems of Neurosis*, by permission of Routledge & Kegan Paul Ltd.

children normally produces the impetus for social man to strive for superiority. The patient's failure to exhibit social concern was viewed as further indication of her personality disturbance.

The dominance of the prototypic attitude in love and marriage is exemplified in the following case. As a girl, the patient was the second child of the family, very weak, very pretty, spoiled by her mother and ill-used by a drunken father. She lost her mother's favoritism at the age of three, when a baby sister was born, and protested by becoming truculent and high-tempered. She was supposed to inherit bad temper from her father, and some psychologists would uphold this mistaken opinion, but any child might take this line of development in such an unfavorable turn of circumstances. Indeed, from the attitudes of aggressive, disobedient, or domineering children we are often able to guess correctly at some salient feature of the home environment, such as this displacement by a younger child.

This girl became an actress and had many love-affairs, which culminated in her becoming the mistress of an elderly man. Such an obvious exploitation of advantage indicates deep feelings of insecurity and cowardice. This relationship, however, brought her trouble: her mother reproached her, and although the man loved her he could not get a divorce. During this time her younger sister became engaged.

In the face of this competition, she began to suffer from headaches and palpitation, and became very irritable towards the man. This was a neurotic impatience, and it was the cause of her coming to consult me. In a certain type we find that headaches are regularly produced by severe tensions of anger. The emotion accumulates, so to speak, during a period in which the patient shows no symptoms. The emotional tension may actually result in circulatory changes producing attacks of trigeminal neuralgia, migraine and epileptiform seizures. An illustration of such circulatory disturbances is provided by the well-known respiratory spasms and sensations of choking induced by violent rage.

In those cases of trigeminal neuralgia which have no organic basis I have already emphasized the importance of psychological factors. These may, of course, act through vascular disturbances induced by emotion, and the frequent repetition of such interferences with the blood supply may in the end cause organic damage to the tissues of the nervous system.

The tendency to anger is related to excessive ambition; both of which originate in a competitive striving to escape from a sense of being overcome. They occur in unsocial natures, who feel uncertain of attaining their goal by patient striving, and often try to escape to the useless side upon an outburst of temper. Children make use of such explosions to conquer by terrifying, or at least to feel superior; and in a similar way they use the consequences—their headaches. The neurotic origin of headaches was not known to the scientific world when I first spoke of it in 1910, but it must have been well known in antiquity. Horace, in an ode to Mæcenas, wrote of those ambitious persons who do not want to alter themselves but only to change others; and he refers to their headaches and sleeplessness.

To return to the case: the girl's condition was the result of a neurotic method of striving to hasten her marriage, and was not at all ineffective. The married man was greatly worried by her continuous headaches, and made efforts to get a divorce, but he was not very courageous, and made slow progress against the opposition to it. The girl then broke with him and wanted to marry another man; but she soon discovered he was too uncultured, so she returned to her former lover. He (the married man) then came to see me about my patient, and said that he would hurry on the divorce and marry her.

Treatment of the *immediate* illness was easy—in fact, it would have cleared up without me, for the girl was powerful enough to succeed with the help of her headaches. Her goal was to force the man to get a divorce quickly; it was the goal of her childhood, not to be surpassed by her younger sister; and as soon as the divorce proceedings began the headaches disappeared.

I explained to her the connection between her headaches and the competitive attitude to her sister. She felt incapable of attaining her goal of superiority by normal means, for she was one of those children whose interest has become absorbed in themselves, and who tremble for fear that they will not succeed. She admitted that she only cared for herself and did not like the man she was about to marry.

Her palpitation was due to the fact that she had twice been pregnant and both times had resorted to abortion, when she justified herself to the doctor by saying that her heart was too weak for her to bear children. It was true that her heart was irritated by tense situations and suppressed anger, but she used this symptom increasingly and exaggerated it to justify her intention never to have children. Self-absorbed women generally show their lack of human and social interest by an unwillingness to have children; but sometimes, of course, they desire children for reasons of ambition or for fear of being considered inferior.

A dream of this patient is worth recording. She dreamed that she was well dressed and held a naked baby in her arms. She said to the baby, which was of a brown and jolly complexion, "I cannot take care of you, I must give you up." The baby answered, "Yes, you are right." Then she began crying in her dream, and a man passed her, but she turned her head to avoid being seen. The man, however, wished to see her and looked at her.

By the nakedness of the baby she meant that she was too poor to have children. Her sister was to be married to a rich man, whereas she had only enough money for her own clothes, none to spare for a child. The baby's brown complexion meant that she could have a healthy child, but the dream-child reassured her, by agreeing with her, that everyone could see it was impossible for her to have children. The patient said at this time that she felt perfectly well, but suffered from palpitation of the heart night and morning, which showed she was clinging to the idea that her weak heart would excuse her from having children. She was too egotistical and much too eager to keep in the center of the stage of life, to entertain the prospect of children, and moreover she felt the child as a potential rival, because the tragedy of her infantile life was one of rivalry with her baby sister. The man who passed by her in the dream must have been myself, and her turning away was a sign that she did not wish to be entirely open with me; she was afraid that I would blame her, and as she knew I wished to develop her social feeling, she thought I should wish her to have a child.

The decision whether a woman should or should not have a child, should rest entirely with the woman—such at least is my personal belief. I cannot see the use of forcing a child upon a woman who is without social interest or love for children, for she is almost certain to bring it up badly. In such cases I prefer to adjust the woman socially, and then I am sure she will wish to have a baby without suggestion or pressure from anyone else.

18. The Transition from Organ Neurosis to Conversion Hysteria*

George W. Wilson

Using the concepts of Freudian psychoanalysis, Wilson demonstrates concomitance between stages of psychosexual regression and physical symptoms. The psychoanalytic postulate is that peptic ulcer diagnosed as an organ neurosis (now psychophysiologic disturbance) is reflective of disturbances in the oral-dependent stage, while conversion symptoms in the form of back pain indicate conflict in the phallic stage of development. From the psychoanalytic view, oral regression represents an attempt at a psychological solution from a more infantile state than phallic symptoms of regression. Symptoms originating in the phallic period are concerned with Oedipal relationships and are thus related to problems of heterosexual differentiation.

Wilson viewed his patient, a 41-year-old unmarried female attorney, as making progress in psychoanalytic treatment when her peptic ulcer was replaced by back pain. The peptic ulcer allowed the patient to assume a dependent, infantile role receiving sympathy, medical treatment and general care while at the same time making her dependency "legitimate" through a physical illness. The conversion symptom in the form of hysterical pain is reported to have commenced with the analyst's interpretations of unconscious sexual material and his encouragement that she assume a more heterosexual role. The study demonstrates the differences between two classifications of psychogenic physical symptoms and the psychodynamics involved in each.

*Read before the American Psychoanalytic Association, St. Louis, May 6, 1936. Reprinted by permission of the author and publisher from the *International Journal of Psycho-Analysis*, 1938, **19**, 23-40.

In the course of analyses of patients with gastro-intestinal symptomatology it has repeatedly come to my attention that the symptom for which a patient entered analysis was at times replaced by another symptom or symptoms. Often a conversion symptom of hysterical nature was concurrent with and incident to at least temporary cessation of the original organ neurosis. The present paper represents an attempt to trace the transition from an organ neurosis to conversion hysteria and an analysis of the material at the time of the replacement.

It is realized that such a separation of organ neurosis from conversion hysteria cannot be considered a fixed one. However, it is customary to restrict conversion hysteria to symptoms occurring in the voluntary and sensory systems and to speak of organ neurosis in reference to function disturbances of organs whose functions are autonomic and under normal conditions not subjected to voluntary influences. It has been observed that in organ neurosis the psychological factors involved are usually very definitely pregenital in character,[1] whereas in conversion hysteria later phases of instinctual organization are prevalent, more specifically the phallic phase. I shall attempt to trace the progress of the dynamic structure during psycho-analytic treatment from early pregenital to the phallic level coincident with the change from gastric symptoms (peptic ulcer) to conversion symptom in the following case:

This patient is a forty-one-year-old female attorney who came to analysis for recurrent duodenal ulcer, agoraphobia, handwriting difficulties and a feeling of social maladjustment. She is the youngest of three children, having a brother seven years her senior and a sister five years older. Her brother is a successful attorney. The sister, who was unmarried and with whom the patient made her home, is a forceful, ambitious and competent schoolmistress who married during the analysis. Her father is a well-known rabbi. The mother is an ambitious but entirely ineffective person, who during the patient's childhood suffered continuously from gastro-intestinal symptoms which were diagnosed as psychogenic in origin. She had been very attached to her mother as a child and found it impossible to leave home until after she was thirty years of age. As a child she took great pride in being her mother's nurse, caring for her, waiting on her and rarely leaving her side, for she had fears that her mother would die and leave her. These almost constant fantasies, together with her mother's continuous illness, kept her in a state of anxiety for several years. Her ulcer was inactive at the time of beginning the analysis but became active

[1]Alexander, F.; Bacon, C.; Levey, H.; Levine, M.; and Wilson, G.: "The Influence of Psychologic Factors upon Gastro-Intestinal Disturbances: A Symposium—a report upon research carried on at the Chicago Institute for Psychoanalysis." *The Psychoanalytic Quarterly,* October, 1934, Vol. III, pp. 501-588.

and demonstrable through Rœntgen ray examination in a phase of the analysis which I shall describe later.

This patient exhibited certain personality trends described as frequent in ulcer personalities.[2] Specifically I refer to the intense incorporating tendencies which are repressed and lead to over-compensation through increased activity and ambitious effort in life. She was an aggressive, hard-working, efficient and successful attorney. She maintained a very independent attitude towards other members of the firm and refused to accept favours from anyone. The deeper oral receptive and aggressive tendencies were almost but not entirely denied. In relationship to her sister she did live out some of these tendencies by living with and permitting the sister to feed and treat her as in a distinctly mother-child relationship. That this relationship produced considerable unconscious guilt, and also attempts to relieve the guilt, was demonstrated in her attitude towards her sister and other members of her family. She spent money in entertaining her sister, assumed the financial responsibility for their household and sent money and other gifts to her parents and her brother's children. To these children she felt a particular responsibility and, in addition to her gifts, fantasied financing their musical education, something which she herself had been denied, and their college careers.

Much of the material of her analysis revolved about seduction by her brother. This occurred when she was ten years of age and consisted in her being masturbated by him at irregular but rather frequent intervals until she was fifteen, when he married and left home. Before this rejection she began to masturbate herself, and continued this until just before beginning her analysis. There were many periods during this time when, out of fear and an obsessive belief that she was 'damaging' herself, as she in fact believed herself to have been 'damaged' by her brother, she would discontinue this practice. The same idea was prominent throughout her analysis, for she soon began to accuse the analysis and the analyst of injuring her. Many times she made the accusation that the Institute and the analyst had promised to relieve her of conflicts, and this had not been accomplished. In fact, she found herself much worse than before she began the procedure. Before the analysis everyone thought of her as a well-adjusted person, but after coming to analysis she had great difficulty in handling her work as well as her social adjustments. Although she insisted that her ulcer did not have a psychogenic basis, nevertheless she blamed the analysis for its recurrence. She pointed out that it was healed when she began and became active during the process.

---

[2]Alexander, F.; Bacon, C.; Levey, H.; Levine, M.; and Wilson, G.: *loc. cit.* This patient may be identified as patient 'A' in 'Quantitative Dream Studies,' by Alexander, Franz, and Wilson, George W., *Psychoanalytic Quarterly,* 1935, Vol. IV, pp. 371-405.

During these intervals she consulted countless male and female gynæcologists for the purpose of receiving assurance that she *was not* damaging herself and that she had not been damaged, as well as for a means of aiding her in discontinuing this practice. She received all kinds of advice, ranging from that of using her 'will power' to one suggestion that she undergo an operation which was described as similar to circumcision and consisted in rotating a piece of mucous membrane over the clitoris.

The patient successfully blackmailed her brother during most of her life. It was he who paid for her education, financed her frequent trips to physicians for her gynæcological complaints and her gastric symptom. But more than mere finances were involved in the manner in which she expressed her hatred for him. He was blamed for all her symptoms, as well as her failures in heterosexual adjustments and her lack of success in life. (Actually she was quite successful unless asked to assume responsibility.) Her inabilities in any given direction were directly attributed to her experiences with him and therefore to him. Very early in the analysis she became conscious of the wish to make him suffer as she believed herself to have suffered. She wanted him to feel guilty and was intensely envious of his success and his obviously good adjustment in life. She hated his wife and was pleased when she had a miscarriage. Many times she succeeded in arousing his guilt feelings through complaining of illness, of her inability to concentrate on her work, her need to take vacations, etc. On at least two occasions he was summoned from some distance to her bedside because of somatic symptoms which she admitted were used as a means of punishing him as well as a way of receiving attention.

Although the most of her hostility for men was expressed towards her brother, she frankly confessed a hatred for most men. She constantly depreciated her father and described him as being weak and ineffective, a sentimental old bookworm who was at the same time cruel and sadistic. She complained that he gave her much affection when she was a small child, but later completely rejected her. She complained of his religious intolerance. At the same time the patient greatly admired his intelligence, his knowledge of literature, history and music. She had been very attached to him as a child, followed him about and enjoyed his company a great deal, but later detested him, blamed him for most of the family quarrels, which were frequent, and felt he was the bad influence in the whole family situation. She had fantasies of his beating her, and much of her early material offered a striking example of what Freud has described in 'A Child is Being Beaten'.[3] However, most of this hatred was lived out

---

[3]Freud, S.: 'A Child is Being Beaten,' *Collected Papers*, Vol. II, pp. 172-201 (London, Hogarth Press, 1924).

in reference to her brother. Obviously she turned from her father to her brother for affection and physical contact as well as making him the object of her vengeance. This fact becomes of paramount importance in analysing the development of her conversion symptom.

The stage setting for the seduction is also of importance to the understanding of later developments. She claimed this took place while they were lying on her parent's bed in a room overlooking a hospital watching ambulances going in and out. She said they had spent many hours passing the time this way while alone in the house. Her brother often stroked her back and patted her hip, and it was following such common practice that he, on this occasion, exposed and masturbated her.

From the very beginning she exhibited an intense fear of the analysis. She cancelled the first three hours because of the sudden development of acute respiratory symptoms which resembled a common cold.[4] She was late for her first hour and felt a strong disinclination towards coming. She appeared very frightened and complained of the difficulty about having to talk. She also expressed her dislike of having a male analyst, that she would have much preferred coming to a woman. She thought it would be much easier because many of her difficulties she believed were probably sexual in character and her early training had probably produced inhibitions against telling those things to a person of the opposite sex. Then she immediately referred to fears of her father and said that she had always been afraid of him. She followed this with a confession regarding her masturbation episodes with her brother and her fears of having been damaged. Her early dreams contained distinct references to her castration wishes toward men and her fears of the feminine rôle. This transference situation continued for about forty analytic hours. Then her whole transference attitude changed and she began to neglect her work, her compensatory giving to her sister and other members of her family practically ceased and she began to express with increasing frankness her passive dependent relationship to her sister and to me. She spent entire days in bed, during which time her sister prepared the meals and waited upon her as a mother would a child. She complained bitterly of the necessity of earning her own living and wanted to become totally passive and dependent. For her the ideal solution would be to spend the rest of her life in bed, reading, resting and day-dreaming, removed from all contact with reality. This frankly expressed infantile attitude illustrated a commonly observed fact: that when a symptom or a behaviour pattern

---

[4]In this connection see Menninger, Karl: 'Some Unconscious Psychological Factors Associated with the Common Cold,' *Psychoanalytic Quarterly*, April, 1934, Vol. III; also Saul, Leon: 'Psychogenic Factors in the Etiology of the Common Cold' (to be published).

becomes threatened by the analytic procedure, it may become intensified as a defence reaction.

Obviously beginning the analysis had for her a meaning similar to that of the original seduction by her brother. She was afraid of the analysis, afraid of a male analyst because this constituted to her unconscious a reproduction of the original intimate relationships with her brother. There was not only the fear of having her genital desires aroused as they were at that time but there was the added fear of her castration wishes towards him which she unconsciously realized would be reproduced in the analytic situation. Obviously then she took flight into the mother-child transference relationship.

At this point, because her oral dependent relationship to her sister had been thoroughly analysed in the transference situation, it seemed advisable to recommend the discontinuance in real life of the gratification of these tendencies. The analytic situation seemed opportune for such advice for the reason that these exaggerated indulgences had an obvious defence significance for her. Therefore she reacted violently to this advice, refused to make any change whatever and became more dependent and demanding than before.

Immediately following her refusal to co-operate, she began to have gastric symptoms similar to those which had been active during her 'ulcer' periods. She found it impossible to eat anything except bland foods and began to restrict her diet to milk and soups. Severe epigastric pains were complained of after eating, as well as insomnia, and more or less constant nausea. She consulted her former gastro-enterologist, who advised a rœntgenological examination. This was done and an active duodenal ulcer with pylorospasm was demonstrated. At the same time she admitted an intense jealousy of her sister, who had become interested in a man whom the patient considered inferior. She did everything possible to prevent their proposed marriage. She transferred some of her dependent attitude to other more sympathetic mother-substitutes and succeeded in getting a great deal of attention from them. In this way she offered an excellent demonstration of exacerbation of gastric symptoms coincident with her stubborn determination to hold on to her oral incorporating tendencies, at the moment when the analyst not only through interpretations but through recommendations interfered with their gratification.

She attempted to frighten me with the severity of her gastric symptoms and suggested that she take a vacation both from work and from analysis and remain at home attended by her sister. Coincident with my discouraging this and the actual setting of a wedding date by her sister, she suddenly developed a new symptom. This consisted of intense pain starting in the upper lumbar region, continuing down the spine, and radiating into the left hip. This was accompanied by a lateral scoliosis causing her to lean towards the left. The spinal condition became so painful that she could not walk and had to be assisted from her bed. She consulted several orthopædic surgeons, who expressed varying opinions, but a diagnosis of spinal arthritis was finally made. Her brother was, of course, immediately notified and came to Chicago to aid her. She remained at home for two weeks after the onset of this symptom. During this time she was treated with the common remedies for arthritis—rest in bed and applied heat, but her condition did not improve. On the contrary, the pain and scoliosis became worse, and it was finally decided to take her to the hospital for Rœntgen ray examination, after which she was to be mechanically stretched and a plaster of Paris cast applied to her back. Then all of her gastric symptoms disappeared and she could eat anything, but out of fear restricted herself for the most part to a bland diet.

I was informed of her intention to undergo these drastic therapeutic measures and therefore asked her by telephone if she would like to have me come and see her. Her answer was, 'No,' but that *if* I came she would have to receive me out of courtesy. I called immediately, expressed an attitude of friendly interest in her illness, and then inquired about her mental condition. She replied by telling me a dream of the previous night which had disturbed her considerably.

Dream: She saw several soldiers with fixed bayonets. They all belonged to the same army. Suddenly they began to attack and fight each other. She feared that in the confusion she might get hurt.

Without actual confirmatory associations, I told her I believed the dream represented what she was doing in reality to the several doctors (including myself), playing one doctor against another; and that in the dream there was a fear of being hurt and an obvious need for punishment as a reaction to the wish to injure others. Her reaction to this interpretation was a negative one. She replied that she needed competent medical advice, that analysis could probably straighten her out mentally, but she had a real physical, pathological illness which I was ignoring, or at least minimizing.

I advised an immediate Rœntgen ray examination of the vertebral column to determine further what pathological state actually existed and attempted to discourage both stretching and application of the cast, at the same time offering to have her transported to and from my office each day if she wished to continue her analysis. She reserved her answer and two days later I received a letter from her. She was in the hospital, the Rœntgen ray examination had *not* demonstrated any vertebral lesion whatever, but the stretcher had been applied and the cast was to follow. In the same letter she complained that her friends (mother-substitutes) were really her enemies. I replied to this letter by again recommending that she discontinue her attempts of getting herself 'damaged' and return to the analysis. I also indicated that probably she was her *own* worst enemy. These were only reiterations of former interpretations.

However, this letter seemed to have the desired effect, because she left the hospital and returned to the analysis. Her posture was very stiff with distinct deviation to the left. She walked with difficulty. She gave three definite reasons for returning. The first was my interpretations in regard to her being her *own worst enemy,* the second some insight into the manner in which she was 'fooling' the doctors, and the third was that her gastro-enterologist told her he believed her back symptoms were largely psychogenic and that she had better return to analysis.

For several succeeding hours her material contained repeated accusations that everyone wanted to damage her, that doctors were all incompetent, that the sooner psycho-analysis and medicine got together the better it would be for the innocent victims of both. She insisted her pain and deformity were due to some spinal pathology and that the doctors simply could not find it. However, her condition continued to improve.

The development of the new symptom was coincident with thwarting of her last desperate attempt to maintain her passive dependent relationship to her sister. When I began to force her out of this situation, not only with interpretations but with a recommendation that she discontinue the relationship, she evidently made an emotional effort to abandon the pregenital attachment to the sister and face the problem of heterosexuality. An added incentive for such an attempt was that of the sister's impending marriage which drove her into competition with her sister on an adult feminine level. The internal obstacles to this progress are known from her previous analytic material. The way to a heterosexual adjustment was blocked by the intense hate and fear reactions towards men. The sexual episode with her brother intensified her aggressive and castrative wishes towards men to such a degree that it necessitated a projection of these wishes and she attempted to place all the blame onto men. The projection solution then became: It is not she who wants to castrate men. They damage her. Her brother damaged her. I believe that this muscular spasm had a direct relationship to this conflict, a conflict centering about castration wishes towards men and the resultant fears of retaliation. The psychological circumstances under which the symptom occurred corroborate this belief.

At this time when the symptom was at its height I encouraged her to be more socially aggressive, because I anticipated that she was about ready to face the problem of heterosexuality and assumed that the previous analysis had blocked her escape back to a pregenital dependence upon her sister (and mother). I told her specifically that I thought it expedient for her to seek the company of both men and women but more particularly that of men and to make some overt attempts toward friendly relations with them. She laughed at, belittled and rejected my suggestion. She said she had no friends except women, she was out of touch with eligible men. Then she brought the following dream:

Dream: It was all about beds. They seemed to be on a quiet beautiful street. The streets seemed to criss-cross. One was Willow Street which seemed very soothing to her. It was a little eerie too because of the darkness.

It is interesting that before telling this dream in the analysis, she repeated it to her sister.

> In associating to the dream she stated that her sister said she wanted to retreat. Patient says this is not true. She is only interested in being straight and out of pain again. This is such a blow to her pride. She must wear a support, which she despises. The night of the dream a man and his wife were quarrelling in the next apartment—and a boy had an argument with his parents. She envied this boy his ability to argue with his parents without any apparent fear of retaliation. She was always afraid to argue with her parents. There was all kinds of excitement and a radio was going full blast. The people quarrelling expressed themselves beautifully, but excitedly. It reminded her of the good old days at home and her mother's and father's quarrels. She is disturbed about having so many doctors treat her. Maybe she does play one against another. She can see that she is acting like a prostitute except that instead of men in general she is using doctors. She actually lied to two of them and did not realize at the time that she was attempting to get them to quarrel with each other. She has had the feeling that she would like to sleep with several men, a different one every night. She remembers a song from the Gilbert and Sullivan opera, 'The Mikado,' about a little bird who sat in a tree all day long and sang. When asked why he sits and sings all day, the answer is the same monotonous refrain, 'Tit Willow.' No matter what he is asked, the answer is always 'Tit Willow.' She was greatly impressed by this opera, but could only remember the song of the dickey-bird who sang over and over again the same monotonous refrain.

This dream expresses clearly and dramatically the deeper dynamics of my patient's psychology in this phase of the analysis (i.e. the phase in which the transition from pregenital conflicts corresponding to the emotional background of peptic ulcer and the genital conflicts expressed in the conversion symptom as described, took place). The dream obviously contains a threat which was only partially grasped by me at the time and was followed by the carrying out in reality of the threat contained therein. For these reasons I have chosen to examine and interpret the dream rather thoroughly, not only in relation to its manifest and latent contents but in respect to material previously obtained during the analysis.

The dream expresses an intense spite reaction to my advice that she abandon the oral dependent relationship to her sister and mother-substitutes and that she mix with the opposite sex. To this she reacted as though it were a rejection by me towards whom she had an oral dependent transference similar to the relationship to her sister, and all the fury of a rejected girl is contained in the dream. In the dream she accuses me as a girl might accuse her mother. She says, 'You drive me into the street, into prostitution.' (This is expressed by the beds in the dark street.) The depreciation of a sexual life is clearly shewn in the associations. The criss-cross streets to which she associated the quarrelling couple refer to the parents' quarrels and a sado-masochistic conception of intercourse. At the same time the dream also expresses the wish to regress to the security of the analytic situation which is treated as analogous to a mother caring for her child. Willow Street had for her a soothing significance and the tit willow as well as the monotonous refrain refer to the soothing effects of a lullaby.

It is of interest to observe that every element of this dream contains such a double and opposing meaning. Sexuality is referred to as being prostitution, and at the same time the reference to the security of the parental home and the wish for a mother-daughter relationship is clearly shewn. The dream also contains a reference to another type of reaction, namely, fear of the female sexual rôle as shewn in her identification with the boy previously mentioned in the associations. The main content of this dream is the rejection of heterosexuality because of its danger. Verbalized it would be, 'You refuse me, reject me, want me to become a woman. That means you really want me to be a prostitute like my mother.' The opposing meaning is the wish to retreat from the danger of sexuality to the protection of the mother. Also the analyst's interpretations are felt as soothing lullabies. This is shewn in her association to Willow Street which had a soothing influence.

But this too has a negative meaning. The analyst's interpretations, particularly those referring to her oral receptive and aggressive desires, likewise the monotonous repetition about being damaged by her brother and by the analysis, are monotonous refrains. It is not impossible that she also accuses the analyst as she accused her brother. Verbalized it would be, 'You force sexuality upon me just as my brother did.' This, as we shall see, is at least partially a projection of her own wish to damage first her brother and later men in general. Her fear of the darkness (the street in the dream was eerie too) is a reaction to her fear of seeing her prostitution wishes. This may also express the wish to keep the analyst in the dark.

The dream as well as the symptom expressed a drastic defence against genital desires: desires so active and so feared for the reasons stated that she had to build up some defence which would render heterosexuality impossible for her. The complaint against the brother also contained this defence element.

In this phase of the analysis when she is confronted with the problem of sexuality she feels driven into it. She repeats the same reaction which she experienced when her brother 'forced' a sexual relationship upon her. This reaction was one of retaliation fear because of the castration wish, and resulted in rejection of the feminine rôle and an identification with men to avoid the suffering rôle of a woman. The oral dependent attitude toward the mother was transferred to a wish to incorporate the penis orally. The previous material shewed that the wish to incorporate her father's and brother's penis was due not only to resentment and fear but also to the wish to own something, the possession of which pleased the mother.

We see that she had two methods of escape from the problem of heterosexuality. One was a regression to the oral level, the resumption of the oral receptive, dependent relationship to the mother; the second was an escape on the phallic level, an identification with the man by castrating him and incorporating his penis. As I have pointed out in the first part of the analysis the transference material, dreams, etc., express castration wishes towards men which were later followed by an oral-dependent attitude towards me as well as towards her sister and represented a re-living of the defence against the genital desires. The analyst for a long period represented (in the second instance) the mother who would protect her against heterosexuality, but when the conversion symptom developed, this mother-transference had been abandoned and she not only was expressing frank sexual wishes towards me but this frank expression was followed almost immediately by carrying out of sexual impulses in life. When she was driven out of this oral type of solution, she reacted with attempts corresponding to the second pattern, that of masculine identification. Concurrent with this attempt she developed the hysterical symptom previously described.

The psychological meaning of this conversion symptom cannot be fully reconstructed. However, I am inclined to assume an important relationship between the anatomical localization of the symptom and the erotic pleasure-sensation which she experienced when caressed by her brother. This part of her anatomy which was originally connected with pleasure sensations became the seat of pain. This is obviously due to guilt feelings as a reaction to receiving pleasure from her brother and at the same time out of revenge wishing to castrate him. A complete analysis of the symptom is not of paramount importance to the purpose of this paper. However, it appears that with this symptom she symbolically made of her body a penis, a stiff but damaged one. It is not justifiable, however, entirely to separate the two solutions, masculine identification[5] and regression[6] to the oral level. The conversion symptom which led to the contortion of her body not only expressed the phallic solution but at the same time permitted a regression to early dependent attitudes in life. She became entirely dependent, obtained satisfaction out of being nursed, fed as an infant is fed, and received a great deal of attention. She remained in bed and removed herself from all touch with reality.

That the symptom also had a further defence significance in relation to assuming an adult rôle in life is well illustrated in her material. The symptom developed at the time she wished to indulge her passive dependent wishes but was forced into some activity in the reality situation. She repeated many times that her back was less painful when she remained quiet and inactive, that exertion increased her pain. She reasoned that having to work, to come to analysis, to perform the ordinary daily function of life all contributed to her discomfort. At the same time she reported dreams in which she would be sitting, lying or standing quietly, but in danger of being *injured* usually by something being projected in her direction and there was always the feeling in the dream that she must *not* move. She felt secure providing she made no movement. That these dreams refer to insight in the analysis is obvious, but, in view of the fact that her fears of genitality were so intense and that this symptom was clearly a defence against progression to an adult attitude, I believe we are justified in assuming that it contained quite specifically a protest against adult feminine activity, against walking, standing on her own feet in the sense of psychologically growing up. The projectile nature of the danger in the dreams quite plainly referred to her fears of the feminine rôle in intercourse.

The masculine identification represented a new attempt to solve her Œdipus conflict in relation to her mother on the phallic level. Previously she found a solution through renouncing all competition and assuming towards her mother the rôle of the helpless dependent child. Now she wants to possess a penis with which she can please the mother as the father does and in consequence continue to receive from her. With this new attempt at solution on the phallic level the hysterical symptom develops, whereas during the period of her peptic ulcer symptom the psychodynamic background corresponded to a pregenital, i.e. an oral, solution.

---

[5]Freud, S.: 'On the Physical Mechanisms of Hysterical Phenomena,' *Collected Papers*, Vol. I, pp. 24-42. (London, Hogarth Press, 1924.)

[6]See particularly Lewin, Bertram D.: 'The Body as Phallus,' *The Psychoanalytic Quarterly*, 1933, Vol. II, p. 24.

As previously mentioned, the patient made an attempt to carry out in reality the threat contained in the dream. She managed through her brother to meet a male friend of his in Havana during the vacation period and with this meeting began the realization of her dream.

In the first hour following the vacation period she reported that she had had intercourse with this man and that it seemed a very ugly experience. She stated that he was exactly like her father in every respect, that he liked her, said nice things to her and made love to her. She thought him very intellectual but not very aggressive. She said that they talked for hours about things which she had discussed as a child with her father and that for her it was a real mental feast. He was very kind and understanding and never interpreted anything she said or did. He was very affectionate and she enjoyed kissing him, particularly his hands. They spent whole days together, and after two days decided to sleep together. They planned to stay at her hotel, but when they arrived on this particular evening, she found that she did not possess a key to her room. Afterwards she learned that he had it in his pocket (an obvious reference to her lack of a penis and his possession of one). She began immediately to menstruate, which caused a postponement of the sexual relationship. After menstruation finished, they made another attempt. She was quite frigid and the intercourse was painful. She reported that at one point when he placed her head in his lap it almost queered the whole procedure. She thought that the penis was the ugliest and dirtiest of organs and was both disgusted and mad. She said that she could have died laughing at the analyst's interpretations of penis envy. It was very difficult for her not to shew him how much she hated him. Very sarcastically she referred to herself as having been analysed, and laughingly told him she supposed she envied him his penis, at the same time saying, 'That is all poppycock.' He told her that one organ could not function without the other, which observation she said made her feel just fine and dandy. She said she believed most women felt the same way about intercourse, but would not admit it. It disturbed her when he called her 'pal,' because this had been one of her brother's pet names for her. She told in detail of her preparations for intercourse, how she undressed with a do-or-die precision and laughed hysterically when, after undressing, she ordered the light to be extinguished and he pushed the wrong switch illuminating the whole room. She felt that the room was full of men and women watching them. What she enjoyed most in the whole procedure was his masturbating her. Then she referred to her frigidity and said there must be some anatomical and not an emotional reason for it. Her sister told her that in the beginning of sexual relations frigidity was very common.

Following this episode she became convinced that she was madly in love with this man and wanted to quit her position, move to Havana and live with him. This, however, he quite emphatically discouraged and frankly informed her he had no intentions of getting married and was not at all anxious to be tied down to any permanent affair. Following this rejection she decided she wanted to return home, became very anxious to return to the analysis, and felt that anyway she had made a distinct advance toward successful adjustment. But at the same time she felt this was the only man who could possibly care enough for her to overlook her age and other believed deficiencies. She said she felt quite uninhibited in his presence, that she could 'act' with him, that she enjoyed singing to him and entertaining him in other ways. In many respects their relationship assumed a homosexual flavour. She felt that he was somewhat feminine in his actions; that he was very fixated to his family, that he was passive and indecisive, that he probably was quite neurotic but very good company and that anyway he was exceedingly kind to her. Following this recital of her Havana experiences a major part of the analysis as well as her fantasy life consisted of a repetition of this experience.

It was pointed out to her that she had lived out her unconscious transference wishes in this episode, that she received from this man what she could not get from the analyst, i.e. overt manifestation of affection (physical contact) and that she did not receive the things she disliked in analysis, viz., interpretations and objective behaviour on the part of the analyst. Also the evident hostile castrative wishes were interpreted. She accepted all the interpretations except the one referring to hostility. She even claimed that probably this man was hostile to her, that he used her and that he certainly misused her, but there was no hostility on her part whatever. It is obvious that emotionally she equated three experiences: (1) the masturbation episode with her brother; (2) the sexual experience in Havana; (3) the analytic situation. All three she rejected and maintained that they damaged her.

Following this she became openly hostile toward me in the analysis and at the same time experienced a slight recurrence of her spinal symptoms. As often observed in analysis, after overtly expressing the hostility which is under pressure of intense guilt, she again attempted a flight from making conscious her hostile wishes into a passive receptive attitude. She reported a dream in which she attacked her mother, had the feeling that she had killed her and fled in terror. The dream changed and she was passing around a bottle of liquor which someone had given her. This dream demonstrates how when she was faced with making conscious her hostility for her mother, she again fantasied the original type of solution, i.e. repression of the hostile wishes, and attempted to relieve her guilt through compensatory giving.

The oft-repeated claim that her brother and the analyst damaged her had for her the meaning that her brother in the first instance and the analysis in the second instance stimulated her sexual desires and a need for sexual satisfaction. In neither experience was this need gratified. Therefore the wish to damage, as well as the projection of that wish, became for her not only a rationally justified wish for revenge but also contributed to her difficulties when she attempted a genital solution in the analysis. She reached this level only to be thwarted and left unsatisfied; these intense fears of rejection caused her to vacillate between attempts at solution on the oral and phallic levels. The genital conflict is always active, in the conscious material it forms the centre of organization and the oral helpless dependent attitude is kept in reserve as a defence.

To summarize briefly the observations which I have discussed and the conclusions drawn from those observations: A transitory hysterical symptom characterized by a spasm of the muscles of the lumbar region with the resultant left lateral deviation of the body developed during a critical period of analysis. During this period the patient was forced by analytic insight and some active encouragement by the analyst to face the problem of heterosexuality from which she had previously regressed to a pregenital dependent attitude in relation to older female members of her family (mother and sister). The patient's dreams and the association material which she produced in connection with the conversion symptom dealt with the resentment towards the brother and analyst but more specifically with castration wishes and masculine identification. Although the specific symbolic meaning of the symptom cannot be reconstructed with actual proof as to its correctness, it probably expressed a fantasy of incorporation of the male genital with intense guilt feelings as a reaction to the incorporation. The anatomical localization of the symptom is obviously identical with that part of the body which was connected with erotic pleasure sensations experienced by the patient during the sexual episodes with her brother. If the unconscious material which was presented in connection with the hysterical conversion symptom is compared with material which appeared at the beginning of the analysis in connection with the gastric symptoms, striking differences may be observed. The character of the material connected with the gastric symptoms was preponderately pregenital in character and centered about the dependent, demanding attitude towards the patient's older sister and was highly charged with feelings of guilt and inferiority.

In contradistinction to this, the material which appeared in connection with the hysterical symptom belonged to the phallic period of the instinctual development. The masculine identification and rejection of the female rôle was the paramount aim during this phase of the analysis.

This observation is in accordance with the assumption made by Freud and accepted by most psycho-analytical authors that hysterical conversion symptoms express tendencies belonging to the phallic and genital phases of development. It also indicates that in the neuroses of vegetative organs (organ neuroses) pre-eminently pregenital tendencies are involved. In this case the hysterical conversion symptoms developed and the gastric symptoms ceased coincident with the patient's attempt to renounce the regression to oral dependence and face the problem of heterosexual adjustment.

REFERENCES

1. Abraham, K.: 'Forms of Expression of the Female Castration Complex.' *International Journal of Psycho-Analysis,* 1920, Vol. 1, p. 342.

2. Abraham, K.: 'Manifestations of the Female Castration Complex.' *International Journal of Psycho-Analysis,* 1922, Vol. III, p. 1.

3. Alexander, F.; Bacon, C.; Levey, H.; Levine, M.; Wilson, G.: 'The Influence of Psychologic Factors upon Gastro-Intestinal Disturbances': A Symposium: a report upon research carried on at the Chicago Institute for Psychoanalysis. *The Psychoanalytic Quarterly,* October, 1934, Vol. III, pp. 501-588.

4. Alexander, F. and Wilson, G.: 'Quantitative Dream Studies.' *Psychoanalytic Quarterly,* 1935, Vol. IV, pp. 371-405.

5. Deutsch, H.: 'The Significance of Masochism in the Mental Life of Women.' *International Journal of Psycho-Analysis,* 1929, Vol. XI, p. 48.

6. Ferenczi, S.: *The Phenomena of Hysterical Materialization. Further Contributions to Theory and Technique of Psycho-Analysis.* (London, Hogarth Press, 1926.)

7. Freud, Sigmund: 'The Psychogenesis of a Case of Female Homosexuality.' *International Journal of Psycho-Analysis,* 1920, Vol. I, p. 125.

8. Freud: 'Hysterical Phantasies and their Relation to Bisexuality.' *Collected Papers,* Vol. II. (London, Hogarth Press, 1924.)

9. Freud: 'General Remarks on Hysterical Attacks.' *Collected Papers,* Vol. II. (London, Hogarth Press, 1924.)

10. Freud: 'A Child is Being Beaten.' *Collected Papers,* Vol. II, pp. 172-201. (London, Hogarth Press, 1924.)

11. Freud: 'On the Physical Mechanisms of Hysterical Phenomena.' *Collected Papers,* Vol. I, pp. 24-42. (London, Hogarth Press, 1924.)

12. Horney, K.: 'The Flight from Womanhood. The Masculinity Complex in Women as Viewed by Men and by Women.' *International Journal of Psycho-Analysis,* 1926, Vol. VII, p. 324.

13. Horney, K.: 'On the Genesis of the Castration Complex in Women.' *International Journal of Psycho-Analysis,* 1924, Vol. V, p. 50.

14. Jones, Ernest: 'The Early Development of Female Sexuality.' *International Journal of Psycho-Analysis,* 1927, Vol. VIII, p. 459.

15. Jones, Ernest: 'Notes on Dr. Abraham's Article on the Female Castration Complex.' *International Journal of Psycho-Analysis,* 1922, Vol. III, p. 327.

16. Klein, Melanie: *The Psycho-Analysis of Children.* (London, Hogarth Press, 1932.)

17. Lampl de Groot, A.: 'The Evolution of the Œdipus Complex in Women.' *International Journal of Psycho-Analysis*, 1928, Vol. IX, p. 332.

18. Lewin, Bertram: 'The Body as Phallus.' *The Psychoanalytic Quarterly*, 1933, Vol. II, p. 24.

19. Mason-Thompson, E. R.: 'The Relation of the Elder Sister to the Development of the Electra Complex.' *International Journal of Psycho-Analysis*, 1920, Vol. I, p. 186.

20. Menninger, K.: 'Some Unconscious Psychological Factors Associated with the Common Cold.' *The Psychoanalytic Quarterly*, 1934, Vol. XXI, No. 2.

21. Rado, Sandor: 'Fear of Castration in Women.' *The Psychoanalytic Quarterly*, 1933, Vol. II, p. 425.

22. Sachs, Hanns: 'The Wish to be a Man.' *International Journal of Psycho-Analysis*, 1920, Vol. I, p. 262.

23. Saul, Leon: 'Psychogenic Factors in the Etiology of the Common Cold' (to be published).

24. Van Ophuijsen, J. H. W.: 'Contributions to the Masculinity Complex in Women.' *International Journal of Psycho-Analysis*, 1924, Vol. V, p. 39.

8. Special Symptoms

This category is for the occasional patient whose psychopathology is manifested by a single specific symptom. It includes disorders of speech such as stuttering, specific learning disturbances that may include reading or arithmetic disability, tics (which involve the small muscle groups in repetitious, involuntary and seemingly purposeless movement), sleep disorders, and feeding disturbances.

19. The Function of Choice in the Psychotherapy of a Stutterer*

Louis Diamant

Clinicians working with stutterers can choose from among a number of theories to explain this speech pathology. Some writers have described the etiology of stuttering as physiological; others have said it is learned behavior; and still others have theorized that stuttering is a symptom of emotional conflict. Psychoanalytic theory likens the emotional dynamics of stuttering to obsessions and compulsions with similar psychosexual regression. In the obsessive-compulsive syndrome, the patient tries to avoid both masculine-aggressive and feminine-receptive behavior and, by vacillation, he avoids a fantasied consequence of either aggression or receptivity. Speech may acquire special unconscious, aggressive and sexual properties. In this case study, Bobby's stuttering was believed to be related to emotional conflict and, further, to be the main expression of this emotional disturbance. Psychological examination of nine-year-old Bobby indicated much vacillation between passive and active thoughts and behavior, as well as tendencies toward obsession and compulsion. Observations made in the early play therapy sessions confirmed the diagnostic impressions of psychological testing. The act of choosing was extremely difficult and decision-making was viewed as the cornerstone of treatment. Thus the therapy sessions were designed to maximize opportunities for the patient to make decisions without the approval or disapproval of the therapist. Further, Rollo May's position that decision precedes insight was employed, with the acquisition of insight viewed as a reinforcement. Therapy was successful and two years after treatment no speech or adjustment problems were reported.

Cameron (1963) postulates the importance of decision-making, stating, in effect, that conflict, choice and decision-making are related to the advancement of ego-organization. In psychotherapy, considerable importance is given the patient's capacity for decision-making and the ability to make a choice is frequently viewed as a sign of progress with the assignment of value to this behavior crossing theoretical lines.

In reciprocal inhibition and desensitization therapy (Wolpe, 1958), the capacity for choice and decision-making appear available to the patient after he has undergone the anxiety-reducing exercises involved in treatment. In operant conditioning situations, choice can bring the patient music (Barrett, 1962), attention (Allen et al., 1965), or relief from discomfort (Flanagan, Goldiamond & Azrin, 1958). In dynamic psychiatry, decision-making is considered an ego-function and is commonly viewed as a result of insight gained from the investigation of unconscious motivation during treatment. Humanistic and existential psychologists have equated effective choice with emotional well-being. Rogers (1961) has described choice in therapy as a result of the availability of the elements of experience to awareness.

Rollo May (1958) feels, however, that both knowledge and insight precede decision. The decision-making May describes is related to an attitude towards existence rather than to those choices of which we are more commonly aware (marriage, job change, etc.). He states that the concept of decision preceding insight is crucial and yet has never been taken into account in writings on psychotherapy.

The treatment procedure presented in this paper depends on the hypothesis that decision-making brings on insight, and, further, that the patient's development and confirmation of the new concept is a form of reinforcement (Sawrey & Telford, 1968). That an organism should continue an activity which is rewarded by a strengthening of its biological effectiveness has been demonstrated in a number of situations in the laboratory (Scott & Vernay, 1947). The disturbance of choice by stress-producing stimuli has also been demonstrated (Masserman, 1943).

Although this case study presents no revolutionary approach to play therapy, it does provide a means for examining a concept that could contribute to a theory of differential treatment for one childhood disorder. Human behavior has been assumed to be modified developmentally by decision-making, beginning with primary psycho-biological choices through high-level conceptual ones in later years, and a disturbance in the decision-making function involving psycho-sexual development was believed to have produced symptoms of stuttering in the patient. In this case of stuttering related to an obsessive-compulsive orientation, play therapy designed to encourage a maximum of decision-making was required. Neither approval nor disapproval were used as reinforcements to produce desired behavior nor did the patient receive interpretation.

The patient, nine-year-old Bobby W., had been referred to the clinic by his pediatrician for stuttering and "nervousness." When first seen at the clinic he stuttered severely although he had, for two years previously, been treated by a school speech therapist. Mrs. W. reported that Bobby's stuttering had begun when he was about three years of age, lasted for about a month, begun again in the first grade, and then gotten progressively worse. She stated, too, that he liked to have everything very neat and was, in her words, a "perfectionist." Mrs. W. seemed to have been over-protective but was extremely concerned about Bobby's difficulty in engaging in the usual pastimes and games with boys his age. Bobby's father, a mechanic and part-time farmer, provided an adequate income, and enjoyed hunting and fishing. He was, however, passive in family affairs, usually deferring to his wife on decisions involving Bobby. Mr. W., too, appeared frustrated by his inability to get Bobby interested in outside activities.

Intelligence testing showed Bobby to be of average intelligence, although the examiner did not feel the 107 IQ to be optimal. When asked (from the Wechsler Intelligence Scale for Children), "What is the thing to do if a fellow much smaller than yourself starts to fight with you?" and "Why should women and children be saved first in a shipwreck?" Bobby did not answer nor would he even venture a guess when strongly urged to respond. These questions appeared to touch on Bobby's confusion concerning aggressive and passive, masculine and feminine behavior. Such conflicting themes were seen throughout the Rorschach protocol. For example, on Card VIII he saw "a beaver climbing some rocks" (aggressive and industrious), and then, after a brief pause, he said, "No, it's a squirrel." On Card IV Bobby's first response was "a wild animal or huge monster," but he abandoned this response quickly and said, "No, it's a flower." Psychological and psychiatric evaluations provided strong evidence of an obsessive-compulsive orientation. Fenichel (1945) sees in stuttering much of the regression through phallic, anal and oral stages that is in compulsion neurosis. In the course of this regression, speech acquires certain phallic, aggressive and destructive capabilities. It had apparently become increasingly difficult for Bobby to choose active-masculine or even passive-feminine behavior when appropriate and stuttering seemed symbolic of his vacillation and inability to make choices. Play therapy was recommended.

In therapy he was given maximum opportunity to choose and act. Once a choice of action was made, the therapist did not try to strengthen or discourage the behavior with approval or disapproval since the therapy was based on the belief that decision-making brought its own reward.

In the early sessions Bobby appeared immobilized by his inability to make decisions. Although large and strong for his age, he found it difficult to do such things as tear cellophane wrappings or plastic tape which sealed a box. Neither would he make a fist to hit the punching bag but rather slapped awkwardly at it. He was undecided as to whether he was left-handed or right-handed and stated so. This lateral confusion seemed more related to male-female orientation than to neuro-muscular lag and his development of strong-handedness during therapy subsequently supported this view.

Bobby's development of laterality occurred with a concomitant improvement in his speech. This and his approach to another area of indecision are illustrated by the following session.

Bobby entered my office in a rather aggressive, almost swaggering manner. He immediately set up a target ball game, then sat in my swivel chair and, spinning it, pitched to the target each time he came around. He was throwing considerably better and consistently left-handed. After playing at this for a while he went to the playroom to make a plaster of paris figure. There were aprons for this activity made out of patterned fabric which could have been interpreted as being somewhat feminine. I pointed out the aprons and explained their purpose, but he would not wear one. Ordinarily, children working with plaster of paris were simply told to put on an apron, but I did not say a word in this case. I knew that Bobby had done a great deal of housework and that this decision was important. I recalled an earlier session in which he had very skillfully made a pot holder from loops but stopped before tying up the last loops. When I asked why he had left it untied, he undid this female performance by taking the pot holder apart, loop by loop, putting the loops carefully back in the bag. In the current session he had chosen to make a plaster model for which he had not mixed nearly enough plaster. The model did not come out, and his clothing, shoes and hair were covered with the plaster. Bobby complained bitterly about both conditions. I neither advised nor admonished. He had decided to risk his mother's anger about his clothing and I had let him.

Predominantly, and almost to the closing sessions, the decision-making was largely connected with activities such as throwing, going out to the parking lot to play, going to the vending machines, making models, painting, slopping clay or plaster of paris. Discussions relating to making decisions for outside situations were rare. It seemed that Bobby had first to work through the process of choice and identity in activities which directly involved the therapist. Transference appeared to lend meaning to the acts of choice in fundamental close physical and verbal behavior. However, towards the close of therapy there was a reversal in this tendency and Bobby's play activities were those expected from an eleven-year-old and he increasingly discussed home and school problems. The course of therapy provided a number of excellent opportunities to observe the movement to higher levels of choice. It appeared that earlier discussions of "problems" were used by Bobby to maintain the conflict between his mother and the therapist and that they had little chance of solution through advice or approval. It seemed that Bobby did not seek answers to these outside situations, but more often than not sought to maintain the externalization of his own male-female identity conflict as a tussle between his therapist and his mother.

As decision-making brought on ego growth, Bobby sought action in reality. An example of higher-level decision-making may be seen in a session near the end of the therapy.

Bobby had maintained, with Mrs. W.'s insistence and encouragement, a belief in Santa Claus until almost the closing sessions. When he had discussed this topic in an early session it seemed then that he had presented the question of Santa's existence as a challenge to his mother's dictum and, with the decision left up to him at that time, it remained unresolved for almost two years. In the 69th session, which followed the Christmas holidays, he once more brought up the Santa Claus theme. The crux of the matter was, as Bobby expressed it, that Santa Claus had gotten to his house last and had run out of the things Bobby wanted. He seemed torn between the belief that there was a real Santa Claus and that his parents had put the gifts under the tree. He said that a friend had waited up all night and had told him that here was no Santa Claus— that it was really his parents. Bobby did not quite believe this story and his mother had continued to encourage him to believe in Santa Claus. When he asked me directly, I told him that he should consider the evidence and make up his own mind. He made the assessment against Santa, a decision which the case worker reported as upsetting to his mother. But Bobby stuck to his decision and Mrs. W.'s opinion did not drive his belief into an obsessional limbo. The Santa Claus decision was, in some respects, a crucial juncture in therapy for it indicated not only the consolidation of gains for Bobby but seemed to signal the relinquishment of Mrs. W.'s own obsessional concerns with her son's behavior, as well as her own development of broader relationships and interests.

While progress has not been chronicled in this brief paper, Bobby's speech did improve with the course of therapy. Stuttering, the primary symptom of his emotional disturbance, diminished as ego strength obviated this behavior. The gains in psychotherapy are attributed largely to the advancement in ego organization promoted by decision-making and, two years after treatment, no speech or behavior problems were reported. Although laissez-faire play activity has currently lost favor to the more obviously structured and less permissive behavior modification, reality therapy, etc., it could, with appropriate exposition and specific application, regain some of its lost glitter.

REFERENCES

1. Allen, K. et al. Effects of social reinforcement on isolate behavior of a nursery school child. In L. Ullman and L. Krasner (Eds.), *Case studies in behavior modification.* New York: Holt, Rinehart & Winston, 1965. Pp. 307-312.

2. Barrett, B. H. Reduction in rate of multiple tics by free operant conditioning methods. *Journal of Nervous & Mental Disease,* 1962, **135**, 187-195.

3. Cameron, N. *Personality development and psychopathology.* Boston: Houghton Mifflin, 1963.

4. Fenichel, O. *The psychoanalytic theory of neurosis.* New York: Norton, 1945.

5. Flanagan, B., Goldiamond, I., and Azrin, N. Operant stuttering: The control of stuttering behavior through response-contingent consequence. *Journal of the Experimental Analysis of Behavior,* 1958, **1**, 173-178.

6. Masserman, J. *Behavior and neurosis.* Chicago: University of Chicago Press, 1943.

7. May, R. Contributions of existential psychotherapy. In R. May, E. Angel, and H. Ellenberger (Eds.), *Existence.* New York: Basic Books, 1958. Pp. 37-91.

8. Rogers, C. R. *On becoming a person.* Boston: Houghton Mifflin, 1961.

9. Sawrey, J. and Telford, C. *Educational psychology.* Boston: Allyn & Bacon, 1968.

10. Scott, E. M. and Vernay, E. L. Self-selection of diet. VI. The nature of appetites for B vitamins. *Journal of Nutrition,* 1947, **34**, 471-480.

11. Wolpe, J. *Psychotherapy by reciprocal inhibition.* Stanford, Calif.: Stanford University Press, 1958.

9. Transient Situational Disturbances

This category is reserved for more or less transient disorders of any severity (including those of psychotic proportions) that occur in individuals without any apparent underlying mental disorders and that represent an acute reaction to overwhelming environmental stress. Disorders are classified according to the patient's developmental stage; i.e., adjustment reaction of infancy, childhood, adolescence, adult life, or late life.

An adjustment reaction of infancy, for example, might be grief associated with separation from the patient's mother, manifested by crying spells, loss of appetite, and severe social withdrawal. Jealousy associated with the birth of a patient's younger brother, an adjustment reaction of childhood, is manifested by nocturnal enuresis, attention-getting behavior, and fear of being abandoned. An example of an adjustment reaction of adolescence would be irritability and depression associated with school failure and manifested by temper outbursts, brooding, and discouragement. Fear associated with military combat and manifested by trembling, running, and hiding constitutes one example of an adjustment reaction of adult life. An adjustment reaction of late life might be manifested by social withdrawal associated with feelings of rejection in connection with forced retirement.

20. Diagnostic Psychodrama with a College Freshman*

Donald G. Zytowski

The psychodrama is an elaborate method of group psychotherapy which can also be used as a diagnostic device. As a diagnostic instrument it can be considered much the same as a projective technique in that it permits the observer some understanding of a person's behavior and dynamic traits in a situation which, while being organized, is unstructured enough to elicit very revealing responses. In the psychodrama, auxiliaries (usually trained actors) provide the working stimulus and the director is the analyst and psychotherapist. Proponents of psychodrama believe that only through this process is the patient able to express highly personal and emotional thoughts in a setting resembling real life.

Jill, the 18-year-old college freshman described in Zytowski's study, sought help at the University Counseling Center when, for emotional reasons, she could not cope with her English assignments. Except for her difficulties in English she was doing well in school both scholastically and socially, and the focus of her disturbance appeared to be in her composition course. The counselor felt that Jill had overreacted to what appeared to be an ordinary event in college life. He therefore sought a diagnosis on a deeper level and chose psychodrama for this purpose. Although the auxiliaries in this case were untrained, Zytowski was able to encourage Jill to express rather strongly her guilt and hostility to herself for what she believed were her inadequacies. Prior to the psychodrama she had not been aware of this dissatisfaction with herself and had successfully covered these feelings until the time of her failing grade.

---

*Reprinted by permission from Group Psychotherapy, 1964, 17, (2-3), 123-128, J. L. Moreno, M. D., Editor. Copyright 1964, Beacon House Inc., Publishers.

Washington University operates as an adjunct of the Dean's office, a student counseling service where students who are experiencing difficulties in their educational progress are referred or bring themselves for assistance to overcome these problems, and proceed as far towards their goals as is possible.

Jill, the subject of the psychodrama, was first seen approximately two months after the beginning of her freshman term. She demonstrated some anxiety in coming to the counseling service. She inquired about the counseling service first, made an appointment, broke it, and finally appeared for a third time, and was seen in an intake interview. Her complaint concerned her inability to complete papers for English composition, a course required of all freshman students. She was at that time enrolled in a scientific curriculum, because of her interest in high school science courses and her ability in mathematics. She also indicated that high school English had been easy for her, and was interesting in its literature aspects, somewhat more than in its creative composition aspects.

Jill explained that in the first paper she wrote for English class she received a C grade, which was as much as she expected, and seemed to be in line with the achievement of the rest of her class. However, in a series of papers developing on the theme of courage, Jill attempted to use as an example of courage an incident from her own personal life and experience. The teacher rejected Jill's example of courage and this experience so shook her that in subsequent assignments on the same theme, and in new assignments in new themes, Jill had been unable to complete and turn in to the teacher any of the assignments which followed. A number of papers she had written several times but could never satisfy herself with their quality, and could never bear to turn them in.

In the course of relating these events Jill's feelings became so overpowering that she began to weep copiously. The writer felt that it was important to investigate the reasons for such an extreme reaction to what had begun as a small incident which nearly every student of English faces.

HISTORY

Jill is the eldest daughter of a Jewish family living in a southern city. The mother received three years of college, with a major in English, before quitting school to marry. It is the mother's desire that the daughters be able to complete four years of schooling, and receive a degree, as she had not. Jill has three sisters, each spaced roughly a year and a half apart, who follow her and for whom the mother is equally desirous that they receive a college education. In Jill's mind this necessitated on her own initiative the winning of a scholarship aid on the basis of good achievement her freshman year, so that she will not use too large a share of the money which is available for their education.

Jill's father is a physician, who until very recently held a teaching and research post in the local Medical School. According to Jill, he has given up this post to enter private practice, in hopes that he would be able to earn more money, so that all four children might be supported in college. She was aware of the initial expenses of setting up a private practice, and because of her father's limited specialty did not feel that he would be financially successful too soon. She felt very strongly that she wanted to win a scholarship in order to help with the family finances.

Jill enjoyed excellent relationships with peers both in high school and so far in college. She had apparently not experienced any conflicts over Jewish-Gentile relationships as they occur in Southern cities, and had enjoyed sufficiently satisfying relationships with peers of both sex, throughout. She did reveal to the writer that she had influenced a close friend to attend this University on a larger scholarship rather than another school of high renown on a smaller stipend. The obvious implication of this was more than financial, but also to be near Jill in order that they could make overtures to their possible eventual marriage. Both the boy and Jill were cognizant of this relationship but had not verbalized it to each other.

It was decided that Jill should come to see the counselor weekly during the time she attempted to work on her English papers and that she would be seen in a supportive relationship since the counselor felt that she had sufficient ego strength in spite of her present difficulties to recover her former skill. Several weeks of contacts failed to show any change in the situation. At intervals she had worked completely through the night to complete a paper but had not been able to compose her thoughts adequately nor to express herself as she had wanted to, so as to finish any paper.

THE PSYCHODRAMA

Jill was asked if she would like to participate in a rather different kind of experience with several other individuals. It was explained to her that there were several sympathetic people who were counselors-in-training with whom she, under the writer's direction, could attempt to role-play her difficulties and perhaps find some solution or reduction of anxiety accompanying her problem. In her characteristically enthusiastic manner, Jill agreed to participate.

It was decided that since her anxiety had seemed too strong for her situation, the psychodrama would necessarily have to be an exploratory or diagnostic one. Three sectors of her life were selected to be played out for Jill to see more clearly. They were the interactions and feelings about the English instructor, the interactions and feelings over her situation with regard to her family, and finally, her feelings and relationships with the boy friend whom she had attracted into attending the University with her.

The auxiliary egos were three counselors-in-training, mature persons with a background of public school teaching, and present duties as secondary school counselors, two men and one woman, all unsophisticated in the techniques of psychodrama. The warmup consisted of introductions all around and some general conversation about Jill's background and the background and interests of the auxiliary egos. Jill was then asked about some of the events which had transpired between herself and her English professor. As she began to relate the situation in which she had conferred with the teacher over her first failing grade, Jill was asked to show us how she had acted in the situation. The female auxiliary was placed in service as the English instructor and Jill reversed roles in order to demonstrate how the instructor had behaved in the situation. Jill was able to show the group that the instructor had been eminently fair in her handling of Jill's writing and her difficulties following the first incomplete paper, and that she did not harbor any hostile feelings toward the teacher.

The next area into which the group moved was Jill's relationships with her parents. The writer felt that Jill might have a need to compete with an image of her mother's success as a student of English, and roles were assigned and played out to investigate the possibilities. Jill ably conveyed to the group that she felt highly accepted by her mother, whether or not she would fail in her mother's particular field.

A scene was then worked out from a future orientation portraying Jill informing her father of poor grades. Through instructions to the auxiliaries the father was presented as outraged over the failing grade and the necessity of spending more money in order to continue Jill in school when money was obviously at a premium. Jill rejected this scene entirely as she believed it could not happen.

The next material explored the relationship with the boy friend, knowing that Jill had been influential in bringing the boy to this school. It was supposed that she might feel acute guilt should she fail so badly that she might have to leave school, thereby leaving him at a school which was not his first choice but with no alternatives to pursue his former first choice. While Jill did seem to accept the potential for this situation as valid, she was able to convince us that she was not in danger of being removed from the school, and that her failing grades were occurring only in the circumscribed area of English composition.

At this point the psychodrama was nearly concluded as being unuseful, having explored all of the hypotheses of the director without success. It was decided to follow up on one additional hypothesis, concerning the possibility that Jill had considerable inadequacy feelings which she had been veiling successfully until the time of the first failing grade. She had in the intake interview made a point of telling the counselor that she had in high school had an obesity problem over which she had to be careful to exercise control. For this situation an auxiliary was assigned the role to express an "inner voice" which spoke very forcefully but quietly the doubts and fears that nearly any freshman in a new college would experience, had enlarged upon them to the point of asserting that her failure in one course really confirmed her true inadequacy. Jill became quite involved in an active denial that this was the case. While the auxiliary was role-playing an inner voice, Jill was not role-playing, but was expressing feelings as sincerely and with more intensity than she had in either individual interviews or the group technique to this point. Finally, the inner voice role became so distressing to Jill that she shouted out with much emotion that she did not feel inadequacies, that she did not feel guilt feelings toward her parents, or her boy friend, but rather she felt it toward herself.

The writer felt that it was highly possible that Jill's ability to organize her thoughts and express herself on paper had indeed been inhibited by the angry feelings toward herself. It was further decided that some symbolic expression of these angry feelings toward herself was necessary to free her and permit her to be as effective as before the time of the first failure. The scene which followed was very intense. Using only the materials at hand, such as would be found in a group therapy room, Jill's name was written on a paper which was hung on the door.

She was urged not only by the director but by the auxiliaries to commit some act of aggression against the symbolic self. The only available mode seemed to be to throw some object at the name. Her inability to handle her anger with herself was poignantly illustrated by her inability to accept any object for this purpose. Kleenex, pencil, and note pad were all thrust into her hand, and all were promptly dropped by her as she received them.

Finally, she accepted a medium-sized and rather heavy pad of paper. It was realized that she was sitting very limply in her chair and that she would be unable to throw the object with any force while she was sitting. She was urged to stand up and really throw the object at her symbolic self on the wall. This met with the same difficulty as getting her to grasp the object. The director interceded with another auxiliary by assisting Jill to her feet and all four auxiliaries stood closely behind her with at least one hand actively, firmly supporting her back, shoulders, and arms. It was still anticipated by the director at this time that Jill would only make a symbolic effort at throwing the note pad at her name, and that this would have to be sufficient to attempt to provide a dramatic finish to her self-anger. Instead, to the director's and the auxiliaries, surprise, Jill hesitated a few moments and then threw the object with all the force and obvious emotion she could muster. There was sufficient force in the throw to result in a resounding noise, the paper was knocked from the wall and parts of the scratch pad fluttered everywhere as they fell.

Instantly Jill turned to the woman auxiliary and broke into deep sobbing tears, which persisted for several minutes. No words were said and she was offered the physical comfort of this auxiliary until she began to calm herself. She attempted to apologize for her behavior but the apology was hardly recognized by the director or the auxiliaries. Instead, to attempt to capitalize on the gains the scene might have accomplished, Jill was asked to describe her task for her next English class. She sat down calmly and then gave a verbal explanation of the theme plan and content of the next paper which she had been assigned to write. It demonstrated to those present a high degree of understanding and careful planning and tight cogent logic concerning the emotional aspects of the assigned topic. Everyone in the room was impressed with this and tried to convey to Jill their confidence that she would perform adequately, and that she would most certainly be able to complete this paper.

The session having proceeded roughly two hours, by this time, and with the apparent exhaustion of not only Jill but the auxiliaries, it was terminated at this time. There were many repeated "I'm so sorry for troubling you" and "Thank yous" on the part of Jill. It was agreed before she left that she would return in another week to discuss how her school work had proceeded in that time. In that next meeting with the counselor, Jill again wished to convey her thanks and appreciation for the help that had been given her by the group. Without being asked, Jill reported that she had been able to work on her assignment with considerably more ease than she had found since her first failure and that she anticipated that she would be able to continue this through the remainder of this semester.

CONCLUSIONS

It is the opinion of the writer that this psychodrama, originally conceived as a diagnostic session, after a near-concession to failure became a very meaningful and instrumental catharsis. The lack of formal training of the auxiliaries presented no serious problem in the situation because of the intense level of participation which finally evolved. The usefulness of psychodrama in uncovering study inhibitions among college students and its facility for intensifying and accelerating the process was aptly demonstrated by this session.

21.   The Traumatic Neuroses of War*

Abram Kardiner

World War I brought about the first major psychiatric interest in emotional disturbances resulting from combat. Large numbers of military men were incapacitated with psychological symptoms considered, at first, to be indicative of an organic central nervous system disorder resulting from the explosion of gunfire (thus the label, "shell shock"). In the years immediately following the war, investigation frequently produced no evidence of concussion, even though the symptoms greatly resembled an organic disturbance. This selection is from an extensive study of the mental disorder related to the stress of combat, and primarily associated with a particular traumatic or frightening event. The author, Abram Kardiner, was a psychoanalyst and anthropologist personally associated with Freud. Kardiner diverged from the classical analytic view by placing greater emphasis on the role of social conditions in personality development. He believed that the traumatic neurosis was extremely incapacitating, presented extreme difficulties in patient management, and urgently needed differential diagnosis and related therapy.

The 1952 edition of the American Psychiatric Association's Diagnostic and Statistical Manual of Mental Disorders *reclassified traumatic war neurosis as gross stress reaction. This has since (1968) been changed to adjustment reaction of adult life.*

The case study is that of a 33-year-old man who, by his own description, had been a "fearless" soldier until the traumatic episode in

---

*Reprinted by permission of the National Research Council, Washington, D.C., from pp. 99-112, 116-117, of "The Traumatic Neuroses of War," *Psychosomatic Medicine Monograph,* 1941.

274

combat. When seen by Kardiner the disorder had been stabilized for seven years (Kardiner divided the course of the disturbance into acute, transitional, and stabilized stages) and was, from Kardiner's point of view, a difficult treatment prospect. The patient was given to periods of panic, nightmares, acts of aggression, and loss of consciousness. Kardiner saw, in emotional disturbances precipitated by severe traumatic events, dynamics other than those which had been formally postulated in psychoanalysis. It was his belief that the usual assumption of psychoneurosis based on the interference of sexual instincts was not applicable to traumatic neurosis but, instead, the patient's problem of dealing with the environment was central to the disorder. The study presents evidence that in the traumatic neurosis the disorganization is related to an incapacity to maintain normal activity levels and the concomitant frustration.

Now we can approach the question of the character of the neurotic reaction: Is it in the nature of a regression or disorganization? The traumatic neurosis is characterized by the thinness of its psychological fabric and by the absence of those displacement phenomena which make up the bulk of the material in a transference neurosis. This absence makes us suspect that the material of this neurosis is different in character from the transference neurosis. Up to a certain point the two types of neuroses seem to be similar; judging from the amnesia that usually envelopes the traumatic event, the work of repression seems to be exactly like that in the transference type except that it does not seem to involve idea systems nearly as much as it does *action* systems. The repressed ideas are hidden from consciousness and kept there by a powerful force; the repressed affects, however, seem not to have the same leeway in the traumatic type; they cannot be as readily displaced or symbolized, and even in the dream life we find them invariably tied to the traumatic event. The repressed affects, however, are associated with constant inhibitions, and the blocked energies do find their way out again in a form not familiar in the transference neuroses. The outburst of aggression in these neuroses does not have any resemblance to the process in compulsion neurosis; in the latter, the aggression is organized and directed toward specific relations to individuals; in the traumatic neurosis, much more diffuse and disorganized. Another important difference lies in the methods both neuroses employ in handling the anxiety. It seems much more difficult in the traumatic cases. In connection with the disposal of the anxiety, the work of repression shows a departure from the psychoneurosis. In fact, after a certain point the work of repression seems to cease altogether, and the ego itself disintegrates from that point on. We have already indicated that the conflict is about the outer world and concerns certain specific instruments of mastery.

Let us first examine a case which has much in common with the ordinary neuroses:

The patient was thirty-three years old, fifth child of a family of ten, three of whom were dead. His mother had died when the patient was nine years old. This latter event, according to the patient, did not affect him very much.

At the age of twelve the patient, who did not wish to live with his brother after his father broke up house, ran away from home and became a mess boy on board a sailing vessel. His schooling was interrupted at that time and was never resumed. He never learned a trade, although he had had a large variety of occupations prior to service. Between his twelfth year and the present time the patient had spent about three years with his father, worked for a while as a sailor, then as a stove mechanic, and finally as a truckman, which occupation he continued until he entered service.

Of his history prior to service nothing definite could be established but that he had epileptiform seizures following an attack of diphtheria, which continued for an indeterminate period.[1] The character of his infantile convulsions could not be ascertained and was probably denied because he thought it would impair his status as a government claimant. His parental attachments were not unusually strong; his reaction to his mother's death was quite normal. He was emotionally a rather shallow individual; he was never in love with anyone, though he married after he returned from service a woman many years older than himself. Toward her he was very ambivalent. As a soldier he distinguished himself by extreme bravery in situations of danger.

When the patient was first seen, in March, 1925, his neurosis was seven years old. It might, perhaps, be best to tell the story as he told it himself in the course of treatment. When he entered the room he sat down rather stiffly; the expression of his face was hard, immobile, and Parkinsonian, most lines of expression being obliterated. He answered in monosyllables and seemed to have an attitude of defense. He volunteered no information and made no complaints. In looking over his previous records, I noted that the patient was suffering from spells of some kind. I

---

[1]The patient could not have had the seizures very often in service without being discharged. This fact is important, however, since it shows that the patient had proclivities for reacting with loss of consciousness. In view of the fact that the patient was not a typical epileptic, this early history does not vitiate the merits of the case. For purposes of this essay, the clinical diagnosis is immaterial.

proceeded, therefore, to make the usual inquiries about his war experiences and the traumas to which he had been subjected. At this point I began immediately to encounter a great deal of resistance and anger. He explained his anger on the basis of an unwillingness to talk about the war and especially about a certain event which had occurred in service. This particular event, he said, was the starting point of his neurosis. When his anger was abated to some extent and he was encouraged to talk about it, anxiety set in. We see, hence, that it did not take very much to uncover the anxiety underneath his superficial aggressiveness and his defensive attitude toward the environment. At this point the patient became very plaintive and pleaded for help, but insisted that concerning the traumatic event he remembered absolutely nothing. The patient was then asked to describe the fainting attacks or spells and every detail in connection with their onset which he could recall. He said everything grew dark, and he sometimes saw shadows in this clouded state. When asked to pursue the subject of shadows, he remembered that on the night he was blown up he was crawling on the ground on a scouting expedition, about seven o'clock, in pitch darkness, and that while thus engaged, searchlights began playing on the party and caused shadows on the ground. At this point the patient became very agitated and begged to be relieved from further pursuit of the subject at that time.

His following appointment was two days later. He came about two hours late and stated that for the past two days he had been in a constant state of panic, that he hardly knew where he was, that he could not sleep at night, that he was disturbed, that he had distressing dreams, and that he was afraid to move out of the house for fear he would get an attack and have to come up to the clinic in a taxicab.

This state of anxiety persisted throughout the greater part of the hour, although, when the patient first came, his anxiety was slightly covered by a series of defenses seemingly directed toward the external environment.

The task of recovering the traumatic event consumed a period of several months but was never completely accomplished. After violent upheavals and a great many distressing dreams, the patient would recall some little minor detail in connection with the frightful event. All of this was exacted from him in the face of persistent and violent resistance, in quite the same manner as the hysteric struggles to bring out the details or interpretation of some painful experience. The difficulties he had in recalling these details of the traumatic event would sometimes result in an attack of vomiting, as if he wished to vomit forth this foreign body buried in his mind. The spells came at varying intervals, sometimes twice a day, sometimes after a remission of four or five days. The occasions on which he got the spells seemed to be such as resembled or symbolized some detail of the original traumatic event. For example, he would very often have a spell just as he reached the top of the staircase and when he would enter a dark room. By the "spells" the patient intended to describe a loss of consciousness not accompanied by convulsions—a syncope without relaxation of sphincters but with occasional biting of his tongue and grinding of his teeth. This latter fact was evidenced by his many teeth broken from chewing clothespins to vent the violent aggression during his attacks. The oral character of his aggression is self-evident.

The loss of consciousness was always complete although occasionally more like a petit mal and sometimes took the form of a fugue with an outburst of violence. Of this latter type of spell, the patient described a state in which he would seize any near-by object, his shirt collar or necktie or an article of furniture, and proceed to tear or break it. On such occasions he has been known to assault any person who came into his immediate vicinity or who dared to touch him. On these occasions also he would chew his clothes and masticate them into fragments. Formerly he was precipitated into these spells by any sudden or persistent noise. The only aura which the patient had was a gradual blindness and the seeing of shadows. The major spells lasted from fifteen minutes to two hours, and he always woke up with a feeling of confusion and disorientation followed up by a stuporous sleep.

The patient stated that he was a fearless soldier, never subject to anxiety states during the war. The traumatic event took him entirely by surprise, and at the first sitting he remembered nothing but that, confined in a straitjacket, he woke up in a field hospital a long time afterwards. From his story it would seem that for a few days or possibly as long as a fortnight, the patient had been in an acutely agitated hallucinatory state. He would recall nothing more at this stage of the treatment.

After the first few sittings the repetition mechanism was explained to him, and insofar as it was possible, he was directed to see that the spells were repetitions of the original traumatic event and that in his original reaction he also lost consciousness. Furthermore, he was told that all the auras he described were hallucinatory sensory reproductions of the experience immediately preceding the first loss of consciousness on the battlefield and that he was protecting himself with all his might against any repetition in the outer world of the original trauma and against any recollection of the event.

After the first few sittings then, the patient's reactions were extremely violent and distressing. This phenomenon has been observed by some other authors, who state, therefore, that such a practice of permitting them to recall the original trauma is wrong in these traumatic cases. With this view I cannot concur, for this recollection is a means to an end. This attitude of alarm, when the patient shows an aggravation of symptoms, speaks for a lack of experience and an ignorance of the psychopathology of the disease. Any form of anxiety that the patient expresses is, from the point of view of therapy, a much more benign reaction than any of those which set in as a result of complete suppression of the anxiety. Whereas the patient may complain and may appear, for the time being, to those which set in as a result of complete suppression of the anxiety. is the kernel of the therapy. One must not be alarmed by it. The patient's immediate reaction was that he had seven spells within a period of a week after his first visit to me; that he spent two sleepless nights; and that, although he had been having anxiety dreams for the past seven years, they did not compare in terror with those he had had since his first visit to me.

He then said that ever since the traumatic event he had suffered from insomnia, from the typical anxiety dreams. The content of these dreams was that something horrible was happening to him or that he was in the rôle of the aggressor by killing some man and was punished as a result, or finally that some person very dear to him was dead. Immediately after the treatment was begun, the patient brought two dreams: "I dreamed that I was killing a man and then that I was being electrocuted. I really felt the electric shocks going right through me. I couldn't sleep for a long time. Then I had another dream in which I was murdering a man. The horror of these dreams was so great that I had to get up and walk the floor until seven o'clock in the morning. Then I tried to go to sleep again, but I was awakened this time by a dream that the enemy was after me. Then I found I couldn't sleep any more, and during the following four days I had dreams in which I tore my hair and my clothes."

The remarkable feature of all this was that, together with a dependency upon me for help, a vast amount of anxiety was released.

The dreams brought by the patient were that he was being tortured, killed, persecuted by people around him with weapons, or that he was being annihilated by the elements, that thunder and lightning were raging around him, or that he was falling from great heights. He also dreamed that people to whom he was much attached were being killed. This sometimes concerned his wife and sometimes his father. These latter dreams were extremely distressing, and whenever he had one of this variety, the patient came with a profound feeling of guilt and with the same kind of conflict found in the transference neurotics when they discover their hostile wishes and death fantasies about some person whom they presumably love. The type of dreams in which the patient was the aggressor was usually the more distressing. In fact, one could hardly perceive any difference in affect toward the dreams in which he was the aggressor and those in which he was being annihilated. As we shall later show, the dream of annihilation and the dream of aggression are complementary parts of the same nuclear complex.

A dream in which he was killing his wife obsessed him for days. After such a dream he would walk around the next day crying, but he did not know about what. When asked to associate with it, he said that his wife, the most valuable person in the world to him, had helped him through all his difficulties, and yet he had dreams of murdering her, of seeing her casket being carried out, and so on. The guilt which obsessed the patient often took the form of hypnogogic hallucinations, in which someone, usually in uniform, would point a finger at him and shout, "You killed me!" This type of experience would often repeat itself several times during the same night. These aggressive dreams almost always brought associations about his mother. She usually was encouraging him, advising him not to be afraid, and assuring him that she was in her resting place. In association with these sadistic dreams, the patient mentioned that prior to service he had frequent occasion to witness accidents. This he did with perfect equanimity; he had several times seen men killed in the railroad yards, he saw a lion escape in Central Park from the Zoo, he saw operations performed on animals; but he was never fearful.

Prior to the war he was never afraid of death; even now, when directly questioned, he said that he did not fear death, but that he rather wished for it as a release from his difficulties. He narrated, moreover, that before service he was a gentle and agreeable person but that now he was always looking for trouble, carried a chip on his shoulder, and was always ready to pick a quarrel. This notwithstanding, the patient was very easily frightened by anything which suggested fighting. If he chanced to be at a motion picture with a war scene or a battle or a gun in action, he would go into paroxysms. Whenever a loud noise occurred on the street, he either would be thrown into a panic, a paroxysm, or would start running wildly for blocks at a stretch, finally ending up some alley. On one such occasion he ran for about ten blocks from the original scene, then up three or four flights into a hallway, and landed, exhausted, in a factory. This is very like the running amok observed among the Malays. When asked why he ran, he said that he did not know, that he could not stop running; it was, indeed, very much like the reaction of a frightened horse.

The patient had several displacement symptoms. He feared going uphill or downhill. We shall see presently that this going up- and downhill was associated with the original trauma. He feared falling; he feared riding in a subway train; he feared a collision or the train's jumping the track. He was mortally afraid of street traffic. When he came home and found nobody there, he feared that there had been burglars in the house or that the house was on fire. He feared diving into water or climbing a pole, both of which he had done with bravado as a child. An important displacement was the fear that somebody was following him on the street. This did not have the character or the persistence of a paranoid delusion but seemed a part of his general fearful adaptation to the environment, and he knew that these ideas of being followed were imaginative. He did not take any of the usual paranoid defenses against pursuit.

Concerning his minor spells, the patient often described phenomena of transient blindness. These he got most often when stepping out of a car or a vehicle or out of a house, or when he would see someone being hurt. On several such occasions he had to be taken home by some passer-by. Another form his behavior took was fugues of violence, in which he tore bedclothes to strips, chewed up clothespins, tore his collars, and struck people. Compulsive and senseless laughter and nonsensical talk, of which he was entirely unaware, were also the content of these spells.

As regards the original trauma, the patient did not, during the period of observation, succeed in completely recalling and reconstructing the event. With a great deal of effort, however, he was able to put together some of the fragments sufficiently to indicate some of the conditions under which he lapsed into the state of unconsciousness. His attacks of violence and transient blindness were associated with the trauma. He was able to recall that it took place in 1918; twenty-three kilometers from Metz. He remembered also that he got the command at seven o'clock in the evening, twilight being the time when he got the largest number of spells. He remembered also being in very good spirits. A short while after being given the command it was revoked. He recalled stopping for dinner and having carrot soup. It was stormy and dark, and shells were bursting around him. He climbed up a hill, then heard the word, "Duck, duck!" This latter detail of being on the verge of an incline and hearing the word "duck" recurred in several dreams. He also remembered that the terrible night was Monday and that he woke up two days later in a straitjacket, a considerable distance away from the original site. This was in a dressing station. When the patient first woke out of his unconscious state, he said he was "like a rubber ball." When anybody touched him he "would jump sky-high." Completely disoriented, he did not know his name, could not walk, fell over objects, stuttered, vomited, and talked in a childish gibberish. His reactions were those of a severely frightened child about two years of age. He did not have any persistent paralysis. The whole world seemed to be full of danger; he showed a trait very commonly found in these cases, also in certain cases of epilepsy. He readily identified himself with anyone meeting with an untoward accident. Thus, on one occasion, the patient was on the street when somebody was struck by an automobile. He immediately began to run as though pursued by someone. He ran for blocks and then dashed into a hallway, where he recovered enough to ask for some water. He was in no danger at all; the other fellow was being hurt.

He recalled that, after being confined in a straitjacket for some time, he was released, whereupon he ran away. He did not know where he was running nor why. He was caught and taken back to the hospital, where he said someone tried to reassure him by showing him a dead man—a most inappropriate piece of active therapy.

Concerning the original trauma, a few more details were uncovered. He remembered that he was in the second line trenches; that a dud came over, fell near him, and threw a great deal of mud on him; and that he was, in all likelihood, trampled over by his comrades who were running away from the dud. Many other details he could not unite with the original trauma, but, as far as could be learned, the patient was not blown up by a shell. What had probably happened was that he was given a command to go over the top, which he did; that, as he landed in a second line trench, a shell came over but did not explode, landed near him, and splashed him with mud; that in the confusion he was thrown down and trampled upon by those around him.

Furthermore, the patient's attitude toward work is notable. He could not resume his former occupation, and all his efforts at rehabilitating himself in a new occupation were unsuccessful. He had the typical attitude of inadequacy to work. The accuracy of manipulation of his hands and fingers and his ability to coördinate them in any form of manual work were markedly impaired. He described a phenomenon I have encountered frequently in the dreams of traumatic neurotics, namely, certain days occurred on which everything would go wrong, on which he was incapable of holding objects in his hands; he would stumble over everything and would break things, very often to the detriment of his employer. Extremely slow at work, he would labor for hours over something which normally should consume only a few minutes. Needless to say, the patient was able to bestow but little interest upon his working activities. An interesting feature about this case was that the words most common in the patient's vocabulary were those describing combat and struggle. He was always "fighting something through," "winning something." The successful accomplishment of a task was described as "murdering it." This is also an interesting specimen of the preseverative tendency of the traumatic case and also of the epileptic.

Thus, in the patient's adaptation we see a tremendous battle against the environment and a complete inability to exert a high degree of control over part of his personality—that part concerned with the mastery of the environment, even in the form of a feeling of security or in the ability to perform any persistent work. Accordingly he endured the frustrations impatiently; impediments to the ease and comfort of his external existence were tolerated with particular difficulty. He responded with exaggerated and disorganized affect to physical hurt. Any trifling scratch or slight to his person would throw him into a panic. He suffered extreme fluctuations of temper from great violence and anger to maudlin tenderness. For example, he cried for three days when he had to have his dog killed, and he melted with tears when he witnessed a funeral procession. His emotional ties had a conspicuous poverty; but this impression may have been produced by his conflict with the external environment which, for the time being, overshadowed his social relations with people. All his reactions were either sadistic or masochistic. Moreover, the patterns of his love life and social life were probably drawn from those of his relations to the outer world.

After observation for about a period of five months his nightmares of sado-masochistic content ceased, and he was able to sleep the greater part of the night, and his spells had subsided to a large extent. The issue of compensation was, however, a great obstacle to the cure of this patient. He frequently understated his improvement, for fear that if I reported him well, he would lose his compensation. Thus, after an absence of seven months, the patient alleged that he continued to have spells; but on inquiry his wife informed me that he had not had a spell for five months. One must, furthermore, note that during the early course of the treatment the symptoms increased in severity. By that I mean his anxiety and distress became much more severe. The capacity for displacement, anxiety, and transference were the means of his partial rehabilitation.

Most of the patient's symptoms were reactivated on the occasion of a mild trauma. One evening he was in a taxi which collided with another vehicle. His old panicky reaction returned. All his symptoms, dreams, spells, and secondary defenses recurred. He was in such a disturbed condition that he had to be taken to Bellevue Hospital and kept there for several days. Prior to this time he had had no spells, slept well, ate well, had ceased his vomiting, was free from cardiospasms, and was becoming much less sensitive to noise. This new trauma, however, did not have any lasting effect; after a short period his condition was about the same as before discontinuance of treatment.

We must emphasize especially the existence of defects in the patient's adaptation prior to the onset of his illness. They existed together with a pronounced poverty of achievement. He had many vocational difficulties and educational handicaps. I was not able to elicit, during the time of treatment, any reasonable account of why he left home at an early age, except that it followed the death of his mother and that he did not want to live with his father. His early epileptiform attacks indicate already a marked constitutional factor and the projection of the bulk of his conflict with the outer world.

When the patient first presented himself, we found a neurosis with the following characteristics. The patient was evidently in severe conflict which he had partly succeeded in repressing. The only ideational representation of the repressed material was to be found in the conscious recollection of the trauma. Against this and against any situation which resembled it, he directed all his energy. He had almost a complete amnesia for the traumatic event and the reactivation thereof was met with the same resistance we encounter in the transference neuroses when a deeply repressed factor is approached.

The content of the material which the patient was trying to keep from consciousness was chiefly the traumatic event. This need not be inferred; he was quite explicit about it. When his vigilance was somewhat relaxed as in sleep, he was disturbed by hallucinatory reproductions or faintly disguised and displaced representations of this experience.

He had several typical types of dreams: a) the dream of annihilation; b) the dream of aggression with punishment; c) the dream of cruel activities or hostile wishes against those whom he loved best, associated with strong guilt affect.

In the dreams of annihilation he was awakened, as usual, by the desire to evade the threat of extermination. In the dreams of punishment we have a replacement of the aggression onto another object; the aggression is now turned upon the patient himself. This is a complicated phenomenon to be treated at length later. The hallucinations of fingers pointing at him also belong in this category. In the third type of dream the transformation of this aggression toward the love object occurs with the accompaniment of intense guilt which is unbearable and tortures him throughout the day. To note the point at which these guilt dreams occurred in the course of the neurosis is very important. They were most persistent during the time when the patient made an active transference onto me and became dependent upon me for help. Thus the patient is trying to repress an instinctive urge, which to the outer world expresses itself as either aggression or fear of annihilation but, when directed toward his love objects, takes the form of cruelty with the corresponding reaction formation of great tenderness and pity. Thus, he cries when his dog dies.

What the patient expresses in the form of guilt to his love object he expresses to the outer world as a fear of annihilation. The guilt is, thus, the expression of the aggressive impulse directed toward an object whom the patient needs for his protection. On the other hand, the aggression itself is apparently caused by the failure of the object (mother) to intervene between him and the hostile environment. In either case he feels helpless, and devoid either of resources to master the world or of a protector who will do it for him, he is justified in feeling the world to be a hostile place. This fear of the outer world is really another way of indicating that he has lost the means of mastery. Such a state of affairs we showed to be the case in the dreams of a man who was suffering from a vascular disease which he knew to be progressive and fatal.

Hence the conflict in the annihilation dreams is, therefore, the repression of the persistent urge to master the world, at least sufficiently to be able to live comfortably in it, and the patient's incapacity to do so by virtue of the inhibitions initiated by the trauma. The patient thus makes a compromise with the assumption toward the environment of a passive attitude which cannot be represented in another way than by annihilation. In his behavior toward the environment the individual has not the leeway that he has in the sexual domain, where the repressed aggression takes the form either of guilt or of the assumption of a feminine attitude. In this instance we see a familiar phenomenon in the compulsion neurosis in which the guilt feeling the patient has to his love objects is due to the expectation of being loved by those objects toward whom he has repressed, however, a strong aggressive tendency based on the frustrations. Hence the reaction formation in the guise of excessive tenderness. But the passivity to the outer world cannot be thus elaborated. If his aggression—by which is meant merely organized mastery—to the outer world is inhibited, he can only remain in contact with it at all by compelling it to maintain him without his own efforts, just as it did when he was an infant. But then the entire outer world was encompassed in the mother. In this way he re-established, to a degree, his shattered relations to the external world. The dependency upon compensation is thus a defensive measure. By his infantilism he wants to compel the mother to pity him and thus force her to take him to her again. His normal aggression to the outer world being blocked, he reinstates a childish attitude of dependency on his wife, mother, physician, government. That the trauma symbolizes birth in this case, there can be no doubt; for under no other conditions is there such a sudden release of aggression due to helplessness and so extreme an attempt at mastery by way of the oral zone.

The inhibitions to maintaining a normally aggressive attitude, which means just normal activity, to the outer world shows itself in tremors, slowness of motion, vertigo, clumsiness, inability to hold objects in his hands, spells, and so on. As secondary defenses against this repressed aggression we see a reaction not unlike the feeling of guilt. He defends himself against the onslaught of the environment by a sensitivity to stimuli, by a rigidity to posture and motion, by a complete disorganization of his responses, and by an attempt to exclude the outer world by means of attacks of transient blindness or spells of unconsciousness, in which state alone the patient is able to carry out the mastery in the form of disorganized activity by breaking, tearing, smashing, and so forth. One must especially note the tendency which this patient has toward oral destruction. He tears objects not only with his hands, but he takes them into his mouth, he grinds clothespins, he tears sheets with his teeth. All these defenses cover up an anxiety which, however, remains accessible. This anxiety is, *par excellence,* an indication of the amount of organization which remains in the ego. We shall return subsequently to deal with this problem at length. Whereas this patient's anxiety is always at hand, in other cases we find that the anxiety once present has completely disappeared beyond resuscitation. Yet clinical symptoms exist not unlike those described in this last case.

We can attempt to evaluate the pathological processes in this case from the viewpoint of 1) discharge phenomena and 2) regression. If we consider the aggressive outbursts as discharge phenomena, we must first account for the tensions which accumulate. These give no direct evidence. We know only of certain things which the patient has lost the capacity to do. Can this be the source of the accumulated tensions? They cannot possibly come from any other source. For these activities are slow, gradual, integrated release phenomena which make up the bulk of sheer existence. The evidence for their contraction exists in the form of the lost aptitudes to work and activity generally. We can say, therefore, that these normal activities are organized, integrated, and purposeful discharge phenomena which, being blocked, are now replaced by disorganized, purposeless, unintegrated activities like discharge phenomena in appearance. So the problem of discharge reduces itself to a problem of form, organization, and purpose. The purpose is gone because the utility or pleasurable objective seems to have vanished.

The question about whether these phenomena are to be regarded as disorganized or regressive will be taken up later. Meanwhile it is essential to recognize the difference between these phenomena and those encountered in the transference neuroses. Here we find no slow, gradually integrated use of a type of adaptation used in infancy, and which yields gratifications similar to those earlier ones. If we predicate a regression we must, moreover, be able to identify the infantile prototype. In infancy there is a stage of mastery which consists of tearing, breaking of objects, prior to the development of dexterities which extract a higher pleasure or utility value from the organized manipulation. The child gets much satisfaction from these early activities. One could, therefore, say that these disorganized aggressive phenomena represent a regression. If so, it must be added that there is no such gratification in the traumatic neurosis, because the utility of the object and the utility function of the executive apparatus cannot be exploited. It produces nothing but frustration. On the other hand true regressive phenomena do occur in the acute phases of traumatic neurosis. . . .

To recapitulate: The traumatic event creates excitations beyond the possibility of mastering, inflicts a severe blow to the total ego organization. The activities involved in successful adaptation to the external environment become blocked in their usual outlets. These activities are executive in character and take in the entire apperceptive and executive apparatus, the sensory-motor, the higher intellectual centres, and the autonomic system. These activities are consummated in some form of *aggression*. This *aggression* is expressed in every function of the sensory-motor apparatus and its adjuncts, the central and autonomic nervous systems. This aggression is, moreover, capable of infinite degrees of refinement and is progressive with the growth of the child. The adaptation to the external world is the result of a complicated series of integrations, which owe their existence in part to the narcissistic gratification of success. As a result of the trauma, that portion of the ego which normally helps the individual to carry out automatically certain organized aggressive functions of perception and activity on the basis of innumerable successes in the past is either destroyed or inhibited.

The adaptation to this situation takes on various aspects in accordance with different factors. A diminished capacity to exercise the functions that can yield gratifications in the world exists, together with a constant desire to have done with the world completely and, at the same time, to adapt the self on a level compatible with these altered resources. In the paralytic types (sensory or motor) such adaptation is most successful and consists of an obliteration of only a portion of the world, namely the offending part; but the rest of the world can still yield its gratifications. This is really a negative form, autoplastically done, of mastering the world or rendering it harmless. The patient throws away or sacrifices a piece of his ego, the introjected world, to maintain a certain equilibrium.

The wish to have done with the world in many instances takes on a phobic form, with the constant but ineffectual effort to re-establish harmonious relations with it. This is affected by a regressive process of a) making fewer demands on it, b) by re-establishing an infantile relation to it. This means that the higher, more elaborate adaptations are so inhibited while the more primitive ones are so reactivated that in the end only two modalities exist: mastering the world or being annihilated. The phobic character is emphasized by the higher investment of all seismic and sensory apparatus, irritability, and the lower types of mastery, disorganized aggression. In this type the attitude to the world is ambivalent, if one may so describe it.

In another type the wish to obliterate the world and to re-establish amicable relations with it takes the form of a total obliteration of the world episodically or periodically, in the form of syncopal attacks and a renewal of the whole process of attaining from the beginning gratifications from the world. The syncopal attacks not only symbolize or enact death but also rebirth. The process of obliterating the world is here complete as well as renewal of the whole process of adaptation.

10. Behavior Disorders of Childhood and Adolescence

This major category is reserved for disorders occurring in childhood and adolescence that are more stable, internalized, and resistant to treatment than *Transient Situational Disturbánces* (Chapter 9) but less so than *Psychoses, Neuroses,* and *Personality Disorders* (Chapters 4, 5, and 6). This intermediate stability is attributed to the greater fluidity of all behavior at this age.

Subcategories include the hyperkinetic reaction of childhood or adolescence, characterized by overactivity, restlessness, distractibility, and short attention span; the withdrawing reaction, characterized by seclusiveness, detachment, sensitivity, shyness, timidity, and general inability to form close interpersonal relationships; the overanxious reaction, characterized by chronic anxiety, excessive and unrealistic fears, sleeplessness, nightmares, and exaggerated autonomic responses; the runaway reaction, in which individuals characteristically escape from threatening situations by running away from home for a day or more without permission; the unsocialized aggressive reaction, characterized by overt or covert hostile disobedience, quarrelsomeness, physical and verbal aggressiveness, vengefulness, and destructiveness; and the group delinquent reaction, in which individuals have acquired the values, behavior, and skills of a delinquent peer group or gang to whom they are loyal and with whom they characteristically steal, skip school, and stay out late at night (more common in boys than girls).

22. Awakening into Consciousness of Subconscious Collective Symbolism as a Therapeutic Procedure*

Ernest Harms

Fundamental to the analytic psychology of Carl Jung is the concept of a universal, collective unconscious. Unlike the personal unconscious, which contains memories repressed in the individual's lifetime, the collective unconscious holds memories and ideas that are common and shared, can be expressed symbolically and are rooted in the history of man. It is possible, under some circumstances, that the conscious may be invaded by forces of the collective unconscious, resulting in mental disorder. The Jungian analyst feels that by bringing into the conscious certain symbols of the collective unconscious in a meaningful way, creative forces are liberated, with a positive effect on adjustment.

In the case study presented by Harms, a pre-adolescent boy, appearing to be mentally retarded and diagnosed as a behavior disorder, is treated by being given an opportunity to express, through his drawings, the disturbance caused by his pervasive collective unconscious. Harms theorized that the symbolic content of the boy's drawings was identical to the medieval alchemists' symbol. From Jung's model he hypothesized that the drawings were representations of a sexual unity theme found in the symbolic alchemical concept of the squared circle, the symbol of wholeness and the union of opposites. Harms felt that the boy's behavioral and intellectual problems (he had almost abandoned previously acquired educational tools such as writing and speaking) were related to the invasion of his conscious by this unconscious material. Furthermore,

---

*Reprinted by permission of the author and publisher from the *Journal of Child Psychiatry*, 1948, **1**, 208-238.

he felt that by making the symbols conscious, the patient's mind would be released from the medieval imprisonment and returned to the premorbid level of intellectual and social functioning.

CASE REPORT

The case of M. is one of the seldom observed occurrences of subconscious collective symbolism, the bringing of which into the sphere of interest and research in abnormal psychology has been one of the great achievements of Carl Gustav Jung. When Jung first pointed out the appearance of such symbolism as a deciding factor in the mental life of the insane, his colleagues ridiculed the idea, but since then the importance of his entire theory of collective subconsciousness has been recognized by many serious students of normal and abnormal psychology.

In the case to be described special emphasis is placed upon the role of the symbol in the inner life of the patient and on the therapeutic procedure employed to free him from a pathological subconscious collective symbolism.

M. was born in May 1935. His parents were immigrants from Eastern Europe. The father is a psychoneurotic who works only part of the time, as a taxi driver. The mother is also a neurotic bearing stigma of a difficult family life. The elder son of the couple, born in 1928, has been in a mental hospital for many years diagnosed as a schizophrenic. There is a record of mental illness among the relatives of both parents.

Because she had already had one mentally diseased child, M.'s mother had taken "abortion pills" during her pregnancy, but M. was born at term. He was not breast fed, and an incorrect formula caused diarrhea lasting several months. He had whooping cough at 18 months, and chicken pox when he was two years old. He started to walk and talk at the normal age. According to his mother, he fell at the age of 18 months, striking his head on the floor, and she states that from this time his growth was retarded. She reports that he was always a sickly child; he had "running" ears when he was four weeks old. As he grew older he became more and more difficult to manage: "He never obeyed and was very wild and demanding." He was sent to school for a short time but the principal requested that he be kept at home. Apparently school disturbed him a good deal; however, he managed to pick up a considerable amount of elementary knowledge. In the period between school and institution he became more and more uncontrollable. "He fought with everyone, he hit himself, he made an attempt at suicide"—the latter not completely proven —"he began to fear the dark and to talk about ghosts."

In 1943 he was brought for observation to the Psychiatric Division of Bellevue Hospital, New York City, where he received 19 electric shock treatments. Since his mother refused to take him home he was admitted to Kings Park State Hospital with a diagnosis of mental deficiency with behavior disorder. The behavior symptoms consisted of constant restlessness and teasing the other children. He talked constantly, either to himself or others, expressing his distrust, aggressive demands, and restless paranoic curiosity. The only way to control his physical restlessness was to give him a piece of paper and a crayon or pencil. He filled the paper with small drawings using the pencil so violently that it frequently pierced the paper. These drawings were the feature which attracted my attention for the boy. Most of them were symbolic in character: flags, national emblems, religious and other symbols which would be familiar to simple minded people.

In my study of the case I did not start with any preconceived pathological or psychological theories; my aim was simply to discover the impulses which called for such intensity in the boy's pictures and why he expressed himself in such symbolism. There was no specific intention of inaugurating a cure by art therapy; the idea, at first, was to let the boy express himself and to observe developments.

The first approach was rather difficult. When invited into the small office he became suspicious. He looked under the paper which was given him for drawing, and under the table, and ran like a caged animal up and down the room. After vain attempts to explain that we only wanted him to enjoy himself drawing, he had to be sent back to the ward.

The second attempt, a week later, was more successful. He understood what to do, hastily drew first his usual small symbols, and then continued to write nonsense syllables to which he gave his own meaning which changed from one reading to another, and hieroglyphic representations of his own name and address. When he jumped up and became restless again he was sent back to the ward.

The third time his behavior was quite different. He came eagerly into the room and sat down immediately at the table as if expecting to be given pencil or crayon. When he entered the room he was engaged in an incoherent conversation about fighting the Japanese and Germans, which he continued after sitting down. When given drawing material he drew in rapid succession several unarticulated war pictures of the type of Figure 6. Between the drawing and the conflict in his mind he grew more and more excited, until suddenly he addressed me as follows: "Getting after me, getting me killed," and with increasing excitement he began to repeat over and over a vulgar word referring to intercourse, which he wanted to have with me, with his nurse, the attending doctor, and also with his father. This was followed by violent jerks of his whole body, during which

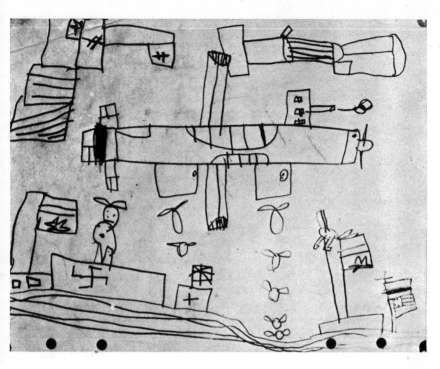

FIGURE 6

he hurt himself so severely that he fell down crying. As a consequence he was sent back to the ward.

During a fourth session, at which he produced the same type of drawing and exhibited the same type of release attack, an attempt to calm him down with kind words and petting produced the reverse of the desired effect, only making him wilder.

During the following session (there was always an interval of one week between sessions) I changed my attitude. In general M. presented the same behavior pattern although he was somewhat less excited. In the course of the first drawings he roused himself to a similar attack but when he started to hit himself I stepped behind him and with gentle force held both his arms while talking to him quietly. After the first violent resistance, he suddenly calmed down, discarded the last unfinished drawing and started another on a fresh sheet. The drawing which he produced rapidly, without saying a word, is shown in Figure 7. After completing the drawing he was so exhausted that he had to be led back to the ward where he sat in a corner without moving or talking, with his hands pressed between his knees, for about an hour.

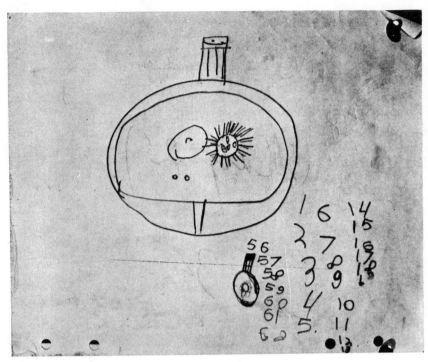

FIGURE 7

His drawing was an amazing presentation of a very common medieval alchemical symbol representing, in the alchemical bottle, a picture of the sun and the moon in a relationship of what can only be called cosmic sex communication. The literature of the Middle Ages contains a great number and a considerable variety of such symbols. There are even entire series expressing the contemporary conception of the creation and constitution of the cosmos, the earth, and the physical and mental nature of man. In particular, the inner change and development, healthy as well as unhealthy, were expressed in this symbolic language which, because it represented the psychology and even psychiatry of that period, has attracted the interest of students of modern analytical psychology. From this standpoint I devoted considerable attention to these documentations of the Middle Ages, especially during the time when I was a collaborator of Carl Gustav Jung. His book, *"Psychologie und Alchemie,"* contains not only a great number of such sun and moon intercourse drawings of alchemical origin but an introduction to the meaning of this psychology and philosophy. . . .

The patient's drawing represented the sun and moon in the magical bottle, together with two very small circles such as are found in similar alchemical drawings. In addition to this main concept there was a smaller bottle apparently showing sun and moon in completed relation as in many of the original old drawings. There were also two sets of numbers similar to those known as number symbolism, for instance in the so-called "Hexen-Einmaleins," one of which appears in Dürer's famous etching *"Melancholia."* It is not our present task to interpret the meaning of this entire symbolism and its apparent role in the patient's subconsciousness, but to present actual occurrences. Interprètation will be attempted in the second part of this paper.

During the rest period which the boy took after completing the drawing just described he sat in the occupation section of the ward which could be seen from the experiment room. As soon as he showed a tendency to activity he was called back to the experiment room and asked to continue making pictures. He accepted this suggestion willingly, drew first a few forms of alchemical bottles, none of which he completed, and

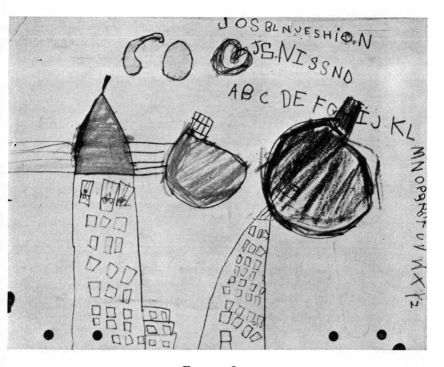

FIGURE 8

finally drew the picture reproduced as Figure 8. Clearly recognizable are two bottles with the sun and moon apparently in a reproductive union. This drawing proves beyond doubt that Figure 7 also represents the sun and moon inside the bottle. An interesting feature of Figure 8 is the set of nonsense letters and, below, the attempt to remember letters of the regular alphabet.

There can be no doubt that these alchemical symbols were recalled to the boy's mind by some kind of abnormal remembrance as an expression of the collective subconscious and that they had some connection with a pathologically precocious sex consciousness. An investigation of these relationships was attempted in the next session.

When, a week later, the boy saw me enter the ward, he hurried to me and wanted to be allowed to draw immediately. He was rather active but his mind seemed clearer and he had more self control. He did not talk in his former incoherent fashion. Before being given paper, his drawing of the magic bottle (Figure 7) was shown him and he was asked: "Who did this?" and "What does it mean?" He smiled for the first time and answered: "You know I did that." When asked again what it meant he would answer only: "You know." When praised for his good work but asked to tell why he had done it he became aggressive, saying: "Was this good? I fucked you a good one. . . ." When finally given paper, the following remarkable symptom appeared: for the first time since the observation began he was able to write actual words and even his name, eagerly filling two sheets. He then drew several confused lines, but he also tried to draw several bottles containing nothing symbolic. For experimental purpose he was shown several photographs of nude Greek statues of both sexes and was asked to tell which were men and which women. He mixed them up completely, showing that he understood nothing of the actual physical sex characteristics. Immediately after this experiment he produced in Figure 9 a version of sex difference in the form of outer dress. However, it may not be exaggeration to designate the design beside the woman a vaginal symbol.

By this time there was definite evidence that M. was better able to express himself by drawing than by intellectual expressions. It was also obvious that if given the opportunity to express himself by means of such drawings he would release such subconscious symbolic elements and thus free the mental parts of his psyche. Apparently through such activity he was liberated from the pattern of "hauntedness" and "possessedness." (This unusual language is used for the purpose of a connection with the later interpretation of the case.) There was overwhelming evidence that such release of subconscious symbolism had an amazing influence on his entire existence. Not only was he less restless, but he began to remember incidents of his earlier life before he had been overcome by this

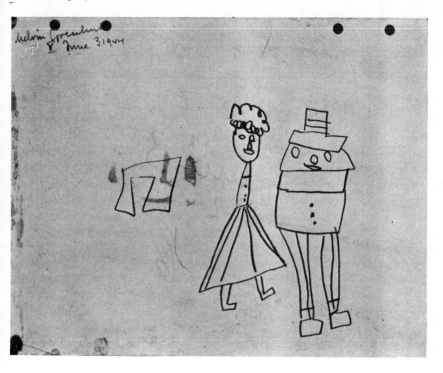

FIGURE 9

condition of almost total amentia. He was also able to understand and remember what the other boys in the same ward said.

The beneficial effect of his drawing activity became increasingly evident during the following weeks. Figure 10 shows how purpose slowly emerged from chaos. His drawings also became more organized and better planned. He began to print his whole name on his pictures. The inscriptions on Figure 10 are mostly more or less incorrect names of the other boys in the ward. The intensity of his subconscious preoccupation with sex also finds expression in one of the inscriptions and in this connection one observation must be made here, since it will be of great importance later. Practically all the drawings have as the central or dominant element either a long form, designed as an airplane, or tree stump, etc., or a wider oval or rhomboid form, mostly designed as a ship. When asked the meaning of these two forms, the most intelligent answer he could give was to call the long form "He" and the rhomboid form "She." There is little doubt that these forms represent roughly symbolized sex patterns which in their physical appearance the boy would not recognize. Some kind of symbolic expression is doubtless involved in each of these draw-

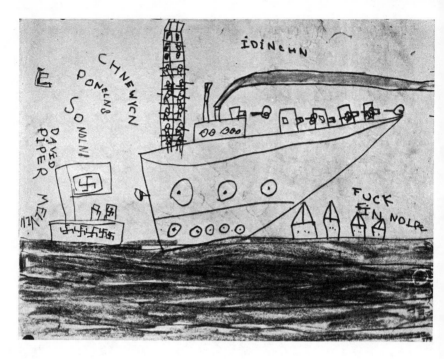

FIGURE 10

ings, working itself from the subconscious to an individualized expression.

After the production of Figure 10, the sessions were discontinued for three months. The report of his behavior during this interim was not satisfactory. He soiled himself again, was aggressive and disagreeable with his ward companions, and extremely noisy. However, he did not seem so mentally disturbed as before the sessions were started nor did he run around aimlessly but spent most of his time looking over the same comic magazines. The supervisor reported that occasionally M. asked the attendant the meaning of a picture or word in the magazines. When I entered the ward he recognized me at once and evidently expected to be called to the experiment room.

In resuming the sessions with him, the former attitude was used. He was asked whether he would like to draw and he responded with great eagerness. At first he produced the same motives, mainly the two major symbolic forms, but there was a fundamental difference from his earlier pictures (Figure 11). They are much simpler, clearer, less confused and less violent, although during the first session he began to excite himself

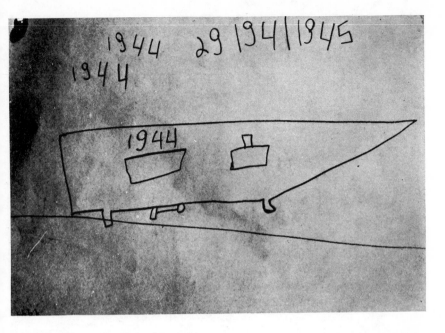

FIGURE 11

again to the verge of an attack of aggressiveness which, however, did
not reach its full development.

At the beginning of the second session he was shown his original
sun and moon drawing (Figure 7). His reaction was quite unexpected:
he burst out crying, saying that he did not want that again. When asked
why, and whether he knew who drew the picture, and why he was afraid
of it, he stopped crying, looked at it with interest, and replied hesitatingly,
"I guess I did it." Without any further remarks he started to draw. The
first picture (Figure 12) has an interesting inscription doubtless derived
from his reading of the comics, together with one of his typical attempts
to clear his intellectual restraint by writing the alphabet. The next drawing (Figure 13) again shows the sun and moon symbolism, but in a more
natural, realistic setting. They are placed in the sky and a star is added.
However, he apparently had to overcome some resistance in producing a
materialistic setting for this symbolic expression, as evidenced by his crying at the beginning of the session. Frequently he wrote the word "moon"
on the drawings, later substituting the word "sun."

The change from a "moon predominance" to that of the "sun" became increasingly important in the boy's developmental experience during

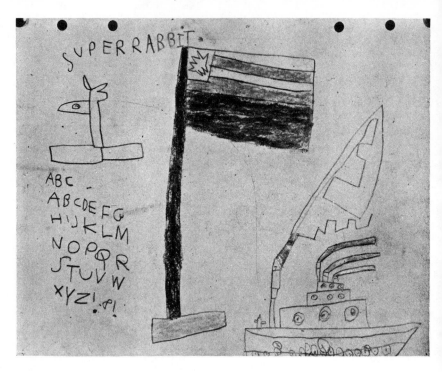

FIGURE 12

the next few weeks of our working with him. The day after he drew Figure 13 he suddenly remarked that he wanted to draw a man and demanded colored crayons which had always been on his desk but which he had hardly ever used. The result was Figure 14, a figure in which the hat and abdomen are colored yellow. The inscription, of course, derives from the comics, but another experience seemed to be involved whose meaning later became clearer.

During the new series of weekly sessions in which he was merely urged to draw what he pleased a profound change occurred in his entire behavior. This was so obvious that it was reported spontaneously by the ward attendants. He almost completely abandoned his attitude of restlessness and usually sat alone in a corner, leafing through the comic books and magazines provided for the children. Occasionally he asked the attendant or the nurse questions regarding the pictures he had just looked at or about the simple facts of life in his present environment, expressing the greatest astonishment at what he was told. One of the most impressive of his questions was "Are not all these boys sick?" He seems

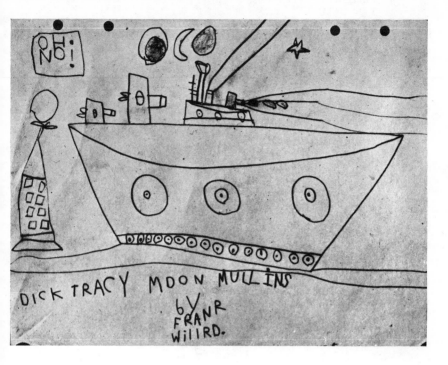

FIGURE 13

to have suddenly become aware that he was in an atmosphere of insanity. This and other questions indicate that at this time he began to emerge from the darkness of his condition of dementia or amentia and to waken to a new mental life.

Figures 15, 16, and 17 were drawn during the next session. They show an increase in the entire mental awakening process. The first drawing (Figure 15) shows, in the middle, a strongly emphasized sun attacking a half moon. The inscriptions are still chaotic but a careful analysis would probably find some meaning in them, proving as does the total character of the drawings, a slow intellectual recovery. In Figure 16 attention should be given to the inscription which contains the word "today," with the boy's own name "Melvin" and the word "man," which seems to express the assurance of progress toward the "end" which is also in the inscription. This "end" is clearly expressed in Figure 17 where we find the inscription "Scott—end." Scott was the name of the head nurse in M.'s ward. The boy expressed a definite feeling that he was drawing near the end of his illness of which he was now aware, or at least his mental

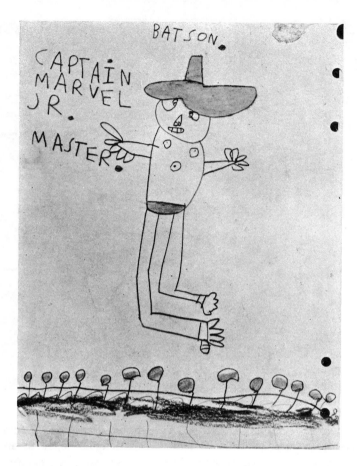

FIGURE 14

awakening had progressed to the point where he was aware of his condition and aimed toward its ending. Figure 17 also contains the sun picture as do almost all of this new series, but here it can be clearly recognized in its symbolic character. It is not the sun in the sky, but the sun in some kind of symbolic action which is definitely expressed in the way the sun and moon pictures are placed in the drawing. Incidentally no more nonsense syllables are present. No more periods of excitement occurred during the sessions, only a slight intellectual struggle when he was asked to leave the experiment room and return to the ward, which is readily understandable. Finally, the ward attendants reported that he was behaving well and seemed to be improving rapidly.

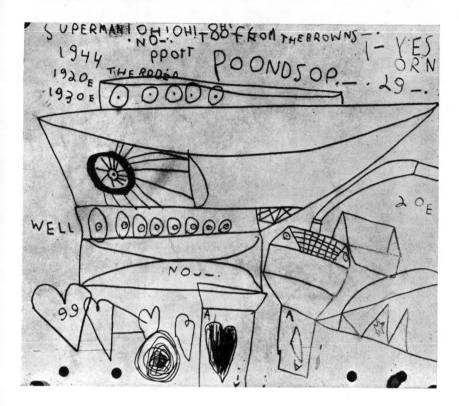

FIGURE 15

During the last two reported sessions the boy had wanted to fill all the drawing sheets with words instead of "doing pictures." Only by special urging and even threatening to send him back to the ward induced him to do what we were interested in, but this tendency was not only a specific indication of what was going on in his mind but an important part of the entire process. Drawing was for him now "always doing the same" while the ability to rationalize and express himself by writing words meant much more to him. In studying these word-filled sheets . . . we first notice a steady advance to clearer and more correct reproduction of the intellectual content. Another interesting feature was the tendency to produce series of words which had a certain connection in their meaning, such as the days of the week and the names of the months. There were also words of closely connected things, such as domestic animals, and words with the same rhyme endings. These obviously represented the boy's desire to reconstruct his former systematic and organized knowledge which he had

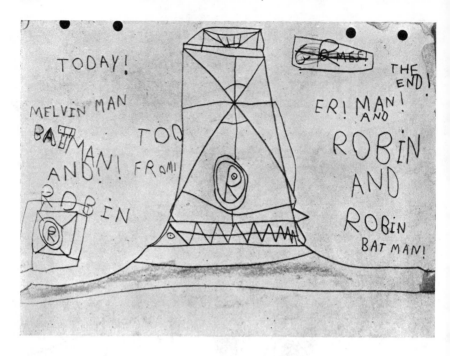

FIGURE 16

lost during his illness. However, it should be mentioned that such systematic series are very common in the medieval pictorial philosophies in which the sun-moon symbol had its actual role.

The boy seemed to feel the importance to his inner development of this knowledge of the word series. [In one case he] started a week series but "got lost"; he therefore writes "lost job." Under the correctly completed series he gives himself the evaluation "good work." The difficulty of his struggle to find the way back to consciousness is shown by his search for the right word. First he writes "Goodness"; then a little later his slowly awakening mind finds the right expression, "Good work."

Figures 18, 19, and 20 represent the last period of my work with the boy and all show clear signs of a clearing up of his disordered mind. Figure 18 expresses clearly his urge for an "exit" from what he now considered a kind of imprisonment. Some days earlier he had asked a nurse whether being in this ward meant being in prison. In this drawing, sun and moon are again represented in the basic connection but predominance is given to the sun. In several earlier drawings (Figures 16 and 17) the sun is alone. The predominant role of the sun in the development of the

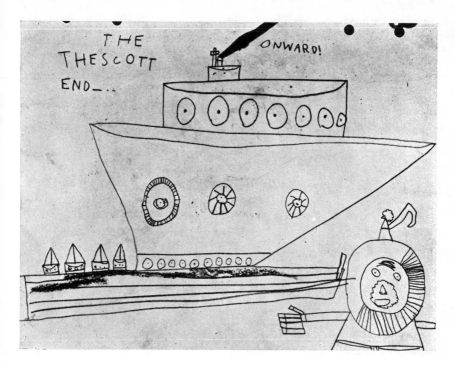

FIGURE 17

boy's mental concept is more and more evident in these last drawings. Figure 19 again shows the sun and moon relationship but, at the same time, the sun as a dominant factor alone. Figure 20 is an example of the final development, showing the sun only. An entire series of such drawings was produced during the final weeks of the collaboration. He even signed the drawings with a sun, adding a few little strokes instead of his name. Once he even pointed to such a sun signature, saying: "That is me."

During these final weeks his entire personality structure changed: he even showed a little friendliness and cheerfulness. The specific earlier symptoms of behavior disorders and dementia faded away. His behavior pattern was still one of insecurity which can be easily accounted for by his years of mental confusion and the divergence of age and mental status. His mentality was still retarded and he spent most of the time sitting around and looking through magazines and comic books. He asked the members of the staff many simple questions characteristic of the infantile "question age."

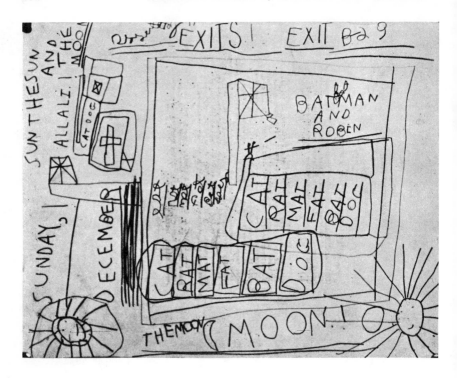

Our report and the reproduced drawings show without a doubt that these drawing exercises produced a fundamental change in the boy's pathological condition. Furthermore, we believe that our method of applying the drawing exercises—of which we shall speak later—improved his mental status. There can be no doubt that we freed his intellectual abilities which had been submerged in a dementia which our treatment did much to improve. Our previous presentation gives no indication as to the actual abnormal process in which the boy was found or the background of our therapeutic influence. In the following pages we shall attempt to clarify these problems.

SOME METHODOLOGICAL CONSIDERATIONS

The use of so-called art expression in work with children has become a very common procedure. It is applied for occupational and pedagogical purposes, as well as for the diagnosis of normal abilities and abnormal traits, and particularly as a psychotherapeutic media. In comparison to

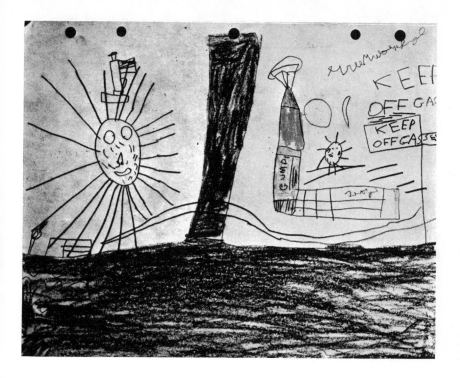

FIGURE 19

the tremendous quantity of its application, the amount of thought, or even philosophy or psychology, devoted to it is infinitesimal. Naturally, theories have been developed regarding the value of child art but these theories have nothing to do with its actual role in the mind and life of the child. Some of the best known general theories are the most impossible, such as Goodenough's attempt to evaluate children's art in accordance with the degree of reality attained. It is amazing that a professor of child psychology should not realize that a child's mental world is not one of natural science based on experience but is one based on imaginative fantasy. Another theory is that which attempts to explain every child's drawing. The worst of these concepts is Lauretta Bender's in the application of a Freudian super-sexual theory to explain children's imaginative play drive. To really understand children's art and its psychopathic deviations, it should not be approached with theories outside its own world. We must understand the psychology and esthetics of children's formal desires because they alone provide a sound background for understanding such utterances. Few workers in this country have attempted what the great

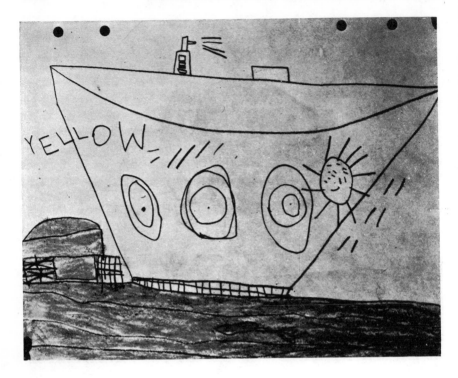

FIGURE 20

founders of these studies undertook 25 years ago—a fundamental study of art and child art and the art expression connected with abnormal behavior. At the time when G. F. Hartlaub, in *"Der Genius im Kinde,"* made the unique attempt to understand the genesis of infantile art expressions, and Prinzhorn published his books on the art of the insane and criminal, I started my study of child art by attempting to combine the ideas of both. However, not until recently have I felt justified in publishing my conclusions on pre-esthetic form types. Really serious research in this field as in any other takes a lifetime to produce valid results. Many papers have been published describing the various aspects of such a basic issue and attempting preliminary or final solutions of specific questions. My studies of children's humor and children's religious expressions have tried to clarify the preliminary problems of the infantile creative effort. Only if we discover how a child really expresses elements which he cannot express rationally in words shall we find the clue to the formal and pictorial sense of the child. We are far from a final understanding of these facts.

We have already explained that our case of a demented child's unusual pictorial expression is not presented merely as an interesting case history but for the purpose of a basic consideration of the involved scientific aspects. Methodological aspects are first considered; they concern the relationship of such expressions and similar ones from an earlier period of human development. For this purpose we put aside the question whether our patient's drawings should be called art or evaluated esthetically. We may call them child art but we are only interested, in addition to their psychological and psychopathological significance, in their anthropological or rather anthropological-historical relationship. In the first place, these drawings *were not merely play*; they meant something very serious and unusual to the boy, expressing elements in which he released inner experiences which he was not able to express in other ways. For some reason he had lost the capacity for intellectual expression normal for a child of his age. His first drawings were of a definitely symbolic character. They expressed—or tried to express—ideas (flags, emblems, etc.) which are difficult to say in words.

Some anthropologists have studied such pre-intellectual expressions of prehistoric and primitive men who had a similar symbolic and pictorial language long before our letter languages were developed. Some modern students have tried to compare these primitive drawings with those of children. A very simple test shows that there is little to gain by comparing such anthropo-genetic products with infanto-genetic ones. To be scientifically exact we can only compare works by children of primitive people with those of our own children. Those who have made such attempts have presented some rather amazing results. They found that the products of children of primitive tribes (Eskimo, African, Indian) were of much higher quality than those of our children of the same age. Excellent studies have been made by Lauge, Koch, Rivers, Malinowski, Westermark, Landman and others. They explain the technical and esthetic maturity as well as strength of expression in such primitive children's drawings by the training they receive in handiwork almost from the day they are able to hold an implement. It has been repeatedly emphasized that the expressive force of primitive child drawing follows the line of primitive adult art. We vainly strive for such qualities in modern art. While children's art is acknowledged to have some of these "primitive" qualities, they are not similar to those which we consider valuable in our adult art; the two sets of values do not match.

This makes it clear that we cannot find by this way a methodological basis of evaluation in the field of juvenile art research. It is equally difficult, even in comparing the products of a living individual with those of a culture dating back at least six hundred years, to apply any of the anthropological and historical methods which have been developed for the study of primitive forms of language. This is because we are not dealing with a formal expression but with a kind of religious symbolism which, as such, has never been studied in such a way that its content was made the central object of investigation.

This explanation is necessary in order to eliminate the misunderstandings which quite naturally arise if juvenile art works are offered as a medium of psychological or educational studies. For our purpose it is unessential whether these drawings are made by a child of five, ten or fifteen years of age, whether the child is of Negro, Jewish or British descent, or whether his capacity for formal expression corresponds with his natural age. We are mainly interested in the content of his experience and the unusual products he creates. We are also interested in what goes on in his mind regarding this content during our work with him. Although in the preceding case report the boy developed a simpler and clearer presentation, these formal elements are not the object of our study; they are secondary characteristics.

We should not have been obliged to eliminate all possible formalistic considerations if we had not feared that the essential problems of our case would be misunderstood. We can find a methodological starting point in C. G. Jung's work on collective subconscious symbolism. Almost four decades ago, Jung attempted a psychological study of the processes involved in our use of symbolic expressions for the kind of experiences for which we have "no words." His attempts at a psychology of the symbolic picture language which is found in any period of human development and in any national group have been very little understood and less acknowledged. His psychology of symbolism centers in his explanation that just that part of our inner life which never comes to the surface and knowledge of our consciousness and our rational and intellectual experience, and which we now call our subconsciousness, makes various use of symbolic language as its actual form of expression. In this respect symbolism is the language of the non-rational sphere of our inner life. Jung's achievements along these lines afford a methodological key to the understanding of the means of symbolic expression of the demented boy in our case report and of the amazing fact that he reproduced and actually lived with a symbolism typical of the religious experience and expression of the European Middle Ages. . . .

ATTEMPT AT AN INTERPRETATION OF THE
PATHOLOGICAL STATUS OF OUR CASE

The present interpretation is not a theoretical concept which could be applied to cases of a similar type. It is a pioneering voyage toward almost undiscovered countries. I hope that other workers will look for similar cases and make their own interpretations. If results similar to mine should be found and my interpretation should be confirmed, this alone would give them a general theoretical importance. . . .

The severity of his mental disablement may be judged by the fact he did not call himself "I," using his first name instead. He had regressed to the mental pattern of a baby before the development of the ego. The first time he used "I" was when he identified his first alchemical drawing. In a very real sense he had been pushed back to an "ego-less" stage in which he had to seek the language of collective expression, which we have given in symbolism. . . .

Our patient also tended to express his few remaining intellectual or semi-intellectual activities in the crudest sex language and continued to do so even during the course of our collaboration. However, this sex language was not related to a concrete understanding of the sexual functions but was merely an inherited knowledge of the elements of sex, as shown by the two basic forms which recurred repeatedly as the center of his imaginative expressions. Some may call such sex knowledge "instinctive"; I prefer to call it "hereditary," which I believe does not contradict the idea of instinct since this must also be hereditary.

There is no doubt that the sun-moon relationship drawn by the boy falls into the class of phallic and vaginal symbols of hereditary sex imagination. But WHY he produced these alchemical symbols and no others we are unable to explain except by the simple statement that he had just this hereditary connection and disposition. Some children reproduce various religious concepts and we have no better explanation for this than for why adults choose any particular religion or philosophy. Our patient simply had a tendency or disposition to these alchemical concepts as a hereditary feature of his personality.

This disposition undoubtedly supplied the background for his mental disorder. If he had been a fairly normal boy he would have played with a chemistry set or joined a junior astronomer's club and made weekly visits to the Planetarium. . . .

One more aspect of this case remains to be discussed and it is the one most difficult to understand. How could this medieval imagery appear in such a perfectly clear and complete form in the mind of this demented child? Most products of the demented, the half-mad, and even of the fairly normal who draw such symbols, are distorted or fragmentary. We can only suppose that he had become so little involved in real mental life that he had become a pure transmitter for such hereditary symbolism. This unusual case gives us a real opportunity for insight into the appearance of subconscious hereditary elements.

THE THERAPEUTIC PROCESS

In our psychopathological report we declined to give any theoretical aspects and we emphasize this still more strongly in our interpretation of the definite improvement and change in attitude of our patient during the period we worked with him. While there is no doubt that our influence upon him was of a therapeutic character, it was not intended in the usual sense as a definite cure. It was more or less an experiment carefully carried out to be sure that the patient's condition would get no worse. We simply wanted to discover what a simple release by means of drawing would accomplish in a demented child who evidently had an obsessive desire to express himself in a pictorial form.

After we had, in this simple way, set the scene for a release, our object was to see whether such release methods would supply diagnostic as well as therapeutic procedures. When we realized that it was a case of hereditary symbolism, we applied the knowledge we had acquired from a study of Jung's viewpoints and methods. Most of the material presented here is the author's own opinion and, as said before, he regards it more as a venture in pioneering than an attempt to set up standards.

The basis of a therapeutic approach to such a case is AN UNDERSTANDING OF THE MEDIEVAL OR ANCIENT CONCEPT OF WHICH THE SYMBOL IS THE EXPRESSION AND A KNOWLEDGE OF THE PSYCHOLOGICAL ROLE PLAYED BY SYMBOLISM, AND THE DYNAMICS WHICH ARE THE BASIS OF THIS ENTIRE CONCEPT. It was clear from the beginning that the boy must be given the opportunity to live out the relationship with this symbolism and to express it with absolute freedom. As has been mentioned before, whenever the sun-moon relationship occupies the middle place of the concept, it represents the fertilizing of the moon by the sun and the eventual victory of the sun forces over those of the moon. This aspect had to be carefully watched and represented the chief part of the attempt to free the boy from his obsession.

The first step was to test the reality of the concept in the boy's mentality and the various angles of the problem. The results of the tests showed that this symbolism was a very real factor in his mentality and subconscious. One of the earliest drawings (Figure 8) proved that he had only a symbolical understanding of the sex processes; they were only a "symbolic concept of hereditary pattern" to him. His mind became clearer almost immediately after a therapeutic situation in regard to this symbolic process was established.

This therapeutic situation had to be established according to the medieval concepts of such obsessive factors. A study of such concepts reveals that a drawing of a symbol calls forth the subconscious forces concerned. Since the boy was evidently an individual of this medieval mentality this method was applied, not by giving the boy a general drawing of the sun-moon symbolism but by showing him *his own* concept. This assured me that I remained within the circle of his own concept, but it also called for his own ego and consciousness. During all of the following exercises his own drawing was held before him. The most important element in the entire therapeutic procedure was that he subconsciously realized that I understood him and his problems. Of course, during the first eight or ten sessions nothing occurred that could be described as intellectual or conscious understanding by the boy of his problem such as doubtless developed during the later period of our collaboration. His reply of "You know" to my question of what the symbol meant was evidence of his subconscious knowledge that I understood him and his resistance to my repeatedly showing him his drawings was evidence of the inner struggle with the obsessive forces to becoming conscious and of the release of those vectors of the psyche which they had completely overpowered.

This method of making the symbolism conscious was amazingly successful. The ability to write and think and count slowly returned. The drawings themselves became simpler and more organized even after the intermission of a summer vacation. In continuing my treatment for the release of his consciousness from its medieval symbolic imprisonment I carefully followed the technique of demanding more and more conscious and thinking activity. However, I adjusted myself as much as possible to the momentary status of the boy's mind. For instance, I never mentioned the real meaning of the drawing of the sun and moon until he himself stated that it was the sun and moon. From that time I spoke of them repeatedly although I never mentioned the esoteric meaning of the symbolic relationship which was an "understood" factor between me and his subconscious. *This kind of "esoteric" behavior seems to me essential in all such therapeutic procedures.* They all move in a sphere of "tabu" which must be maintained if the therapy is to succeed. Children's minds are not ready and often not willing to intellectualize and such methods often do considerable harm. On the other hand, they react naturally to a symbolic approach in tabu form.

There is, of course, a difference between the general tabu situation and one where the object is to free a consciousness from being overpowered by such subconscious symbolic tabu elements as was the case in our patient. His was a case of "historic backwardness" which threatened to overpower the small modern consciousness which he had been able to develop. Therefore I had to fight these symbolic elements by eliminating them altogether. This I accomplished by allowing it to work itself out in its own pattern and at the same time assimilating it to a conscious intellectual pattern by talking about it.

We already know the result. The boy underwent an "alchemistic transformation" of the moon forces into sun forces in his consciousness. Finally he drew the powerful sun and even signed his name symbolically as a sun. But after I had helped him to work out this "alchemistic transformation," what emerged was a reawakened modern consciousness as it had been before his mind had become darkened.

Again I wish to state that I hesitate to designate this procedure as a definite therapeutic method. It proved to be the right thing in this case and may be so in others. Further attempts of the same kind will show whether it is justified.

REFERENCES

1. Harms, Ernest: The normal genius. *Centralbl. f. Psychotherap.*, 1932.
2. Harms, Ernest: Kinderkunst als diagnost. *Hilfsmittel. Zeitchr. f. Kinderpstchtr.*, 1940, **4**, 129-143.
3. Harms, Ernest: Child art as an aid in diagnosis of juvenile neuroses. *Orthopsychtr.*, 1941, **2**, 191-209.
4. Harms, Ernest: Korrektur des Begriffes der infantilen Sexualitaet. *Zeitschr. f. Kinderpsychiatrie*, 1935, **2**, 1-13.
5. Harms, Ernest: Prolegomena of monistic aesthetics. *J. Esthetics*, 1941, **1**, 96-104.
6. Harms, Ernest: Psychology as an autonomous science. *J. Gen. Psychol.*, 1943, **38**, 81-94.
7. Harms, Ernest: The development of humor. *J. Abn. & Soc. Psychol.*, 1943, **38**, 351-369.
8. Harms, Ernest: The arts as applied psychotherapy. *Occupt. & Rehab.*, 1944, **23**, 51-71.
9. Harms, Ernest: The development of religious experience in children. *Am. J. Soc.*, 1944, **50**, 112-122.
10. Harms, Ernest: Childhood schizophrenia and childhood hysteria. *Psychiatr. Quart.*, 1945, **4**, 242-257.
11. Harms, Ernest: The social implications of mentally disadvantaged children. *School & Society*, 1946, **63**, 291-292.
12. Harms, Ernest: Paternus and materna. *The Nervous Child*, 1946, **5**, 146-164.
13. Harms, Ernest: Psychology of formal creativeness: Six types. *J. Genet. Psychol.*, 1946, **69**, 97-120.
14. Harms, Ernest: Ego-inflation and ego-deflation. *The Nervous Child*, 1947, **6**, 284-300.

23. Patterns of Acting Out of a Transference Neurosis by an Adolescent Boy*

S. R. Slavson

In this paper, Slavson deals with some important clinical aspects of delinquency. The etiology of delinquency is considered from an intrapsychic perspective, certain dynamics of group psychotherapy are examined and the limitations of group psychotherapy in dealing with such phenomena as transference neurosis are discussed. Slavson was a pioneer in group psychotherapy for children and adolescents. While holding the view that psychoanalytic principles could be applied to the group treatment process, he doubted that psychoanalysis or psychoanalytic therapy could be accomplished in the group. Basic to the concept of psychoanalytic therapy is the development and working through of the transference neurosis (in transference, the role of parent or parent substitute is projected onto the therapist and the patient reacts emotionally to this child-parent fiction).

Frank, the delinquent boy discussed here, apparently made a number of positive attitudinal changes and adjustments as a result of his participation in group psychotherapy within a residential treatment setting. He had begun to relate better to both his peers and authority figures. There was some reduction in anxiety and hostility and a more realistic expression of anger. The author felt, however, that the development of transference neurosis to the group leader persisted after Frank's discharge from the institution. Slavson predicted that the transference, expressed in both aggressive attacks on the group leader as well as in a suppliant attitude (e.g., Frank's offer to shine the therapist's shoes), would present future difficulty. Slavson believed his prediction was substantiated by

---

*Reprinted by permission of the author and publisher from the *International Journal of Group Psychotherapy*, 1962, **12**, 211-224. Copyright 1962, S. R. Slavson.

Frank's later acting out in a series of serious antisocial acts. Acting out, in the transference, is a process by which unconscious and unverbalized impulses and feelings directed toward the therapist are translated into symbolic and usually unrealistic behavior.

Frank, a fourteen-and-a-half-year-old boy, was committed to residential treatment because of neglect and because of a charge of continued truancy, petty larceny both in and outside his home, and unmanageable, disruptive behavior at school. He had received brief treatment in a community clinic, which seemed to quiet him down to some degree, but the recurrence of his behavior and its violence made it necessary to commit him to a county hospital for observation. A social study of the family and the findings of the hospital staff resulted in a recommendation that he be removed from home and placed in a treatment setting.

Frank was the third of four children. At the time of commitment both his older sister, 26, and older brother, 24, were married and out of the home. The family consisted of father, mother, Frank, and a girl two years younger than he. The father, a truck driver on a transcontinental route, was absent from home for weeks at a time, and since his trips were frequent he spent very little time with the children. He was described as an easy-going, ineffectual, quiet man who exercised little control over his family. The mother, on the other hand, was authoritarian, tyrannical, promiscuous, and a chronic alcoholic. Frank had witnessed at least one episode of sexual intercourse between his mother and one of her paramours. During one of the prolonged absences of her husband the mother "settled down" with one of her "boy friends" in a more or less permanent relationship. Upon his return, the husband gave her a choice between himself and the other man. She decided to return to her husband.

One of the persons who had had an influence on Frank's early life was his maternal grandmother, who had been very protective of Frank and favored him greatly. She had been in charge of the home while the mother was at work, but this arrangement no longer prevailed when Frank was committed as the grandmother had died in the interim.

Frank was an unplanned child and his mother had been extremely upset when she discovered her pregnancy. She had attempted to abort, and later claimed that her drinking bouts began at the time of his birth. One of the significant events in Frank's life was his brother's marriage when Frank was eleven years old. This brother and Frank had shared a room, and after the brother's departure from home, Frank developed a fear of the dark which persisted for several months and necessitated that a light be kept on in his room. During an interview in the community clinic, after describing the beatings he received from his parents, he stated that the brother had protected him against the mother's cruelties. But at the termination of the interview, when he was leaving the room, he turned back and said, "I don't like my brother, John, best; I like my dog, Rex, best."

Frank's adjustment in the Village was described as "decisively poor." The noisy, unco-operative, pugnacious behavior which he had manifested in school before coming to the Village reappeared. He was described as being "provocative, manipulating, scornful, contemptuous, and condescending." He was "cynical, pedantic, pseudointellectual, with grandiose attitudes, and aroused universal antagonism among his cottage mates." Toward adults he was "sarcastic, critical and demanding, and provoked punitiveness from them in return." His female caseworker made every effort to establish a relationship with the boy; she even saw him daily at first because of his extreme separation anxiety. But the outcome after a year's effort was disappointing. "While there was some superficial understanding," wrote the caseworker, "there was very little basic change in Frank over the period of a year of individual casework treatment."

Frank, now fifteen and a half years old, was placed with several other boys in an analytic therapy group which met for a period of six months. This was the first group in our project to test the response to group therapy of court-committed boys in residential treatment. During the first six sessions of the group there were the usual gripes against the institution, the staff, and adults in general. Frank, among others, expressed suspicion that the group was being watched and the conversations recorded. He was the most aggressive and the most disturbing member in the group. During the third session he screamed at the therapist: "I don't like you, I never would and never will like you!" At another time he threw an ashtray into the therapist's lap. His all-out efforts to create disturbances were resented by the other boys, who suggested that he be dismissed from the group. However, Frank's behavior was accepted with tolerance by the therapist, a fact that surprised the other boys greatly. After the third session, Frank asked to stay with the therapist for a while and revealed that he was very upset because his mother had been drinking heavily again and was very ill. It must be noted that when the mother drank she remained in a stupor for days on end, lying about sloppily on a couch, screaming vituperations at anyone who approached her.

When Frank came for his fourth session, he took a seat next to the therapist. When one of the boys mentioned sexual urges toward women, Frank suggested that "we leave sex out of this for awhile." This session, like the preceding ones, was characterized by a great deal of restlessness and complaints against adults taking advantage of the boys.

During a discussion in the seventh session, Frank revealed that he had recently been bothered by the thought that something was going to happen to his brother. He dreamed about his brother getting hurt. He had had this dream twice before, and once his brother actually did get hurt. As he was saying this, Frank became very anxious and restless and walked aimlessly around the room. When this distractibility was called to his attention by the therapist, Frank said, "I am angry because they won't let me call my brother," and he continued his roaming around. This type of behavior was characteristic of Frank and was in striking contrast to that of the other boys. They also had resisted treatment for a long period, but they expressed their resistance verbally. Frank, however, was given to much greater anxiety than were the others and was the only boy who acted it out motorically.

Frank's complaints about his mother reappeared frequently during the group discussions. In the eleventh session, when the boys talked about stealing and homosexual activity, Frank remained silent. At another session he spoke of his acting up in the gymnasium because he felt "kind of miserable inside." He said he had had to do it even though he knew he was doing wrong. He claimed that one of the coaches had slapped him, but he seemed to accept this punishment with equanimity. He said, "You know where you stand [when one is punished], and that is okay with me if I cross the line."

A degree of calm became noticeable in Frank as the group sessions proceeded, but in the thirteenth session, Frank became very upset and attacked two of the more passive boys. His restlessness increased even more when the group started talking openly about their parents. His distractibility and disruptiveness mounted and he moved up and down the room. At one point he drew his cigarette lighter from his pocket and threw it out of the window. It landed on the slanting roof, and Frank attempted to crawl out through the dormer window. Because of the danger involved, this was prevented by the therapist, who promised that after the session he would help Frank retrieve the lighter. Frank quieted down, but when the other boys began to speak, he vehemently pounded on the table with the blade of his knife. Concerned that the knife might ricochet and hurt someone, the therapist suggested that Frank be careful. But Frank ignored this, screaming that the Village was a jail and that he was in it for punishment. He repeated that he hated the therapist, used abusive language toward him, and carved the letters f-u-c-k into the polished top of the table. This startled and upset the other boys. The therapist attempted to encourage Frank to talk about what was bothering him, pointing out that this behavior must stem from some inner turmoil. Frank burst out that he felt like running away and proceeded to narrate how he had received a letter from his mother with a newspaper clipping about an unmarried girl who had become pregnant and that he was angry because this was a girl he could have "gotten into." The girl, recently released from an institution, was the daughter of a woman who had accused Frank's sister of being a whore.

When the group left, Frank remained to retrieve the lighter, and the therapist took this opportunity to talk to him. Frank began by referring to the mother's letter but proceeded at once to discuss his fears about his brother. The brother had not come to visit him and he was afraid that the brother was angry with him.

In the next session the therapist found Frank to be much quieter. During the early part Frank commented· that he didn't like his haircut and added that the therapist, too, needed a haircut. Another boy was discussing his mother, whom he had hardly known and who had abandoned him when he was a small child. The boy said, among other things, that he would beat her if he ever saw her. Frank said he didn't think the boy should ever do anything to his mother. When asked why by the therapist, he said, "After all, my mother was drunk all the time and it is just something I have to live with. I used to knock the shit out of her, but that didn't do any good." When the boys questioned him, he corrected himself smilingly, "Maybe I didn't really hit her, but I wanted to at times." He proceeded to say that sometimes he thought it might be better not to have a mother around; he had one and she had not done him any good. He could not understand the attitude toward mothers because his mother drank and did not give him anything, "so why should there be anything in return?"

As the discussion progressed the therapist commented that sometimes people cling to feelings of guilt. Frank was the first to agree with this statement and elaborated that he always felt unhappy when he saw his mother drunk and that at times she accused him of doing things that "made her that way." At other times he felt guilty because his family worried about him because of his behavior.

It should be noted that Frank invariably chose a seat next to the therapist.

At the fifteenth session the conversation among the boys led Frank to confess that he had stolen money from a boy in his cottage. He claimed that he did it in retaliation for the theft of some objects from his personal locker. On the basis of previous discussions as to why people steal, one of the boys explored with Frank other reasons for his stealing, but Frank repeated that it was a retaliatory act. The effort on the part of other boys and the therapist to explore the meaning of his act did not prove fruitful.

At one point of emotional tension generated by the discussion, Frank said, "I know that I was mixed up and maybe I am getting unmixed, but it takes a long time, and it is hard to stay away from your family." When the therapist responded that the aim of the institution was to help the boys with these problems, Frank, for the first time, spoke favorably of it. He said, "Some people in the Village are all right and maybe they want to help us, but it is still a long way from home." He then turned to the therapist and said, "Do you remember when I tried to give you some money to hold? That was the money I stole. You did not report me, but somebody heard me asking you for the money and that is how I got caught." After a brief silence he added, "Changing takes a long time and sometimes moves too slow."

At the close of this session, as at many of the others, Frank lingered on after the group had left, but when he saw that another boy wished to talk to the therapist too, he left the room.

The theme of the next session was parents and the boys' relationships with them. Frank said resentfully, "Kids shouldn't feel that way about things." He stalked up and down the room and again proceeded to open the window. He conveyed his great yearning to go home during the holiday vacation that was coming. He revealed that during the previous week he had lain awake at night, unable to fall asleep; he had roamed around the cottage, occasionally meeting the watchman on his tour. When asked by another boy why he couldn't sleep, Frank answered curtly, "It's obvious: home." Another boy asked Frank why he didn't talk about it because, "when you talk you don't feel so tense." Again Frank burst forth with preoccupations about his mother being drunk, especially since the father would not be home this time of year. He said that he felt guilty about his mother and recalled that she always blamed him for her drinking. She never drank when the other children were born; she took to drink after his birth, she said. "I always think about it, and when I think about it I feel rotten inside," he declared. Several of the boys expressed sympathy with him and one of them suggested: "You know that it isn't true." Silence fell upon the group. When the group left Frank remained behind to tell the therapist that he would stay with his brother on his visit home if he found his mother drunk.

The next session was held after the Christmas visit home. Frank came in particularly disturbed and immediately went to the window. The therapist warned him about leaning out. He challenged the therapist by asking: "What are you going to do about it?" The therapist told him that he would send him out of the room. Frank sat down at the table with the other boys, and during the discussion he talked about his brother for a minute and then about a spider he had brought in a tin can. The spider's name was Herman. At first Frank threatened to release Herman so he could sting the other boys, explaining that Herman was poisonous. After a while he said that Herman was getting on his nerves and that he would burn him. He lit a match and threw it into the can, but the fire quickly went out. Frank then stuffed paper into the can and set it on fire.

Recognizing Frank's agitation, the therapist asked him to tell the group about his holiday vacation. At first he refused to talk about it and the therapist asked him, "Do you mean your mother was drunk again when you went home?" Frank exclaimed piteously: "I couldn't even get into my mother's apartment because she was out [in a stupor] on the couch again, plastered, so I went down to my brother's house and spent the weekend there." He then proceeded to describe how he had gone back and forth between the brother's and the mother's apartments, but she remained in a continuous stupor during the three days he was home. Further discussion about mothers ensued as a result of Frank's narration, which was terminated by his saying: "I will just have to accept it and work out something for myself as long as it does not hurt me." After this, he grew less agitated but was apparently unable to continue talking. When the session ended he asked the therapist's permission to sit for a while in the waiting room downstairs, apparently to collect himself, before returning to his cottage.

For a number of sessions the boys' discussion had turned to girls and women, with some members of the staff being mentioned as possible sexual objects. When a boy jokingly spoke of a social worker with large breasts, another said, "She always seems to be walking around stretching her arms so that people can measure her to see how much she's got." Frank identified her as his social worker and said, "I could measure her any time." *Soon after this Frank declared that if his brother beat him up he would accept it "because it is in the family."* One of the boys changed the subject. Frank agreed with still another who wanted to return to the discussion of women and said, "Let's talk about women, it's a more interesting subject." At one point the therapist remarked on the naturalness of sexual urges in adolescent boys. Frank misinterpreted his statement with the following remark: "You mean you really want us to go home and feel them [girls] up and do things to them?" When the group's laughter had subsided, Frank said: "I'll go around telling everybody that you told me it was all right for me to do it." Again there was an outburst of laughter. When the therapist questioned Frank if he really thought that this was what the therapist had meant, Frank said, "I was only kidding." Frank did not remain with the therapist at the end of this session.

In the next session an interesting episode occurred. Frank, who was a member of the ROTC, brought his boots and some shoe polish and proceeded to shine the boots in preparation for inspection. He asked the therapist if he could shine his shoes as well. The therapist asked him why he wanted to do it, and Frank's response was that he had some polish left. The therapist said that his shoes were new and did not really need a shine but thanked him for the offer. This incident is rather significant in terms of Frank's nuclear problem.

The next session, the twenty-third, Frank brought with him a book of pictures of nude men and women and loaned it to another boy who wanted to look through it. The matter of sex was brought up again, along with the fact that living in an entirely masculine environment caused some of the boys to be preoccupied with sex. Frank said, "Well, you know what to do about it," and made a motion with his hand indicating masturbation. When the discussion turned to heterosexual intercourse, the therapist explained the function of marriage as a means of satisfying the sex urge and ended by saying that he was aware that boys always wonder about these matters and the feelings involved and that they sought means of doing something about it. Again, Frank said that he knew what to do and indicated by his hand the act of masturbation.

One of the boys volunteered that his father had once caught him masturbating and was very angry with him. Frank suggested that the father may have thought that it was something wrong and harmful to the boy. This remark was probably the result of a discussion in which the therapist had conveyed to the boys that masturbation, of which the boys were very much afraid, was harmless if indulged in moderately. When one of the boys introduced the subject of the cottage parents checking up on the residents of the cottages during the night, Frank said, "You know, there are a lot of queers around." The discussion seemed to have met some need in Frank, for he spontaneously said, "Well, we talked today."

In a supervisory discussion of the episode in which Frank offered to shine the therapist's shoes, it was suggested that the therapist's refusal be aired with Frank. The therapist therefore found an opportunity to ask Frank what he thought about the incident. The boy's response to this was that he tried to find ways of getting the therapist angry. One of the boys, Albert, remarked that Frank had made himself angry instead since he had been rebuffed by the therapist. At this point Frank lost his temper with the boy. The therapist intervened by saying that Frank was really angry with the therapist rather than with Albert. He further stated that Frank was trying to show the therapist that he liked him and instead the therapist had pushed him away. "Like you?" exclaimed Frank, "Enough to kill you!" However, the statement sounded more like, "I like you very much," than one of hostility. Frank again left with the rest of the group.

At the twenty-fourth session Frank once more appeared very disturbed and described a conflict he had had with his cottage mother because of her slight of a Negro resident. During this recital Frank touched one of his arms and said that he was getting "boils" again and that it was the cottage mother who was "giving them" to him. The therapist stated that the boils might be caused by his own mother rather than the cottage mother. This sparked Frank's exclamation that he knew his mother was drunk again and "it is driving me nuts!" He had received a letter from her and from the manner of her writing he was sure that she was in a drunken state, and there was no one to take care of her because his father was away again. "If she would only stop for awhile!" he screamed. "If I was only home to take care of her!" He added that if he returned home he would have to stay with his brother, who would take care of him. His brother would never hit him. As the discussion progressed, Frank remarked that he really didn't need his mother any more, he was just concerned about her because there was nobody around to take care of her.

The next session, the twenty-fifth and last for this experimental group, Frank was in a euphoric state. He chatted with people on the stairs and greeted effusively one of the group members who had been away for a few weeks because he participated in the varsity ball games. As the group was discussing these games, Frank jumped up and began to juggle ashtrays. The therapist suggested that he put them down and that his behavior seemed to show that there was something bothering him. Frank said that he was going to throw an ashtray at the therapist, and he looped it into the therapist's lap. The group was startled by this, and some of the boys reprimanded him for doing "such a crazy thing." Frank said, "I told him [therapist] I was going to do it. You dared me to." He then rose from his seat and moved to another close to the therapist. The therapist suggested that Frank was upset about something and that talking about it would make him feel better. While group members expressed indignation at his behavior, the therapist repeated that Frank probably had acted the way he did because something was disturbing him.

Later, the boys were discussing termination. One of them, a newcomer, asked about having candy and ice cream. The therapist asked what they sounded like when they asked for candy and ice cream. "Babies," said Frank; "we are babies when we want candy." He then proceeded to nag the therapist to swap wrist-watch bands. "I want that band," he said, and then rhythmically repeated, "I want your wrist-watch band; I want your wrist-watch band; I want your wrist-watch band." The therapist told Frank that he could not have his band, since it was a gift, and several members of the group told Frank to "shut up," but he continued. The therapist asked Frank what it was he was trying to tell the group by his behavior. Instead of answering, Frank said, "I will count to thirty, and at that time I am going to take that band from you." A self-conscious hush settled over the group. One of the boys broke the silence, telling Frank that he better not try anything on the therapist. Nonetheless, Frank began to count, and the therapist turned to John, asking why he wanted to protect him. John said that no one should throw things at the therapist since he "didn't do anything to anybody." The therapist asked him what he thought Frank should do about his conduct. At this point Frank stopped counting, smiled, broke into laughter, and said, "Fooled everybody. I wasn't going to do anything to Mr. S."

Having broken through Frank's anxiety, the therapist again asked what was upsetting him. Frank said, "I am in trouble again." His grandfather had died and he had gone home on a weekend pass. At his uncle's home he convinced his small cousin to sell him a wrist watch for a couple of dollars. The wrist watch was worth much more, and he was sure that when his uncle found out there would be trouble. He knew that his cousin had gotten it from his uncle as a present and, therefore, he wanted it. John said, "But this is no reason for going around throwing ashtrays at people." Frank agreed and said he just did not know what to do with himself. He had gotten into trouble with his cottage parents the day before and a few days earlier. He struck his hand against the table in a manner that obviously hurt him. The boys minimized the importance of the events and tried to console Frank.

Later, when some of the boys asked the therapist for help in getting discharged from the Village, Frank said that he wanted to be around his sisters because "they are nice to me and take care of me." James said, "When Frank grows up and meets some girls, he will not always be talking about his sisters. There will be other people." Frank grew livid with rage, grabbed James' shirt at the neck, and threateningly shouted, "Buddy, don't ever say that again!" Questioned by the therapist, Frank responded, "I have no such ideas about my sisters and it is a dirty thing to say." James broke in and said that he had had nothing like that in mind at all and elaborated that, as Frank grew up, he would get married and would be thinking about his wife and family and "everything else." Frank, however, remained crestfallen and dejectedly murmured: "I just can't stand it any more. It is not the watch that is bothering me; it is what happened on the weekend." He grew very quiet, his face became very tense, and he said: "It is my brother. When I went home for the weekend I told my brother that I got smacked by the cottage father and he said he'd take care of the cottage father for me." But when, later, the brother and Frank were at the cottage, the brother said to him, "Straighten up!" Frank said: "My brother didn't give me a chance. He just told me to straighten up, and he didn't listen to my side of the story." Frank again violently banged his hand against the table, screaming, "My brother betrayed me!" Questioned by the therapist, he asserted that his brother was "the one person I could trust, the one person I could turn to. Now I have no one to turn to," and proceeded to blame himself for everything that occurred in his life. When the therapist said, "You blame yourself for everything that happened and maybe when something like this happens you get yourself in trouble at school, throw ashtrays at people, hoping that someone will eventually hit you. This seems to be what you are doing to yourself now because of what your brother said."

The boys attempted to persuade Frank that his brother might have meant well. The therapist added, "Perhaps your brother in his ignorant way tried to help you." Frank burst out in intense rage, screaming, "Don't say that about my brother! He is the smartest man in the world!" The therapist explained that he had used the word in a different sense than it sounded. He meant to say that his brother did not have all the facts. John now began to quiet Frank down.

Frank grew more cheerful toward the end of the session. As the boys were leaving, Frank was with Charles, the most recent arrival and toward whom Frank had been very antagonistic at first. They went out together, talking about Charles' brother who once beat him severely but whom he now loved because he felt that his brother was interested in him.

Symptoms and Functioning after Twenty-five Sessions of Analytic Group Psychotherapy

The cottage parents described Frank as more direct, less evasive, and less manipulative in dealing with them. He was less provocative with his cottage mates and was capable of acquiring and sustaining friendships. While six months before he had been described by his cottage parents as the "lowest of the low," they now spoke of him favorably and thought that he had carved out for himself a "niche in the cottage group." He frequently took responsibility for the conduct of the whole cottage and even for the cottage parents' children.

Similarly, the school reported that he caused "much less trouble than in the past" and that he was willing to wear glasses to correct his unilateral strabismus, something which he had vehemently resisted before. He was still distractible and finished his tasks only with considerable difficulty. He still provoked other boys occasionally, but this had been greatly reduced in frequency, intensity, and duration.

The female caseworker who saw Frank during and at the termination of group treatment (not the same whose report was quoted) stated:

> Frank is now freer and more open in his expression of anger toward his mother and is able to accept the fact that she neglected him. While in the past he denied this, he now recognizes more objectively his mother's personality and problems as separate from his own. His verbalizations and attitudes reflect more trust of adults than prior to group therapy. He is now able to speak in a more factual way of "being wanted" at home and to say that he was "not too unhappy" at the Village. He recognizes Children's Village, not as a punitive

agent, but as an instrument for help with some of his problems at home. The group acted as a catalyst for individual therapy.

The caseworker's findings were confirmed independently by the group therapist, who found evidence in Frank's productions in the group that he now recognized that his acting out was a result of inner turmoil rather than being due to purely external circumstances. He permitted himself positive feelings for the therapist and recognized himself as being "mixed-up" and having an unfounded mistrust of adults.

A memo from a top administrative staff member who spoke to Frank before his discharge from the Village a year after termination of group therapy stated:

> I think you will be pleased to know that before Frank left I asked him what he thought counted most in his stay at the Village. Somewhat hesitatingly he stated: "My cottage parents and Mr. G. [the Protestant chaplain]." We explored with him what was important to him about his association with these staff members, but he was quite unclear on the subject. After we shook hands, I said, "Good luck," and he was walking out of my office when he turned back and added, "It was really the discussion club with Mr. S. that was the most important thing." Frank then explained this by adding that the "kids could really talk about their real problems to each other, with those who understood them best, and it wasn't adult-dominated."

DISCUSSION

There is plenty of evidence of the parents' neglect of Frank and of serious prenatal and postnatal rejections. The mother tried to abort him, considered him very ugly, and refused to believe that he was a normal-looking baby. She seemed incapable of tender feelings toward him, blamed him for her alcoholism, beat him, and finally placed him in an institution. Despite all this rejection, Frank was strongly tied to his mother. She was the focus of his libidinal strivings, and she created a void in him which only she could fill. At the same time, he felt himself responsible for her rejection of him and saw himself as unworthy of her love. This contributed to his weak ego organization and his incapacity to mobilize resources to meet the demands of his life. His distractibility derived from this, as well as from his deep inner yearning for love and from the tensions generated by unfulfilled needs, which he vicariously satisfied by petty stealing from his mother.

Equally clear is his lack of identification with and support from his father. Because of the father's long absences from home, Frank was unable to achieve the identification that would permit internalization of the masculine traits of his father and his ego strengths, whatever they were.

Only one person seemed to play a constructive role in Frank's life, his brother, who was seen by the boy (in actuality or in fantasy) as one whom he "likes." Even this, however, he denied by the feelings toward his dog. An important factor in this relationship may be the fact that Frank and his brother shared a room. It is not known whether or not they shared the same bed. The boy's reactions to his brother, his continued reference to and dependency upon him, would point to a homoerotic or even homosexual tie. The circumstances of this patient's life favored such a development from every point of view. The castration by, and masochistic submission to, his mother, the lack of opportunity for identification with his father, the mother's preference for her daughter, and the physical proximity of the brother at times of affect hunger, all would favor such an eventuality.

This hypothesis is supported by Frank's adjustment to life. His provocativeness with peers which led to rejection and physical punishment was a continuation of his masochistic submissiveness to a (sexually) castrating mother. His placating and devious approach to adults as stronger persons can be understood as sexual submission, and his aggressiveness and attack upon the group therapist can be seen as a defense against his homoerotic feelings toward him. Frank usually stayed after the sessions so as to have at least a brief time alone with the therapist, and his offer to shine the therapist's shoes can be construed as his assuming the submissive, catering (female) role in relation to a strong (mature) male. His intense restlessness during the sessions, evidenced by frequent and impulsive standing up and walking around the room (the only boy in our analytic groups who did this), lighting matches, burning paper, scorching the table, carving on it, throwing things out of the window and perilously leaning out of it (symbolizing an attempt at suicide), all point to a homoerotic panic which gradually subsided.

That Frank came to terms with himself to some extent is evidenced by the report of the caseworker: "There is even more telling confirmation of this in his behavior and relatedness in school, the community, and casework. These changes can be attributed to the help he received from the group in overcoming his guilt and emerging from the tragic sense of life that was his." This was achieved by universalization and reduction of guilt, objectification, and reality testing. It was also sponsored by ventilation of feelings, discharge of hostility, and by being accepted. There were improved feelings of self-worth and an improved self-image. Group therapy thus affected ego strength and personality integration both structurally and behaviorally. What is yet to be established in this case is the libidinal modifications effected by group therapy.

Here we need to view the problem both from its nonsexual and sexual aspects. The centripetal flow of the primitive libido brings expansion and growth of the personality in numerous directions, but only if there are appropriate stimuli and opportunities in the environment. The capacity of the child to utilize opportunities for growth is derived from the support he receives from key persons in his life. They can either enhance his growth, restrict it, or block it off. When not too crippling damage has been inflicted upon the growth urge in these primary circumstances, it can later be reawakened by stimuli from extrafamilial sources, such as school, friends, and other individuals and groups. But if the restrictive and crippling forces in the home have been of great intensity, the personality becomes impoverished, and compensatory and defensive adaptations and behavior patterns arise. One of the forms this took in Frank, for example, was stealing.

The comments of the various staff members pointed to unmistakable improvement in this boy's social adjustment and capacity for relating to other people, but at the time of his leaving the institution, we noted that this improvement was only partial and might not be sustained under the inordinately stressful circumstances of his life at home. This prophecy was based upon our recognition that Frank was acting out a "transference neurosis" developed in the group. This transference neurosis stemmed from his homoerotic (or homosexual) tie to the older brother, displaced (transferred) upon the therapist. A transference neurosis cannot be worked through in group therapy; its resolution requires an extensive libidinal transference upon an individual therapist.

Our prophecy unfortunately came true. Shortly after Frank left the institution, he experienced a traumatic event which added to his distress and ego strain. His father took him along on a cross-country trip, and upon arrival at their destination, introduced his son to his common-law wife and asked Frank to live with them as a member of this duplicate family unit. Frank instead returned to New York and obtained a job in a spray paint plant where his brother was employed. He stayed on that job for several weeks, after which he tried to enlist in the Navy but was rejected because of his defective eyesight. He then returned south, where he worked on a part-time basis in an amusement park and lived with friends of his father; we do not know whether this was the woman involved or whether it was a family of the father's acquaintance. While there, he met a girl and decided to marry her. He was at this time between 17 and 18 years old. Not having any funds, he returned to New York with the intention of earning and saving a sufficient sum of money so that he could go back and marry the girl.

Unsuccessful at obtaining the kind of job that he wished and that would pay him enough, he broke into an office building, stole some money, and later passed a bad check, apparently on a blank acquired during his illegal entry into the office building. When he learned that he was being sought by the police, he started south, hitch-hiking and stealing on his way. He was apprehended and returned to New York, where he was sentenced to a four-year prison term on a charge of unlawful entry. All this transpired within one year of his discharge from the Village.

11. Conditions without Manifest Psychiatric Disorder

This category is for individuals who are psychiatrically normal but who nevertheless have severe enough problems to warrant clinical examination. These conditions may either become or precipitate a diagnosable mental disorder. Categories include marital maladjustment, social maladjustment (culture shock), and occupational maladjustment. Also classified here are individuals exhibiting dyssocial behavior; i.e., those who are predatory and follow more or less criminal pursuits, such as racketeers, dishonest gamblers, prostitutes, and dope peddlers.

24. Excerpts from the Case of Mrs. O.*

Carl R. Rogers

Carl Rogers, apparently convinced that neither the probing and uncovering methods of the Freudians nor the objective variable manipulations of the behaviorists gave satisfactory results in psychotherapy, developed client-centered therapy. Basic to this view is the belief that the human organism is intrinsically oriented towards love, self-regard and self-actualization. Rogers feels that destructive and primitive behavior is not an inherent part of the human condition, but rather an outgrowth of frustration related to interference with the development of positive self-regard. He has become identified with the school of "humanistic psychology" and has taken a position against what he considers the dehumanizing effects of objectivity in behavioral science. Although eschewing diagnostic labels, his theory and techniques have been applied within a broad range of nosology.

The case presented in this paper is one with marital problems and no manifest psychiatric disorder. The excerpts from the therapy sessions with Mrs. O., a housewife in her mid-thirties, present excellent illustrations of Rogers' nondirective technique. Throughout the sessions, the therapist's interested and reflective attitude maintains an environment designed to give the client an opportunity to understand her own feelings, observe her defenses, and develop a more realistic and satisfying view of herself as a person. It is important to note the regard that Rogers has for

---

†Carl R. Rogers, "Some Directions and End Points in Therapy" in *Psychotherapy: Theory and Research*, edited by O. Hobart Mowrer. Copyright 1953, The Ronald Press Company, New York. Reprinted by permission.

the "feeling" aspects of relationships and how the value of feeling is emphasized in these sessions.

THE EXPERIENCING OF THE SELF (OR POTENTIAL SELF)

One aspect of the process of therapy which is evident in all cases might be termed the awareness of experience, or even "the experiencing of experience." I have here labeled it as the experiencing of the self, though this also falls short of being an accurate term. In the security of the relationship with a client-centered therapist, in the absence of any actual or implied threat to self, the client can let himself examine various aspects of his experience as they actually feel to him, as they are apprehended through his sensory and visceral equipment, without distorting them to fit the existing concept of self. Many of these prove to be in extreme contradiction to the concept of self, and they could not ordinarily be experienced in their fullness, but in this safe relationship they can be permitted to seep through into awareness without distortion. Thus they often follow this schematic pattern: "I am thus and so, but I experience this feeling which is very inconsistent with what I am." "I love my parents, but I experience some surprising bitterness toward them at times." "I am really no good, but sometimes I seem to feel that I'm better than everyone else." Thus at first the expression is, "I am a self which is different from a part of my experience." Later this changes to the tentative pattern, "Perhaps I am several very different selves, or perhaps my self contains more contradictions than I had dreamed." Still later the pattern changes to some such pattern as this, "I was sure that I could not be my experience—it was too contradictory—but now I am beginning to believe that I can be *all* of my experience."

Perhaps something of the nature of this aspect of therapy may be conveyed from two excerpts from the case of Mrs. O. Mrs. O. was a housewife in her late thirties, who was having difficulties in marital and family relationships when she came in for therapy. Unlike many clients, she had a keen and spontaneous interest in the processes which she felt going on within herself, and her recorded interviews contain much material, from her own frame of reference, as to her perception of what was occurring. She thus tends to put into words what seems to be implicit, but unverbalized, in many clients. For this reason, most of the excerpts in this chapter will be taken from this one case.

From an early portion of the fifth interview comes material which describes the awareness of experience which we have been discussing.

C.[1]: It all comes pretty vague. But you know I keep, keep having the thought occur to me that this whole process for me is kind of like examining pieces of a jigsaw puzzle. It seems to me I, I'm in the process now of examining the individual pieces which really don't have too much meaning. Probably handling them, not even beginning to think of a pattern. That keeps coming to me. And it's interesting to me because I, I really don't like jigsaw puzzles. They've always irritated me. But that's my feeling. And I mean I pick up little pieces [she gestures throughout this conversation to illustrate her statements] with absolutely no meaning except I mean the, the feeling that you get from simply handling them without seeing them as a pattern, but just from the touch, I probably feel, well it is going to fit some place here.

T.: And that at the moment that, that's the process, just getting the feel and the shape and the configuration of the different pieces with a little bit of background feeling of, yeah they'll probably fit somewhere, but most of the attention's focused right on, "What does this feel like? And what's its texture?"

C.: That's right. There's almost something physical in it. A, a—

T.: You can't quite describe it without using your hands. A real, almost a sensuous sense in—

C.: That's right. Again it's, it's a feeling of being very objective, and yet I've never been quite so close to myself.

T.: Almost at one and the same time standing off and looking at yourself and yet somehow being closer to yourself that way than—

C.: M-hm. And yet for the first time in months I am not thinking about my problems. I'm not actually, I'm not working on them.

T.: I get the impression you don't sort of sit down to work on "my problems." It isn't that feeling at all.

C.: That's right. That's right. I suppose what I, I mean actually is that I'm not sitting down to put this puzzle together as, as something, I've got to see the picture. It, it may be that, it may be that I am actually enjoying this feeling process. Or I'm certainly learning something.

T.: At least there's a sense of the immediate goal of getting that feel as being the thing, not that you're doing this in order to see a picture,

---

[1]In these excerpts, C. stands for client, T. for therapist.

but that it's a, a satisfaction of really getting acquainted with each piece. Is that—

C.: That's it. That's it. And it still becomes that sort of sensuousness, that touching. It's quite interesting. Sometimes not entirely pleasant, I'm sure, but—

T.: A rather different sort of experience.

C.: Yes. Quite.

This excerpt indicates very clearly the letting of material come into awareness, without any attempt to own it as part of the self, or to relate it to other material held in consciousness. It is, to put it as accurately as possible, an awareness of a wide range of experiences, with, at the moment, no thought of their relation to self. Later it may be recognized that what was being experienced may all become a part of self.

The fact that this is a new and unusual form of experience is expressed in a verbally confused but emotionally clear portion of the sixth interview.

C.: Uh, I caught myself thinking that during these sessions, uh, I've been sort of singing a song. Now that sounds vague and uh—not actually singing—sort of a song without any music. Probably a kind of poem coming out. And I like the idea, I mean it's just sort of come to me without anything built out of, of anything. And in—following that, it came, it came this other kind of feeling. Well, I found myself sort of asking myself, is that the shape that cases take? Is it possible that I am just verbalizing and, and at times kind of become intoxicated with my own verbalizations? And then uh, following this, came, well, am I just taking up your time? And then a doubt, a doubt. Then something else occurred to me. Uh, from whence it came, I don't know, no actual logical kind of sequence to the thinking. The thought struck me: We're doing bits, uh, we're not overwhelmed or doubtful, or we can show concern or, or any great interest when, when blind people learn to read with their fingers, Braille. I don't know—it may be just sort of, it's all mixed up. It may be that's something that I'm experiencing now.

T.: Let's see if I can get some of that, that sequence of feelings. First, sort of as though you're, and I gather that first one is a fairly positive feeling, as though maybe you're kind of creating a poem here—a song without music somehow but something that might be quite creative, and then the, the feeling of a lot of skepticism about that. "Maybe I'm just saying words, just being carried off by words that

I, that I speak, and maybe it's all a lot of baloney, really." And then a feeling that perhaps you're almost learning a new type of experiencing which would be just as radically new as for a blind person to try to make sense out of what he feels with his fingertips.

C.: M-hm. M-hm. [Pause.] . . . And I sometimes think to myself. well, maybe we could go into this particular incident or that particular incident. And then somehow when I come here, there is, that doesn't hold true, it's, it seems false. And then there just seems to be this flow of words which somehow aren't forced, and then occasion-ally this doubt creeps in. Well, it sort of takes form of a, maybe you're just making music. . . . Perhaps that's why I'm doubtful today of, of this whole thing, because it's something that's not forced. And really I'm feeling that what I should do is, is sort of systematize the thing. Oughta work harder and—

T.: Sort of a deep questioning as to what am I doing with a self that isn't, isn't pushing to get things *done, solved?* [Pause.]

C.: And yet the fact that I, I really like this other kind of thing, this, I don't know, call it a poignant feeling, I mean—I felt things that I never felt before. I *like* that, too. Maybe that's the way to do it. I just don't know today.

Here is the shift which seems almost invariably to occur in therapy which has any depth. It may be represented schematically as the client's feeling that, "I came here to solve problems, and now I find myself just experiencing myself." And as with this client this shift is usually accompanied by the intellectual formulation that it is wrong, and by an emotional appreciation of the fact that it "feels good."

We may conclude this section by saying that one of the fundamental directions taken by the process of therapy is the free experiencing of the actual sensory and visceral reactions of the organism without too much of an attempt to relate these experiences to the self. This is usually accompanied by the conviction that this material does not belong to, and cannot be organized into, the self. The end point of this process is that the client discovers that he can *be* his experience, with all of its variety and surface contradiction; that he can formulate himself out of his experience, instead of trying to impose a formulation of self upon his experience, denying to awareness those elements which do not fit.

THE FULL EXPERIENCING OF AN AFFECTIONAL RELATIONSHIP

One of the elements in therapy of which we have more recently become aware is the extent to which therapy is a learning, on the part of the client, to accept fully and freely and without fear the positive feelings of another. This is not a phenomenon which clearly occurs in every case. It seems particularly true of our longer cases, but it does not occur uniformly in these. Yet it is such a deep experience that we have begun to question whether it is not a highly significant direction in the therapeutic process, perhaps occurring at an unverbalized level to some degree in all successful cases. Before discussing this phenomenon, let us give it some body by citing the experience of Mrs. O. The experience struck her rather suddenly, between the twenty-ninth and thirtieth interview, and she spent most of the latter interview discussing it. She opens the thirtieth hour in this way:

C.: Well, I made a very remarkable discovery. I know it's—[laughs] I found out that you actually *care* how this thing goes. [Both laugh.] It gave me the feeling, it's sort of well—"maybe I'll let you get in the act," sort of thing. It's—again you see, on an examination sheet, I would have had the correct answer, I mean—but it suddenly dawned on me that in the—client-counselor kind of thing, you *actually care* what happens to this thing. And it was a revelation, a— not that. That doesn't describe it. It was a—well, the closest I can come to it is a kind of relaxation, a—not a letting down, but a— [pause] more of a straightening out without tension if that means anything. I don't know.

T.: Sounds as though it isn't as though this was a new idea, but it was a new *experience* of really *feeling* that I did care and if I get the rest of that, sort of a willingness on your part to let me care.

C.: Yes.

This letting the counselor and his warm interest into her life was undoubtedly one of the deepest features of therapy in this case. In an interview following the conclusion of therapy, she spontaneously mentioned this experience as being the outstanding one. What does it mean?

The phenomenon is most certainly not one of transference and countertransference. Some experienced psychologists who had undergone psychoanalysis had the opportunity of observing the development of the relationship in a case other than the one cited. They were the first to object to the use of the terms "transference" and "countertransference" to describe the phenomenon. The gist of their remarks was that this is something which is mutual and appropriate, while transference and countertransference are phenomena which are characteristically one-way and inappropriate to the realities of the situation.

Certainly one reason why this phenomenon is occurring more frequently in our experience is that as therapists we have become less afraid of our positive (or negative) feelings toward the client. As therapy goes on, the therapist's feeling of acceptance and respect for the client tends to change to something approaching awe as he sees the valiant and deep struggle of the person to be himself. There is, I think, within the therapist, a profound experience of the underlying commonality— should we say brotherhood—of man. As a result he feels toward the client a warm, positive, affectional reaction. This poses a problem for the client, who often, as in this case, finds it difficult to accept the positive feeling of another. Yet, once accepted, the inevitable reaction on the part of the client is to relax, to let the warmth of liking by another person reduce the tension and fear involved in facing life.

But we are getting ahead of our client. Let us examine some of the other aspects of this experience as it occurred to her. In earlier interviews she had talked of the fact that she did *not* love humanity, and that in some vague and stubborn way she felt she was right, even though others would regard her as wrong. She mentions this again as she discusses the way this experience has clarified her attitudes toward others.

C.: The next thing that occurred to me that I found myself thinking and still thinking, is somehow—and I'm not clear why—the same kind of a caring that I get when I say "I don't love humanity." Which has always sort of—I mean I was always convinced of it. So I mean, it doesn't—I knew that it was a good thing, see. And I think I clarified it within myself—what it has to do with this situation, I don't know. But I found out, no, I don't love, but I do *care* terribly.

T.: M-hm. M-hm. I see. . . .

C.: . . . It might be expressed better in saying I care terribly what happens. But the caring is a—takes form—its structure is in understanding and not wanting to be taken in, or to contribute to those things which I feel are false and—It seems to me that in—in loving, there's a kind of *final* factor. If you do that, you've sort of done *enough.* It's a—

T.: That's *it,* sort of.

C.: Yeah. It seems to me this other thing, this caring, which isn't a good term—I mean, probably we need something else to describe this kind of thing. To say it's an impersonal thing doesn't mean anything because it isn't impersonal. I mean I feel it's very much a part of a whole. But it's something that somehow doesn't stop. . . . It seems to me you could have this feeling of loving humanity, loving people, and at the same time—go on contributing to the factors that make people neurotic, make them ill—where, what I feel is a resistance to those things.

T.: You care enough to want to understand and to want to avoid contributing to anything that would make for more neuroticism, or more of that aspect in human life.

C.: Yes. and it's—[pause]. Yes, it's something along those lines. . . . Well, again, I have to go back to how I feel about this other thing. It's—I'm not really called upon to give of myself in a—sort of on the auction block. There's nothing final. . . . It sometimes bothered me when I—I would have to say to myself, "I don't love humanity," and yet, I always knew that there was something positive. That I was probably right. And—I may be all off the beam now, but it seems to me that, that is somehow tied up in the—this feeling that I—I have now, into how the therapeutic value can carry through. Now, I couldn't tie it up, I couldn't tie it in, but it's as close as I can come to explaining to myself, my—well, shall I say the learning process, the follow-through on my realization that—yes, you *do care* in a given situation. It's just that simple. And I hadn't been aware of it before. I might have closed this door and walked out, and in discussing therapy, said, yes, the counselor must feel thus and so, but, I mean, I hadn't had the dynamic experience.

In this portion, though she is struggling to describe her own feeling, it would seem that what she is saying would be characteristic of the therapist's attitude toward the client as well. His attitude, at its best, is devoid of the *quid pro quo* aspect of most of the experiences we call love. It is the simple outgoing human feeling of one individual for another, a feeling, it seems to me, which is even more basic than sexual or parental feeling. It is a caring enough about the person that you do not wish to interfere with his development, nor to use him for any self-aggrandizing goals of your own. Your satisfaction comes in having set him free to grow in his own fashion.

Our client goes on to discuss how hard it has been for her in the past to accept any help or positive feeling from others, and how this attitude is changing:

C.: I have a feeling . . . that you have to do it pretty much yourself, but that somehow you ought to be able to do that with other people. [She mentions that there have been "countless" times when she might have accepted personal warmth and kindliness from others.] I get the feeling that I just was afraid I would be devastated. [She returns to talking about the counseling itself and her feeling toward it.] I mean there's been this tearing through the thing myself. Almost to—I mean, I felt it—I mean I tried to verbalize it on occasion—a kind of—at times almost not wanting you to restate, not wanting you to reflect, the thing is *mine*. Course, all right, I can say it's resistance. But that doesn't mean a damn thing to me now. . . . The—I think in —in relationship to this particular thing, I mean, the—probably at times, the strongest feeling was, it's mine, it's *mine*. I've got to cut it down myself. See?

T.: It's an experience that's awfully hard to put down accurately into words, and yet I get a sense of difference here in this relationship, that from the feeling that "this is mine," "I've got to do it," "I am doing it" and so on, to a somewhat different feeling that—"I could let you in."

C.: Yeah. Now. I mean, that's—that it's—well, it's sort of, shall we say, volume two. It's—it's a—well, sort of, well, I'm still in the thing alone, but I'm *not*—see—I'm—

T.: M-hm. Yes, that paradox sort of sums it up, doesn't it?

C.: Yeah.

T.: In all of this, there is a feeling, it's still—every aspect of my experience is mine and that's kind of inevitable and necessary and so on. And yet that isn't the whole picture either. Somehow it can be shared or another's interest can come in and in some ways it is new.

C.: Yeah. And it's—it is though, that's how it should be. I mean, that's how it—has to be. There's a—there's a feeling, "and this is good." I mean, it expresses, it clarifies it for me. There's a feeling—in this caring, as though—you were sort of standing back—standing off, and if I want to sort of cut through to the thing, it's a—a slashing of—oh, tall weeds, that I can do it, and you can—I mean, you're not going to be disturbed by having to walk through it too. I don't know. And it doesn't make sense. I mean—

T.: Except there's a very real sense of rightness about this feeling that you have, hm?

C.: M-hm.

May it not be that this excerpt portrays the heart of the process of socialization? To discover that it is *not* devastating to accept the positive feeling from another, that it does not necessarily end in hurt, that it actually "feels good" to have another person with you in your struggles to meet life—this may be one of the most profound learnings encountered by the individual, whether in therapy or not.

Something of the newness, the nonverbal level of this experience is described by Mrs. O. in the closing moments of this thirtieth interview:

C.: I'm experiencing a new type, a—probably the only worth-while kind of learning, a—I know I've—I've often said what I know doesn't help me here. What I meant is, my acquired knowledge doesn't help me. But it seems to me that the learning process here has been—so dynamic, I mean, so much a part of the—of everything, I mean, of me, that if I just get that out of it, it's something, which, I mean— I'm wondering if I'll ever be able to straighten out into a sort of acquired knowledge what I have experienced here.

T.: In other words, the kind of learning that has gone on here has been something of quite a different sort and quite a different depth; very vital, very real. And quite worth while to you in and of itself, but the question you're asking is: Will I ever have a clear intellectual picture of what has gone on at this somehow deeper kind of learning level?

C.: M-hm. Something like that.

Those who would apply to therapy the so-called laws of learning derived from the memorization of nonsense syllables would do well to study this excerpt with care. Learning as it takes place in therapy is a total, organismic, frequently nonverbal type of thing which may or may not follow the same principles as the intellectual learning of trivial material which has little relevance to the self. This, however, is a digression.

Let us conclude this section by rephrasing its essence. It appears possible that one of the characteristics of deep or significant therapy is that the client discovers that it is not devastating to admit fully into his own experience the positive feeling which another, the therapist, holds toward him. Perhaps one of the reasons why this is so difficult is that essentially it involves the feeling that "I am worthy of being liked." This we shall consider in the following section. For the present it may be pointed out that this aspect of therapy is a free and full experiencing of an affectional relationship which may be put in generalized terms as follows: "I can permit someone to care about me, and can fully accept that caring within myself. This permits me to recognize that I care, and care deeply, for and about others."

THE LIKING OF ONE'S SELF

In various writings and researches that have been published regarding client-centered therapy, there has been a stress upon the acceptance of self as one of the directions and outcomes of therapy. We have established the fact that in successful psychotherapy negative attitudes toward the self decrease and positive attitudes increase. We have measured the gradual increase in self-acceptance and have studied the correlated in-crease in acceptance of others. But as I examine these statements and compare them with our more recent cases, I feel they fall short of the truth. The client not only accepts himself—a phrase which may carry the connotation of a grudging and reluctant acceptance of the inevitable—he actually comes to *like* himself. This is not a bragging or self-assertive liking; it is rather a quiet pleasure in being one's self.

Mrs. O. illustrates this trend rather nicely in her thirty-third inter-view. Is it significant that this follows by ten days the interview where she could for the first time admit to herself that the therapist cared? What-ever our speculations on this point, this fragment indicates very well the quiet joy in being one's self, together with the apologetic attitude which, in our culture, one feels it is necessary to take toward such an experience. In the last few minutes of the interview, knowing her time is nearly up she says:

C.: One thing worries me—and I'll hurry because I can always go back to it—a feeling that occasionally I can't turn out. Feeling of being quite pleased with myself. Again the Q technique.[2] I walked out of here one time, and impulsively I threw my first card, "I am an at-tractive personality"; looked at it sort of aghast but left it there, I mean, because honestly, I mean, that is exactly how it felt—a—well, that bothered me and I catch that now. Every once in a while a sort of pleased feeling, nothing superior, but just—I don't know, sort of pleased. A neatly turned way. And it bothered me. And yet—I wonder—I rarely remember things I say here, I mean I wondered why it was that I was convinced, and something about what I've felt about being hurt that I suspected in—my feelings when I would hear someone say to a child, "Don't cry." I mean, I always felt, but it isn't right; I mean, if he's hurt, let him cry. Well, then, now this pleased feeling that I have. I've recently come to feel it's—there's something almost the same there. It's—We don't object when *chil-dren* feel pleased with themselves. It's—I mean, there really isn't anything vain. It's—maybe that's how people *should* feel.

T.: You've been inclined almost to look askance at yourself for this feeling, and yet as you think about it more, maybe it comes close to

---

[2]This portion needs explanation. As part of a research study by another staff member, this client had been asked several times during therapy to sort a large group of cards, each containing a self-descriptive phrase, in such a way as to portray her own self. At one end of the sorting she was to place the card or cards most like herself, and at the other end, those most unlike herself. Thus when she says that she put as the first card "I am an attractive personality," it means that she regarded this as the item most characteristic of herself.

the two sides of the picture, that if a child wants to cry, why shouldn't he cry? and if he wants to feel pleased with himself, doesn't he have a perfect right to feel pleased with himself? And that sort of ties in with this, what I would see as an appreciation of yourself that you've experienced every now and again.

C.: Yes. Yes.

T.: "I'm really a pretty rich and interesting person."

C.: Something like that. And then I say to myself, "Our society pushes us around and we've lost it." And I keep going back to my feelings about children. Well, maybe they're richer than we are. Maybe we —it's something we've lost in the process of growing up.

T.: Could be that they have a wisdom about that that we've lost.

C.: That's right. My time's up.

Here she arrives, as do so many other clients, at the tentative, slightly apologetic realization that she has come to like, enjoy, appreciate herself. One gets the feeling of a spontaneous relaxed enjoyment, a primitive *joie de vivre,* perhaps analogous to that of the lamb frisking about the meadow or the porpoise gracefully leaping in and out of the waves. Mrs. O. feels that it is something native to the organism, to the infant, something we have lost in the warping process of development.

Earlier in this case one sees something of a forerunner of this feeling, an incident which perhaps makes more clear its fundamental nature. In the ninth interview Mrs. O. in a somewhat embarrassed fashion reveals something she has always kept to herself. That she brought it forth at some cost is indicated by the fact that it was preceded by a very long pause, of several minutes' duration. Then she spoke.

C.: You know this is kind of goofy, but I've never told anyone this [nervous laugh] and it'll probably do me good. For years, oh, probably from early youth, from seventeen probably on, I, I have had what I have come to call to myself, told myself were "flashes of sanity." I've never told anyone this [another embarrassed laugh] wherein, in, really I feel sane. And, and pretty much aware of life. And always with a terrific kind of concern and sadness of how far away, how far astray that we have actually gone. It's just a feeling once in a while of finding myself a whole kind of person in a terribly chaotic kind of world.

T.: It's been fleeting and it's been infrequent, but there have been times when it seems the whole you is functioning and feeling in the world, a very chaotic world to be sure—

C.: That's right. And I mean, and knowing actually how far astray we, we've gone from, from being whole healthy people. And of course one doesn't talk in those terms.

T.: A feeling that it wouldn't be *safe* to talk about the singing you[3]—

C.: Where does that person live?

T.: Almost as if there was no place for such a person to, to exist.

C.: Of course, you know, that, that makes me—now wait a minute—that probably explains why I'm primarily concerned with feelings here. That's probably it.

T.: Because that whole you does exist with all your feelings. Is that it, you're more aware of feelings?

C.: That's right. It's not, it doesn't reject feelings and—that's *it*.

T.: That whole you somehow lives feelings instead of somehow pushing them to one side.

C.: That's right. [Pause.] I suppose from the practical point of view it could be said that what I ought to be doing is solving some problems, day-to-day problems. And yet, I, I—what I'm trying to do is solve, solve something else that's a great, that is a great deal more important than little day-to-day problems. Maybe that sums up the whole thing.

T.: I wonder if this will distort your meaning, that from a hard-headed point of view you ought to be spending time thinking through specific problems. But you wonder if perhaps maybe you aren't on a quest for this whole you and perhaps that's more important than a solution to the day-to-day problems.

C.: I think that's it. I think that's it. That's probably what I mean.

If we may legitimately put together these two experiences, and if we are justified in regarding them as typical, then we may say that both in therapy and in some fleeting experiences throughout her previous life, she has experienced a healthy satisfying enjoyable appreciation of herself as a whole and functioning creature; and that this experience occurs when she does not reject her feelings but lives them.

Here it seems to me is an important and often overlooked truth about the therapeutic process. It works in the direction of permitting the person to experience fully, and in awareness, all his reactions, including his feelings and emotions. As this occurs, the individual feels a positive

---

[3]The therapist's reference is to her statement in a previous interview that in therapy she was singing a song.

liking for himself, a genuine appreciation of himself as a total functioning unit, which is one of the important end points of therapy.

THE DISCOVERY THAT THE CORE OF PERSONALITY IS POSITIVE

One of the most revolutionary concepts to grow out of our clinical experience is the growing recognition that the innermost core of man's nature, the deepest layers of his personality, the base of his "animal nature," is positive in character—is basically socialized, forward-moving, rational, and realistic. . . .

In psychology, Freud and his followers have presented convincing arguments that the id, man's basic and unconscious nature, is primarily made up of instincts which would, if permitted expression, result in incest, murder, and other crimes. The whole problem of therapy, as seen by this group, is how to hold these untamed forces in check in a wholesome and constructive manner, rather than in the costly fashion of the neurotic. But the fact that at heart man is irrational, unsocialized, and destructive of others and self—this is a concept accepted almost without question. To be sure there are occasional voices of protest. Maslow (1949) puts up a vigorous case for man's animal nature, pointing out that the antisocial emotions—hostility, jealousy, etc.,—result from frustration of more basic impulses for love and security and belonging, which are in themselves desirable. And Ashley-Montagu (1950) likewise develops the thesis that cooperation, rather than struggle, is the basic law of human life. . . . Only slowly has it become evident that [the] untamed and unsocial feelings are neither the deepest nor the strongest, and that the inner core of man's personality is the organism itself, which is essentially both self-preserving and social.

To give more specific meaning to this argument, let me turn again to the case of Mrs. O. . . .

It is in the eighth interview that Mrs. O. rolls back the first layer of defense, and discovers a bitterness and desire for revenge underneath.

C.: You know over in this area of, of sexual disturbance, I have a feeling that I'm beginning to discover that it's pretty bad, pretty bad. I'm finding out that, that I'm bitter, really. Damn bitter. I—and I'm not turning it back in, into myself. . . . I think what I probably feel is a certain element of "I've been cheated." [Her voice is very tight and her throat chokes up.] And I've covered up very nicely, to the point of consciously not caring. But I'm, I'm sort of amazed to find that in this practice of, what shall I call it, a kind of sublimation that right under it—again words—there's a, a kind of passive force that's, it's pas—it's very passive, but at the same time it's just kind of *murderous*.

T.: So there's the feeling, "I've really been cheated. I've covered that up and seem not to care and yet underneath that there's a kind of a, a latent but very much present *bitterness* that is very, very strong."

C.: It's very strong. I—that I know. It's terribly powerful.

T.: Almost a dominating kind of force.

C.: Of which I am rarely conscious. Almost never. . . . Well, the only way I can describe it, it's a kind of murderous thing, but without violence. . . . It's more like a feeling of wanting to get even. . . . And of course I won't pay back, but I'd like to. I really would like to.

Up to this point the usual explanation seems to fit perfectly. Mrs. O. has been able to look beneath the socially controlled surface of her behavior, and she finds underneath a murderous feeling of hatred and a desire to get even. This is as far as she goes in exploring this particular feeling until . . . the thirty-first interview.

[In the thirty-first interview she gives] a clear picture of the fact that underlying the bitterness and hatred and the desire to get back at the world which has cheated her is a much less antisocial feeling, a deep experience of having been hurt. And it is equally clear that at this deeper level she has no desire to put her murderous feelings into action. She dislikes them and would like to be rid of them.

[In the thirty-fourth interview the material] is very incoherent . . . , as verbalizations often are when the individual is trying to express something deeply emotional. Here she is endeavoring to reach far down into herself. She states that it will be difficult to formulate. . . .

Since [it] is presented in such confused fashion, it might be worth while to draw from it the consecutive themes which the client has expressed.

1. I'm going to talk about myself as *self*-ish, but with a new connotation to the word.
2. I've acquired an acquaintance with the structure of myself, know myself deeply.
3. As I descend into myself, I discover something exciting, a core that is totally without hate.
4. It can't be a part of everyday life—it may even be abnormal.
5. I thought first it was just a sublimated sex drive.
6. But no, this is more inclusive, deeper than sex.
7. One would expect this to be the kind of thing one would discover by going up into the thin realm of ideals.
8. But actually, I found it by going deep within myself.

9. It seems to be something that is the essence, that lasts.

Is this a mystic experience she is describing? It would seem that the counselor felt so, from the flavor of his responses. Can we attach any significance to such a Gertrude Stein kind of expression? The writer would simply point out that many clients have come to a somewhat similar conclusion about themselves, though not always expressed in such an emotional way. Even Mrs. O., in the following interview, the thirty-fifth, gives a clearer and more concise statement of her feeling, in a more down-to-earth way. She also explains why it was a difficult experience to face . . . [and while] she recognizes that her feeling goes against the grain of her culture, she feels bound to say that the core of herself is not bad, nor terribly wrong, but something positive. Underneath the layer of controlled surface behavior, underneath the bitterness, underneath the hurt, is a self that is positive and that is without hate. This, I believe, is the lesson which our clients have been facing us with for a long time and which we have been slow to learn.

If hatelessness seems like a rather neutral or negative concept, perhaps we should let Mrs. O. explain its meaning. In her thirty-ninth interview, as she feels her therapy drawing to a close, she returns to this topic:

C.: I wonder if I ought to clarify—it's clear to me, and perhaps that's all that matters really, here, my strong feeling about a hate-free kind of approach. Now that we have brought it up on a rational kind of a plane, I know—it sounds negative. And yet in my thinking, my— not really my thinking but my feeling, it—*and* my thinking, yes, my thinking too—it's a far more positive thing than this—than a love— and it seems to me a far easier kind of a—it's less confining. But it—I realize that it must sort of sound and almost seem like a complete rejection of so many things, of so many creeds and maybe it is. I don't know. But it just to me seems more positive.

T.: You can see how it might sound more negative to someone, but as far as the meaning that it has for you is concerned, it doesn't seem as binding, as possessive I take it, as love. It seems as though it actually is more—more expandable, more usable, than—

C.: Yeah.

T.: —any of these narrower terms.

C.: Really does to me. It's easier. Well, anyway it's easier for me to feel that way. And I don't know. It seems to me to really be a way of—of not—of finding yourself in a place where you aren't forced to make rewards and you aren't forced to punish. It is—it means so much. It just seems to me to make for a kind of freedom.

T.: M-hm. M-hm. Where one is rid of the need of either rewarding or punishing, then it just seems to you there is so much more freedom for all concerned.

C.: That's right. [Pause.] I'm prepared for some breakdowns along the way.

T.: You don't expect it will be smooth sailing.

C.: No.

REFERENCES

1. Ashley-Montagu, M. F. *On Being Human.* New York: H. Schuman, 1950.
2. Maslow, A. H. Our maligned animal nature. *Journal of Psychology,* 1949, **28**, 273-278.

Index

349